Evidence-based Clinical Chinese Medicine

Volume 24

Menopause

Evidence-based Clinical Chinese Medicine

Print ISSN: 2529-7562
Online ISSN: 2529-7554

Published

Vol. 1 *Chronic Obstructive Pulmonary Disease*
by Charlie Changli Xue and Chuanjian Lu

Vol. 2 *Psoriasis Vulgaris*
Lead Authors: Claire Shuiqing Zhang and Jingjie Yu

Vol. 3 *Chronic Urticaria*
Lead Authors: Meaghan Coyle and Jingjie Yu

Vol. 4 *Adult Asthma*
Lead Authors: Johannah Shergis and Lei Wu

Vol. 5 *Allergic Rhinitis*
Lead Authors: Claire Shuiqing Zhang and Qiulan Luo

Vol. 6 *Herpes Zoster and Post-herpetic Neuralgia*
Lead Authors: Meaghan Coyle and Haiying Liang

Vol. 7 *Insomnia*
Lead Authors: Johannah Shergis and Xiaojia Ni

Vol. 8 *Alzheimer's Disease*
Lead Authors: Brian H May and Mei Feng

Vol. 9 *Vascular Dementia*
Lead Authors: Brian H May and Mei Feng

Vol. 10 *Diabetic Kidney Disease*
Lead Authors: Johannah Shergis and Lihong Yang

Vol. 11 *Acne Vulgaris*
Lead Authors: Meaghan Coyle and Haiying Liang

More information on this series can also be found at https://www.worldscientific.com/series/ebccm

Evidence-based Clinical Chinese Medicine

Co Editors-in-Chief

Charlie Changli Xue
RMIT University, Australia

Chuanjian Lu
Guangdong Provincial Hospital of Chinese Medicine, China

Volume 24

Menopause

Lead Authors

Meaghan Coyle
RMIT University, Australia

Jian Liu
Guangdong Provincial Hospital of Chinese Medicine, China

World Scientific

NEW JERSEY • LONDON • SINGAPORE • BEIJING • SHANGHAI • HONG KONG • TAIPEI • CHENNAI • TOKYO

Published by

World Scientific Publishing Co. Pte. Ltd.
5 Toh Tuck Link, Singapore 596224
USA office: 27 Warren Street, Suite 401-402, Hackensack, NJ 07601
UK office: 57 Shelton Street, Covent Garden, London WC2H 9HE

Library of Congress Cataloging-in-Publication Data
Names: Xue, Charlie Changli, author. | Lu, Chuan-jian, 1964– author.
Title: Evidence-based clinical Chinese medicine / Charlie Changli Xue, Chuanjian Lu.
Description: New Jersey : World Scientific, 2016. | Includes bibliographical references and index.
Identifiers: LCCN 2015030389| ISBN 9789814723084 (v. 1 : hardcover : alk. paper) |
ISBN 9789814723091 (v. 1 : paperback : alk. paper) |
ISBN 9789814723121 (v. 2 : hardcover : alk. paper) |
ISBN 9789814723138 (v. 2 : paperback : alk. paper) |
ISBN 9789814759045 (v. 3 : hardcover : alk. paper) |
ISBN 9789814759052 (v. 3 : paperback : alk. paper)
Subjects: | MESH: Medicine, Chinese Traditional--methods. | Clinical Medicine--methods. |
Evidence-Based Medicine--methods. | Psoriasis. | Pulmonary Disease, Chronic Obstructive.
Classification: LCC RC81 | NLM WB 55.C4 | DDC 616--dc23
LC record available at http://lccn.loc.gov/2015030389

Volume 24: Menopause
ISBN 978-981-122-436-2 (hardcover)
ISBN 978-981-122-437-9 (ebook for institutions)
ISBN 978-981-122-438-6 (ebook for individuals)

British Library Cataloguing-in-Publication Data
A catalogue record for this book is available from the British Library.

For any available supplementary material, please visit
https://www.worldscientific.com/worldscibooks/10.1142/11940#t=suppl

Disclaimer

The information in this book is based on systematic analyses of the best available evidence for Chinese medicine interventions, both historical and contemporary. Every effort has been made to ensure accuracy and completeness of the data herein. This book is intended for clinicians, researchers and educators. The practice of evidence-based medicine consists of consideration of the best available evidence, practitioners' clinical experience and judgement, and patients' preference. Not all interventions are acceptable in all countries. It is important to note that some of the substances mentioned in this book may no longer be in use, may be toxic or may be prohibited or restricted under the provisions of the Convention on International Trade in Endangered Species of Wild Fauna and Flora (CITES). Practitioners, researchers and educators are advised to comply with the relevant regulations in their country and with the restrictions on the trade in species included in CITES appendices I, II and III. This book is not intended as a guide for self-medication. Patients should seek professional advice from qualified Chinese medicine practitioners.

Foreword

Since the late 20th century, Chinese medicine, including acupuncture and herbal medicine, has been increasingly used throughout the world. The parallel development and spread of evidence-based medicine have provided challenges and opportunities for Chinese medicine. The opportunities have been evidence-based medicine's emphasis on the effective use of the best available clinical evidence, incorporating the clinicians' clinical experience, subject to patients' preference. Such practices have a patient focus, which reflects the historical nature of Chinese medicine practice. However, the challenges are also significant due to the fact that, despite the long-term development and very rich literature accumulated over 2,000 years, there is an overall lack of high-level clinical evidence for many of the interventions used in Chinese medicine.

To address this knowledge gap, we need to generate clinical evidence through high-quality clinical studies and to evaluate evidence to enable effective use of such available evidence to promote evidence-based Chinese medicine practice.

Modern Chinese medicine is rooted in its classical literature and the legacies of ancient doctors, grounded in the practice of expert clinicians and increasingly informed by clinical and experimental research efforts. In recognition of the unique features of Chinese medicine, for each of the conditions in this series a 'whole-evidence' approach is used to provide a synthesis of different types and levels of evidence to enable practitioners to make clinical decisions informed by the current best evidence.

There are four main components of this 'whole-evidence' approach. In the first component, we present the current approaches to the diagnosis, differentiation and treatment of each condition based on expert consensus in published textbooks and clinical guidelines. This provides an overview of how the condition is currently managed. The second component provides an analysis of the condition in historical context based on systematic searches of the *Zhong Hua Yi Dian* 中华医典, which includes the full texts of more than 1,000 classical medical books. These analyses provide objective views on how the condition has been treated over two millennia, reveal continuities and discontinuities between traditional and modern practice, and suggest avenues for future research.

The third component is the assessment of evidence derived from modern clinical studies of Chinese medicine interventions. The methods established by the *Cochrane Collaboration* are used as the basis for conducting systematic reviews and undertaking meta-analyses of outcome data for randomised controlled trials (RCTs). In addition, the clinical relevance of meta-analysis data is enhanced by examining the herbal formulas, individual herbs and acupuncture treatments that were assessed in the RCTs and the evidence base is broadened by the inclusion of data from controlled clinical trials and non-controlled studies. The fourth component is to determine how the herbal medicine interventions may achieve the effects indicated by the clinical trials. Thus, for each of the most frequently used herbs, we provide reviews of their effects in pre-clinical models and their likely mechanisms of action.

For each condition, this 'whole-evidence' approach links clinical expertise, historical precedent, clinical research data and experimental research to provide the reader with assessments of the current state of the evidence of efficacy and safety for Chinese medicine interventions using herbal medicines, acupuncture and moxibustion, and other health care practices, such as *taichi* 太极.

Since these books are available in Chinese and English, they can benefit patients, practitioners and educators internationally and enable practitioners to make clinical decisions informed by the current best evidence.

These publications represent a major milestone in Chinese medicine development and make a significant contribution to the evidence-based Chinese medicine development globally.

Co-editors-in-Chief

Distinguished Professor Charlie Changli Xue,
RMIT University, Australia

Professor Chuanjian Lu, Guangdong Provincial Hospital of
Chinese Medicine, China

Purpose of the Book

This book is intended for clinicians, researchers and educators. It can be used to inform tertiary education and clinical practice by providing systematic, multidimensional assessments of the best available evidence for using Chinese medicine to manage each common clinical condition.

How to Use This Book

Some Definitions

A glossary is included, containing terms and definitions which frequently appear in the book. It also describes the definitions of statistical tests, methodological terms, evaluation tools and interventions. For example, in this book, integrative medicine refers to the combined use of a Chinese medicine treatment with conventional medical management, and combination therapies refers to two or more Chinese medicines from different therapy groups (Chinese herbal medicine, acupuncture or other Chinese medicine therapies) administered together. Terminology used throughout the book is based on the World Health Organization's *Standard Terminologies on Traditional Medicine in the Western Pacific Region* (2007) where possible, or is from the cited reference.

Data Analysis and Interpretation of Results

In order to synthesise the clinical evidence, a range of statistical analysis approaches is used. In general, the effect size for dichotomous data is reported as a risk ratio (RR) with 95% confidence intervals (CI), and for continuous data, they are reported as mean difference (MD) with 95% CI. Statistically significant effects are indicated with an asterisk*. Readers should note that statistical significance does not necessarily correspond with a clinically important effect. Interpretation of results should take into consideration the clinical significance, quality of studies (expressed as 'high', 'low' or 'unclear' risk of bias in this book) and heterogeneity amongst the studies. Tests for heterogeneity are conducted using the I^2 statistic. An I^2 score greater than 50% may indicate substantial heterogeneity.

Use of Evidence in Practice

The Grading of Recommendations Assessment, Development and Evaluation (GRADE) approach was used to summarise the quality and strength of the evidence ('certainty') for critical and important comparisons and outcomes. Due to the diverse nature of Chinese medicine practice, treatment recommendations are not included with the summary-of-findings tables. Therefore, readers will need to interpret the evidence with reference to the local practice environment.

Limitations

Readers should note some of the methodological limitations on classical literature and clinical evidence.

- Search terms used to search the *Zhong Hua Yi Dian* 中华医典 database may not include all terms that have been used for the condition, which may alter the findings.
- Chinese language has changed over time. Citations have been interpreted for analysis, and such interpretations may be subject to disagreement.
- Chinese medicine theory has evolved over time. As such, concepts described in classical Chinese medical literature may no longer be found in contemporary works.

- Symptoms described in classical literature citations may be common to many conditions, and a judgement was required to determine the likelihood of the citation being related to the condition. This may have introduced some bias due to the subjective nature of the judgement.
- The vast majority of the clinical evidence for Chinese medicine treatments has come from China. The applicability of the findings to other populations and other countries requires further assessment.
- Many studies included participants with varying disease severity. Where possible, subgroup analyses were undertaken to examine the effects in different subpopulations. As this was not always possible, the findings may be limited to the population included, and not to subpopulations.
- The potential risk of bias found in many included studies suggested methodological limitations. The findings for GRADE assessments based on studies of very low to moderate certainty evidence should be interpreted accordingly.
- Nine major English- and Chinese-language databases were searched to identify clinical studies, in addition to clinical trial registers. Other studies may exist which were not identified through searches, and which may alter the findings.
- The calculation of frequency of herbal formula use was based on formula names only. It is possible that studies evaluated herbal treatments with the same or similar herb ingredients, but which were given different formula names. Due to the complexity of herbal formulas, it was considered not appropriate to make a judgement as to the similarity of formulas for analysis. As such, the frequency of formulas reported in Chapter 5 may be underestimated.
- The most frequently utilised herbs that may have contributed to the treatment effect have been described in Chapter 5. These herbs may provide leads for further exploration. Calculation of the herbs with potential effect is based on frequency of formulas reported in the studies, and does not take into consideration the clinical implications and functions of every herb in a formula.

Authors and Contributors

Co-Editors-in-Chief

Distinguished Prof. Charlie Changli Xue (*RMIT University, Australia*)
Prof. Chuanjian Lu (*Guangdong Provincial Hospital of Chinese Medicine, China*)

Co-Deputy Editors-in-Chief

Assoc. Prof. Anthony Lin Zhang (*RMIT University, Australia*)
Dr. Brian H May (*RMIT University, Australia*)
Prof. Xinfeng Guo (*Guangdong Provincial Hospital of Chinese Medicine, China*)
Prof. Zehuai Wen (*Guangdong Provincial Hospital of Chinese Medicine, China*)

Lead Authors

Dr. Meaghan Coyle (*RMIT University, Australia*)
Dr. Jian Liu (*Guangdong Provincial Hospital of Chinese Medicine, China*)

Co-Authors

RMIT University (Australia):
Dr. Mary Xinmei Zhang
Assoc. Prof. Anthony Lin Zhang
Distinguished Prof. Charlie Changli Xue

Guangdong Provincial Hospital of Chinese Medicine (*China*):

Prof. Hongyan Yang
Dr. Guangning Nie
Prof. Xinfeng Guo
Prof. Chuanjian Lu

Members of Advisory Committee and Panel

Co-Chairs of Project Planning Committee

Prof. Peter J Coloe (*RMIT University, Australia*)
Prof. Yubo Lyu (*Guangdong Provincial Hospital of Chinese Medicine, China*)
Prof. Dacan Chen (*Guangdong Provincial Hospital of Chinese Medicine, China*)

Centre Advisory Committee (in Alphabetical Order)

Prof. Keji Chen (*The Chinese Academy of Sciences, China*)
Prof. Aiping Lu (*Hong Kong Baptist University, China*)
Prof. Caroline Smith (*Western Sydney University, Australia*)
Prof. David F Story (*RMIT University, Australia*)

Methodology Expert Advisory Panel (in Alphabetical Order)

Prof. Zhaoxiang Bian (*Hong Kong Baptist University, China*)
Prof. Lixing Lao (*The University of Hong Kong, China*)
The Late Prof. George Lewith (*University of Southampton, United Kingdom*)
Prof. Jianping Liu (*Beijing University of Chinese Medicine, China*)
Prof. Frank Thien (*Monash University, Australia*)
Prof. Jialiang Wang (*Sichuan University, China*)

Content Expert Advisory Panel (in Alphabetical Order)

Prof. Rodney Baber (*The University of Sydney, Australia*)
Dr. Carolyn Ee (*Western Sydney University, Australia*)
Prof. Jinfang Lin (*Obstetrics and Gynaecology Hospital of Fudan University, China*)
Prof. Yong Tan (*Affiliated Hospital of Nanjing University of Chinese Medicine, China*)

Professor Charlie Changli Xue

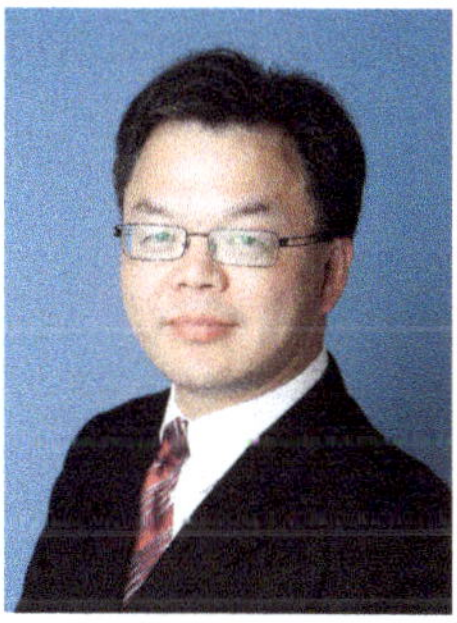

Professor Charlie Changli Xue holds a Bachelor of Medicine (majoring in Chinese Medicine) from Guangzhou University of Chinese Medicine, China (1987) and a PhD from RMIT University, Australia (2000). He has been an academic, researcher, regulator and practitioner for almost three decades. Professor Xue has made significant contributions to evidence-based educational development, clinical research, regulatory framework and policy development, and provision of high-quality clinical care to the community. Professor Xue is recognised internationally as an expert in evidence-based traditional medicine and integrative health care.

Professor Xue is the Inaugural National Chair of the Chinese Medicine Board of Australia appointed by the Australian Health Workforce Ministerial Council (in 2011), and he was reappointed for a second term in 2014. Since 2007, he has been a Member of the World Health Organization (WHO) Expert Advisory Panel for Traditional and Complementary Medicine, Geneva. Professor Xue is also an Honorary Senior Principal Research Fellow at the Guangdong Provincial Academy of Chinese Medical Sciences, China.

At RMIT, Professor Xue is Executive Dean, School of Health and Biomedical Sciences. He is also Director, WHO Collaborating Centre for Traditional Medicine.

Between 1995 and 2010, Professor Xue was Discipline Head of Chinese Medicine at RMIT University. He leads the development of five successful undergraduate and postgraduate degree programs in

Chinese Medicine at RMIT University which is now a global leader in Chinese medicine education and research.

Professor Xue's research has been supported by research grants of over AUD 15 million, including six project grants from the Australian Government's National Health and Medical Research Council (NHMRC) and two Australian Research Council (ARC) grants. He has contributed over 200 publications and has been frequently invited as keynote speaker for numerous national and international conferences. Professor Xue has contributed to over 300 media interviews on issues related to complementary medicine education, research, regulation and practice.

Professor Chuanjian Lu

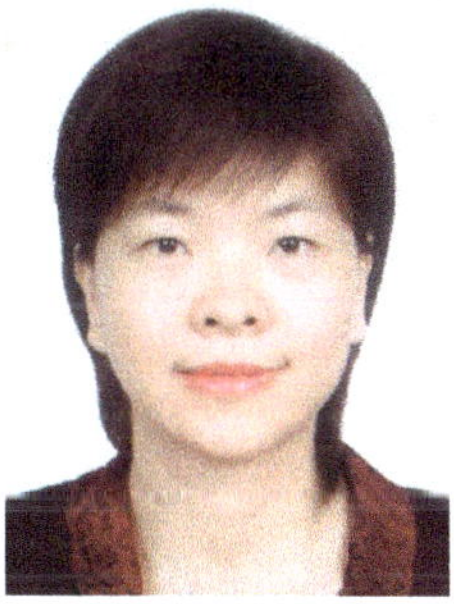

Professor Chuanjian Lu is Vice-president of Guangdong Provincial Hospital of Chinese Medicine (Guangdong Provincial Academy of Chinese Medical Sciences, Second Clinical Medical College of Guangzhou University of Chinese Medicine). She is also Chair of the Guangdong Traditional Chinese Medicine (TCM) Standardisation Technical Committee and Vice-chair of the Immunity Specialty Committee of the World Federation of Chinese Medicine Societies (WFCMS).

Professor Lu has engaged in scientific research into TCM, clinical practice and teaching for some 25 years. Her research has been devoted to integrating traditional and conventional medicine. She has edited and published 12 monographs and 120 academic research articles as first author and corresponding author, with over 30 articles being included in SCI journals. She has received widespread recognition for her achievements with awards for Excellent Teacher of South China, National Outstanding Women TCM Doctor and National Outstanding Young Doctor of TCM. She also received the Science and Technology Star of the Association of Chinese Medicine, the National Excellent Science and Technology Workers of China Award and the Five-Continent Women's Scientific Awards of China Medical Women's Association.

Professor Lu has won the Award of Science and Technology Progress over ten times from Guangdong Provincial Government, China Association of Chinese Medicine and Chinese Hospital Association.

Acknowledgements

The authors and contributors would like to acknowledge the valuable contributions of the following people who assisted with database searches, data extraction, data screening, data assessment, translation of documents, editing and/or administrative tasks: Dr. Jhodie Duncan, Chaoying Guo, Dr. Kevin Wang and Xiaofei Yang.

Contents

List of Figures

List of Tables

1

Introduction to Menopause

OVERVIEW

Menopause, the final menstrual period, signals the end of a woman's reproductive life. This can be accompanied by a range of vasomotor, sleep, psychological and genitourinary symptoms, and can reduce a woman's health-related quality of life. Hormone therapy is the most effective treatment for vasomotor symptoms, which are the most bothersome symptoms for many women. Some women look to complementary medicines for which there is limited evidence.

Definition of Menopause

Menopause marks the end of a woman's reproductive life. The term 'menopause' refers to the final menstrual period (FMP), which is determined retrospectively 12 months from the FMP.[1] Many women experience menstrual, physical and psychological changes leading up to the FMP and beyond, marking the transition from the reproductive to non-reproductive state.[2]

Additional criteria can assist clinical diagnosis and management. Menopause is defined as the permanent cessation of menstruation for at least 12 months.[3] The menopausal transition, also referred to as the perimenopause, describes the time when changes are seen in the menstrual cycle. This phase includes the time preceding the FMP and the first year after cessation of menstruation.[1] The perimenopause may be accompanied by vasomotor symptoms (VMS) of hot flushes and night sweats, vaginal symptoms such as dryness, and mood changes.[2] During early perimenopause, a persistent difference of seven days is seen in the menstrual cycle.[1] In late perimenopause, menstrual cycle length increases to 60 days or more and women may begin to experience characteristic symptoms.[1] Gold *et al.* (2013)[4] offer another definition for late perimenopause: amenorrhoea in the preceding three months but having menstrual periods in the preceding 12 months. A woman is considered to be postmenopausal 12 months after the FMP.[1]

Early menopause refers to the cessation of menstruation in women aged between 40 and 45 years in the absence of other reasons for amenorrhoea.[2] Premature ovarian failure refers to the loss of ovarian function in women aged less than 40 years; however, in these women resumption of menses is possible.[2] Early menopause, premature ovarian failure and menopause after breast cancer are not included in this book.

Clinical Presentation

Symptoms of menopause typically start during the menopause transition and may continue after the FMP. Menstrual cycles become irregular due to declining and fluctuating hormone levels. Vasomotor symptoms are the characteristic symptoms of menopause, although not all women will experience VMS.[2] The sensation of heat in a hot flush usually starts on the upper chest and face, and can become generalised as the flush progresses.[2] Hot flushes can last up to four minutes, vary in severity and frequency, and may be accompanied by sweating, palpitations and anxiety.[2] These can occur at any time of the day or night. Hot flushes during the night can disturb sleep, especially in the first half of the night.[5] Vasomotor symptoms of hot flushes and night sweats are the most bothersome for women[1] and were the main menopausal symptoms American women discussed with their health care provider.[6] Muscle and joint pain is more common than vasomotor symptoms among Asian women.[7]

Genitourinary syndrome of menopause (GSM, an over-arching term that includes vulvovaginal atrophy) includes a range of signs and symptoms arising from decreased oestrogen and other sex steroids.[8] Signs and symptoms include genital dryness, irritation and burning, increased urinary urgency, painful urination (dysuria) and recurrent urinary tract infections.[8] Urinary infections that are not due to oestrogen deficiency do not respond to oestrogen therapy. Sexual symptoms include decreased or a lack of vaginal lubrication, pain or discomfort during intercourse, and impaired function.[2,8]

Musculoskeletal symptoms include pain in joints (arthralgia) or muscles (myalgia), and pins and needles in the hands and feet (paraesthesia).[9] A direct relationship between menopause and fatigue has been suggested,[2] and fatigue was the most frequently reported symptom in Chinese nurses.[10] Similarly, whether there is a direct relationship between menopause and psychological symptoms is unclear.[2] Psychological symptoms include irritability, anxiety and depression, and are reported by many women.[11] Cognitive symptoms such as forgetfulness are also common.[12]

Signs and symptoms of menopause vary and there is no typical 'menopausal syndrome'.[13] Indeed, some signs and symptoms experienced during menopause are common to natural ageing.[14] However, symptom clusters have been described in relation to menopausal transition.[9,15] Recent analysis of data from the multi-ethnic Study of Women's Health Across the Nation (SWAN) shows VMS tended to co-exist with fatigue and sleep disturbance.[15] Four symptom groups were described by Mishra and Kuh (2012)[9] based on data from the British National Survey of Health and Development: somatic, vasomotor, psychological and sexual discomfort. Symptom clusters from the Australian Longitudinal Study of Women's Health included somatic, vasomotor, urogynaecological and physical symptoms.[9]

Epidemiology

Menopause is a natural process experienced by all women,[16] and represents the end of reproductive life. Using the age of 50 as a proxy for menopause, Schneider and Birkhauser (2017)[14] estimate 25 million women will experience menopause each year. Physiological changes begin in a woman's mid-40s, and the menopause transition typically starts around 47 years.[1,4] The age at natural menopause has been reported as between 50 and 52 years among women from 'industrialised' countries.[4] The median age of natural menopause was 52.54 years in a cohort of women from the United States (US).[4] Age at menopause among Chinese women was slightly lower, with a mean age of 48.1 years.[17]

In a review of longitudinal studies, Woods and Mitchell (2005)[12] found hot flushes to be the most prevalent symptom. Hot flushes in reproductive women ranged from 6% to 14% and were as high as 79% in postmenopausal women. In terms of GSM, sexual dysfunction was highest in the late menopause transition (88%). Forty-seven per cent of women reported bothersome vaginal symptoms three years after the FMP, and 57% of women reported incontinence. Reports of sleep disturbance increased linearly, from 31% in late perimenopause to 43% postmenopause. Mood changes, including depressed mood, ranged from 19% in reproductive women to 28.9% in the late menopause transition. Forgetfulness increased from 31.2% in reproductive women to 44.8% in the late menopausal transition. Aching or stiff joints were more frequently reported in postmenopausal women (57% compared to 41% of reproductive women). More recent research has shown the prevalence of vulvovaginal atrophy to be high in postmenopausal women (88%).[18]

One in three women in a British cohort reported sleep disturbance, joint ache or pain, or depression and anxiety.[9] The prevalence of breast tenderness, dizziness, palpitations, forgetfulness and headaches declined over time, while the prevalence of hot flushes, vaginal dryness, sexual difficulties, sleep disturbance, and joint ache and pain increased with advancing age. Vasomotor symptoms were less frequently reported in a cohort of 1,686 Chinese nurses, with hot flushes ranked as 11th in menopause symptoms.[10] The most frequently reported symptoms among Chinese nurses were fatigue (82.7%), irritability (70.2%) and arthralgia/myalgia (69.6%). These findings highlight variation in prevalence of menopausal symptoms in different racial/ethnic groups.

Among women in the US National Health and Wellness Survey who experienced at least one menopausal symptom, the mean number of symptoms was 4.8.[19] Duration of symptoms varies. While early studies suggested menopausal symptoms were present for up to two years, more recent studies have found symptoms may persist for more than ten years.[20] Data from a subset of 1,449 women with VMS included in SWAN showed the median duration of VMS was 7.4 years.[21] Duration of VMS was longest in African-American women (median 10.1 years) and shortest in Japanese and Chinese women (median 4.8 and 5.4 years, respectively).[21] Women who were younger when they experienced their first VMS reported longer duration of VMS. Duration of VMS was also longer in women with a higher body mass index (BMI) and those with anxiety or depressive symptoms. Shorter duration of VMS was found in women who were married or partnered and in women with a higher level of education.

Burden

Menopausal symptoms can have a significant impact on health-related quality of life. Women who experience symptoms of menopause have poorer quality of life than women with no symptoms,[19] and quality of life has been found to deteriorate as women advance through menopause.[22] Unadjusted analyses from SWAN showed that early perimenopausal women reported greater impairment on the five subscales of the Short Form-36 general wellbeing questionnaire compared to premenopausal women.[23] When analyses were adjusted for menopausal symptoms, no differences were seen in impairment between perimenopausal and premenopausal women.

Of all symptoms, VMS are the most bothersome and the most common reason for women to seek advice and treatment.[1] The unpredictable nature of hot flushes and profuse sweating can cause stress and anxiety and reduce quality of life.[24] Vasomotor symptoms have been associated with worse quality of life/health utility score in postmenopausal women.[25,26] Work impairment, activity impairment and menopause-specific visits to physicians have been shown to increase with increasing severity of VMS.[25] The burden of menopause has also been shown for symptoms other than VMS. A diagnosis of vulvovaginal atrophy was associated with a lower quality of life in postmenopausal women.[18] Lower quality of life was seen in domains of emotional wellbeing, sexual function, and self-concept and body image.

The relationship between VMS and menopause is clear, but uncertainty remains as to whether other symptoms, such as mood changes, anxiety and depression, can be attributed to menopause.[2] Unpredictable hot flushes, sleep deprivation and mood swings may contribute to anxiety and stress.[24] Furthermore, the menopausal transition coincides with natural ageing and the time when other life events are common, such as divorce or children leaving home[24] and caring for ageing parents and partners. These and other social, cultural and religious factors can contribute to how women perceive their quality of life during the menopausal transition.[14]

The economic burden from menopause has been estimated in several studies.[19,27] Direct costs for women of menopausal age with self-reported menopausal symptoms, including outpatient, inpatient and emergency department visits, were estimated at USD 248 per patient per annum in 2010–2012.[27] This study found the annual direct costs for menopause were higher than those associated with osteoporosis, lipid metabolism disorders and oesophageal disorders, and were comparable to asthma, anxiety disorder, headache, influenza and essential hypertension. Research by Sarrel *et al.* (2015)[28] found annual direct costs to be considerably higher; costs for women with VMS were USD 423 greater than for women without VMS. Other direct costs, such as prescription and over-the-counter medications, laboratory tests and visits to specialists or complementary and alternative medicine (CAM) practitioners, are likely to increase the financial burden for patients.[24]

Indirect costs relate to lost productivity at home and work, hygiene-related costs and increased energy use for laundry and air conditioning.[24] Data from the US National Health and Wellness Survey found women with menopausal symptoms had significantly higher presenteeism and overall work impairment.[19] Women with menopausal symptoms had higher impairment in daily activities and more physician visits in the previous six months than women without symptoms. From a predefined list of symptoms, depression, anxiety, heart racing and forgetfulness most strongly affected health-related quality of life, lost productivity and health care resource.

Risk Factors

While all women will experience menopause, several factors have been identified that may contribute to the age at FMP and duration/severity of symptoms. Findings from SWAN show that a higher level of education, higher weight, previous use of oral contraception, not smoking, being employed, consuming alcohol, participating in lower levels of physical activity and having higher self-rated health were associated with a later age at FMP.[4] Women who experienced financial stress, smoked, were obese or were of white race/ethnicity were more likely to be moderately to highly symptomatic.[15]

Further findings from SWAN highlight the impact of ethnicity on menopause. When socio-economic, lifestyle and health factors were controlled for, no difference was seen in age at FMP by racial/ethnic group.[4] However, Chinese and Japanese women reported fewer symptoms than Caucasian, African-American and Hispanic women.[13] Caucasian women reported more psychosomatic symptoms such as feeling tense, irritable, blue or depressed, forgetfulness, and headaches than women from other ethnic groups.[13] More African-American women reported VMS compared with other racial/ethnic groups.[13]

Vasomotor symptoms can be triggered by alcohol or spicy food.[2] Younger onset of VMS is associated with longer VMS duration.[20,21] Vasomotor symptoms duration is also longer in women with a greater BMI and those with higher perceived stress, anxiety and depressive symptoms.[21] Ethni city also plays a role in duration of VMS; the median duration of VMS among African-American women was 10.1 years, which was considerably longer than in Japanese (4.8 years) and Chinese women (5.4 years).[21] Duration of VMS was significantly shorter among married or partnered women, women with a higher level of education and less financial worry, and among women who had greater levels of social support.[21] Higher levels of anxiety have been identified as a risk factor for VMS, although it is not clear whether VMS worsens with anxiety or if anxiety is a predictor of VMS.[20] Experiencing hot flushes increases the risk of experiencing other symptoms, including sleep disturbance, anxiety and depression.[15]

Many of the findings from SWAN were also found among women with VMS of hot flushes and night sweats in the Australian Longitudinal Study on Women's Health.[29] Risk factors differed when either symptom was reported alone, leading the authors to suggest that the aetiology of hot flushes may be slightly different from that of night sweats.

Pathological Processes

The loss of ovarian function is the key contributor to reproductive ageing.[30] The pool of non-growing follicles peaks in neonatal life[31] and gradually declines through the reproductive years, before rapidly declining between 30 and 35 years of age.[30] The end of reproductive cycles occurs when the number of non-growing follicles declines to 1,000 or less.[32] The decline in follicle numbers triggers endocrine changes.[33]

The menstrual cycle is a closed-loop feedback system of the hypothalamic-pituitary-ovarian axis,[33] with the endometrium acting as the gonadal steroid end organ.[30] Gonadotropin-releasing hormone (GnRH) produced by the hypothalamus stimulates the pituitary to release follicle-stimulating hormone (FSH). Increasing levels of FSH stimulate the development of follicles, which secrete oestradiol and the inhibins A and B.[31] Inhibin B, a product of follicular granulosa cells,[33] inhibits FSH secretion by the pituitary and the rising oestradiol levels suppress FSH at the hypothalamus (and the pituitary to a lesser extent) in the later part of the follicular phase.[30] Rapidly rising oestradiol levels prompt the pituitary to release a surge in luteinising hormone (LH), triggering ovulation.[31] A mid-cycle peak in inhibins A and B is also seen.[31]

In the luteal phase, the corpus luteum secretes progesterone which inhibits GnRH, along with oestradiol and inhibin A.[31] Degeneration of the corpus luteum breaks the negative feedback loop and waning levels of progesterone and oestrogen secretion allow GnRH production to increase in the hypothalamus in preparation for the next menstrual cycle.[30] Anti-Mullerian hormone (AMH) and inhibins A and B are understood to have a role in preventing follicle development in the luteal phase, although the mechanisms are not clear.[31]

In the late reproductive years, levels of inhibin B and AMH decline.[34,35] Pituitary secretion of FSH is no longer inhibited in early perimenopause and FSH levels begin to rise.[31] Persistently elevated FSH alters cycle length, with some anovulatory cycles.[31] Oestradiol and progesterone levels do not change dramatically in the early menopausal transition,[36] while progesterone levels decline approaching the FMP.[37] In the late menopausal transition, cycles are largely anovulatory due to depletion of ovarian follicles.[31] The levels of FSH are highly variable during the late perimenopause and early postmenopausal period,[31] oestradiol levels are low and inhibin B and AMH are undetectable.[33]

Pathogenesis of Vasomotor Symptoms

The mechanisms underlying VMS in menopause are unclear,[38] but appear to be centrally mediated.[2] Ovarian hormones may influence thermoregulatory mechanisms in the hypothalamus.[24] Core body temperature is maintained within a thermoneutral zone, that is, the zone in which no major thermoregulatory response is required.[38] Minor adjustments within the zone are made by changing peripheral blood flow.[38] Major adjustments occur when core body temperature rises above the upper threshold (sweating) or drops below the lower threshold (shivering).

Core body temperature increases before most (but not all) hot flushes.[39] Warm ambient temperature and warming of the periphery can induce hot flushes, which may indicate that the upper threshold of the thermoregulatory zone is lowered in menopausal women who experience hot flushes.[38] Elevated levels of norepinephrine (noradrenaline) in the brain narrow the thermoregulatory zone (Brück and Zeisberger (1990), cited in Freedman (2014)[38]), and women who experience hot flushes have higher levels of central noradrenergic activation than asymptomatic women.[40] The α-2 adrenergic agonist clonidine reduces hot flushes, while α-2 antagonist yohimbine increases hot flushes.[40] Freedman[38] proposed that elevated levels of norepinephrine in combination with oestrogen withdrawal are involved in the development of hot flushes.

Pathogenesis of Genitourinary Syndrome of Menopause

Oestrogen plays a role in maintaining vaginal lubrication, elasticity and blood flow.[41] The tissues of the female lower urinary and genital tracts share the same embryological origin[42] and are rich in oestrogen receptors.[43] Lower levels of oestrogen seen in menopause result in thinning of the vaginal epithelium, a decrease in vaginal elasticity and rugae, decreased mucus secretion from the Bartholin glands,[44] and decreased vaginal blood flow.[45] This leads to symptoms of vaginal dryness and painful intercourse (dyspareunia).[45] Oestrogen promotes conversion of glycogen to glucose, which non-pathogenic bacteria require for production of lactic acid to maintain vaginal acidity.[45] A decline in oestrogen sees the vaginal pH become less acidic, allowing pathogenic bacteria to grow.[45] The combination of lower vaginal pH, increased residual volume and reduced urinary flow (thus preventing adequate clearance of bacteria) contribute to urinary tract infections seen in menopausal women.[43]

Pathogenesis of Psychological Symptoms

Psychological symptoms during menopause include low or depressed mood, poor concentration and sleep disturbance. It has been postulated that these symptoms can occur as a result of the main physical complaints, such as hot flushes and night sweats.[46] Psychological stressors — loss of fertility, declining physical health associated with ageing, children leaving home and illness or death of family or friends — can also contribute to the development of psychological symptoms in middle-aged women.[46]

Oestrogen receptors can be found in several areas of the brain, including areas that regulate mood, such as the hypothalamus and prefrontal cortex. Oestrogen has been shown to inhibit monoamine oxidases A and B which contribute to degradation of the neurotransmitters including serotonin (5-hydroxytryptamine, 5-HT), noradrenaline and dopamine,[47–50] and can increase the density of receptors for a variety of neurotransmitters.[46] These neurotransmitters are involved in mood and cognitive function. Oestrogen can also increase the activity of the enzyme tyrosine hydroxylase which limits synthesis of catecholamine.[50] The decline in oestrogen that occurs during menopause may decrease 5-HT, adrenergic and dopaminergic activity, leading to altered mood in women with an increased risk of developing depressive illness.[49]

Oestrogen and progesterone contribute to the regulation of circadian rhythms.[51] Decline in oestrogen in the hypothalamus, coupled with age-related sleep changes, can disrupt circadian rhythms and result in sleep disturbances.[52] Furthermore, cognitive decline is often reported in menopausal women.[53] Oestrogen has been shown to influence dendrite growth in areas of the brain related to memory functions and may influence cognitive function through its action on neurotransmitters such as acetylcholine.[46] The evidence of association between cognitive decline and menopause transition is inconclusive.[53,54]

Pathogenesis of Musculoskeletal Symptoms

The main musculoskeletal symptoms reported during menopause are paraesthesia, arthralgia and myalgia. Paraesthesia is a common symptom reported by menopausal women. The decline in oestrogen leads to collagen loss and thinning of the skin.[55] Decreased blood flow to the superficial nerves results in sensations of tingling and numbness (Bensaleh, Belgnaoui, Douira *et al.* (2006) cited in Sharif-Alhoseini *et al.* (2012)).[56]

There is a strong association between musculoskeletal pain/arthritis and declining oestrogen; however, no causal link has been established, likely due to the fact that pain is common throughout life.[57] Oestrogen receptors can be found in joint tissues, including cartilage, subchondral bone, synovium, ligaments and muscles.[58] Chondrocytes in cartilage both express oestrogen receptors and respond to oestrogen.[59] In chondrocytes, oestrogen increases production of proteoglycans, regulates intracellular concentration of calcium, and decreases nuclear factor kappa light chain enhancer of activated B cells, inducible nitric oxide synthase, cyclooxygenase-2, and reactive oxygen species to prevent cartilage damage.[58] Oestrogen therapy is protective at low doses[59] and has reversed spontaneous and interleukin (IL)-1 induced cartilage damage in ovariectomised mice.[60]

Declining levels of oestradiol seen in the menopausal transition increase bone resorption and the risk of fractures.[61] Oestrogen regulates subchondral bone growth and remodelling, regulates development and function of osteoblasts, and promotes mineralisation and matrix production.[58,62] Bone resorption is prevented by 'suppression of receptor activator of nuclear factor kappa-B ligand c-Jun and basal c-Jun N-terminal kinase activity in osteoclast precursor cells'.[59, p. 143]

In muscles, oestrogen promotes proliferation and differentiation of myoblasts, decreases apoptosis of muscle cells, and improves muscle structure and function in women.[58] High levels of oestrogen during the menstrual cycle of female athletes have been associated with anterior cruciate ligament rupture,[58] although conflicting findings have been seen in animal studies.

Oestrogen is known to have anti-inflammatory and mild immunosuppressive effects.[57] These actions have been shown to contribute to protection of cartilage breakdown in animals.[60] Oestrogen stimulates B cell-mediated immune response whilst suppressing T cell-mediated response.[60] Oestrogen also regulates inflammatory cytokines IL-1β, IL-6, tumour necrosis factor-α and transforming growth factor-β.[59] Hormone therapy (HT) and selective oestrogen receptor modulators (SERMs) reduce inflammation, and women in the Women's Health Initiative study who were taking oestrogens had fewer joint replacements.[63] Furthermore, women who receive HT report improvement in joint-related pain or stiffness as well as general bodily aches and pains.[2]

In addition to being found in joint tissue, oestrogen receptors are also present in the dorsal root ganglion, limbic system and hypothalamus.[57] Oestrogen and testosterone activate inhibitory pain pathways;

thus, a decline of oestrogen during menopause may result in greater perception of pain.[57]

Diagnosis

Diagnosis of menopause is made based on the clinical criteria related to the menstrual cycle.[2] Menopause can be diagnosed in women who have not had a period for at least 12 months and who are otherwise healthy, or in women without a uterus who report symptoms of menopause.[3] Measurement of FSH does not add useful information for clinical diagnosis and should not be used for women older than 45 years.[64]

Testing of FSH may be indicative for women between 40 and 45 years of age who report a change in their menstrual cycle or symptoms of menopause, or when menopause is suspected in women under 40 years.[3] If FSH is assessed, it should be measured at the beginning of the follicular phase.[8] Pregnancy should also be excluded.[8] In women who have undergone hysterectomy, menopause can be diagnosed based on symptoms and, if required, two elevated serum FSH tests.[65]

The National Institute for Health and Care Excellence guideline[11] recommends against testing inhibin A, inhibin B and oestradiol, and against imaging tests for antral follicle count and ovarian volume. Ultrasound or pelvic examination should be limited to women at high risk of endometrial or ovarian cancer.[8] Several guidelines recommend against testing for AMH for diagnosis of menopause,[1,11] although this test may be of value to assess ovarian reserve in women with suspected premature ovarian failure.[8]

The staging system for ovarian ageing originally proposed in 2001 was revised in 2011.[66] The Stages of Reproductive Aging Workshop (STRAW) +10 provides nomenclature that allows consistent staging of menopause status. Stages –5 to –3a refer to the early to late reproductive phase. Stages –2 (early menopausal transition), –1 (late menopausal transition) and +1a (early postmenopause) collectively comprise the perimenopause. Stages +1b, +1c and +2 refer to postmenopause. For more information about each stage, see Harlow *et al.* (2012).[66]

Management

Ten clinical guidelines and position statements were reviewed to summarise the management of menopause. These were the North American Menopause Society position statements for hormone therapy[67] and non-hormonal management;[68] the Endocrine Society clinical practice guideline for treatment of symptoms of menopause;[2] the United Kingdom National Collaborating Centre for Women's and Children's Health Clinical Guideline for Menopause;[11] the European Menopause and Androgen Society position statements on management of menopausal health,[8] non-hormonal management of menopausal vasomotor symptoms[69] and menopause for medical students;[70] the American Association of Clinical Endocrinologists and American College of Endocrinology position statement on menopause (2017 update),[71] the statement of the Royal Australian and New Zealand College of Obstetricians and Gynaecologists[1] and the International Menopause Society recommendations on women's midlife health and hormone therapy.[72]

Not all women experience menopausal symptoms and many experience mild symptoms that they are able to manage themselves.[64] Women who seek medical advice should be provided with information and advice about the stages of menopause and common symptoms.[1,3,64] Women's preferences for management should be recorded when taking medical history.[8]

Lifestyle changes to improve general health and wellbeing include dietary and exercise advice, information about smoking cessation,[3,8] weight management, stress reduction, and reducing alcohol and caffeine intake.[1] The risks and benefits of hormonal, non-hormonal and non-pharmacological treatments should be discussed.[3] Advice should be given about contraception and health implications, such as osteoporosis, following menopause.[3] Pharmacological and non-pharmacological treatment options for women experiencing uncomplicated menopause are described hereafter. Further information about management for women with premature ovarian failure or breast cancer can be found in clinical practice guidelines.[2,8,11,67–71]

Pharmacological Management

Pharmacological management for women experiencing uncomplicated menopause includes both hormonal and non-hormonal treatments. Long- and short-term benefits and risks should be explained to women.[3]

Hormonal Management

Many menopausal women seek medical advice for VMS.[1] Hormone therapy is the most effective treatment for VMS[3,67] and GSM symptoms such as vulvovaginal atrophy and some urinary tract infections,[67] and may also improve sleep and musculoskeletal symptoms.[1] Hormone therapy may improve low mood due to menopause.[3]

Oral HT has been shown to increase the risk of thromboembolism.[11] Oral HT is not indicated in women who have suffered a deep venous thrombosis while taking combined hormone oral contraceptives, nor in women with active cardiovascular disease.[11] Non-oral (transdermal) administration of HT at the lowest effective dose is preferred for women with prior history of thromboembolism and those at increased risk.[2] Hormone therapy is contraindicated for women with a past history of hormone-sensitive cancers.[3] Furthermore, the Royal Australian and New Zealand College of Obstetricians and Gynaecologists guidelines state that HT should be used with caution in women with active systemic lupus erythematosus or abnormal liver function.[1]

The benefits to risk ratio for HT is more favourable for women under 60 years of age, or when initiated within ten years of menopause and with no contraindications.[67] When started before 60 years, benefits of HT include VMS improvement and prevention of osteoporosis during systemic treatment.[3] Bone loss will resume once HT has stopped.[8] Symptomatic women with reduced bone density may benefit from HT.[1]

Risks of HT when started before 60 years include unscheduled vaginal bleeding, an increased risk of venous thromboembolism with oral HT, a small increase in the risk of stroke with oral oestrogen, and an increased risk of breast cancer with oestrogen and progestogen combined.[3] Transdermal oestrogen may pose a lower risk of venous thromboembolism and cardiovascular disease than oral oestrogen,[71] and may be a safer option for women at increased risk of venous thromboembolism.[1] Hormone therapy remains an option with cardiovascular risk factors providing these are optimally managed.[3]

After consideration of short- and long-term benefits and risks, women with a uterus should be offered the combination of oestrogen and progestogen and women without a uterus should be offered oestrogen alone.[3,8] Unopposed oestrogen in women with a uterus increases the risk of endometrial cancer[1] when endometrial overgrowth occurs.[67] As such, HT for women with a uterus should include at least ten days of progestogen per month,[1] unless conjugated equine oestrogen (CEE) is taken in combination with the SERM bazedoxifene.[67]

Conjugated equine oestrogens, micronised 17 β-oestradiol, synthetic conjugated oestrogen and ethinyl oestradiol are the most commonly prescribed oestrogens.[67] Custom compounded bioidentical HT is not recommended due to a lack of data to support its safety and inconsistency in product content.[71] Progestins include medroxyprogesterone acetate, norethindrone acetate and native progesterone. Micronised progesterone is considered safer when progesterone is required.[71] The SERM bazedoxifene can be used in combination with CEE in a fixed combination of 0.45 mg/20 mg.[71]

Hormone therapy should start at a low dose[67] and be titrated to achieve symptom relief.[1] Women should be encouraged to report unscheduled bleeding if it persists after three months of HT.[3] The decision to use HT for symptomatic postmenopausal women should be made after considering all risk factors, including cardiovascular disease, time from menopause and age.[71] Annual review of women on HT is recommended.[1] Hormone therapy can be continued as long as is consistent with treatment goals.[72] Providing there are no contraindications, HT can be used for as long as the benefits outweigh the risks.[8]

Low-dose vaginal oestrogen is safe to use long term[67] and may be used for as long as needed to relieve GSM.[3] Vaginal oestrogen is the most effective treatment for women who report vaginal symptoms only.[1] Vaginal oestrogen may improve urinary symptoms where systemic HT has no effect,[67] although there is no evidence of an effect on stress incontinence.[72] Neither vaginal nor systemic HT improve sexual function or interest.[67] Vaginal oestrogen can be combined with vaginal moisturisers and lubricants; it is not required to be used with progesterone[8] and there is no requirement to monitor endometrial thickness during treatment.[3]

Tibolone, a synthetic steroid with both oestrogenic and progestogenic activity, should be restricted to women more than one year postmenopause.[1] Tibolone may increase the risk of irregular bleeding in younger women and may increase the risk of stroke in women over 65 years.[1] Tibolone has a lower risk of break-through bleeding within three months of treatment initiation than combined HT.[73]

Non-hormonal Management

Non-hormonal treatments may offer symptom relief for menopausal symptoms and can be considered for women at higher risk with HT.[71] The selective serotonin reuptake inhibitor (SSRI) paroxetine salt has been approved by the US Food and Drug Administration (FDA) at low doses for moderate to severe VMS.[68] Other SSRIs, such as citalopram and escitalopram, and serotonin and noradrenaline reuptake inhibitors (SNRIs), such as venlafaxine and desvenlafaxine, are effective for hot flashes but are less effective than oestrogen.[8]

Clonidine, an α-2 adrenergic agonist, has a modest effect on VMS.[68] Adverse events include hypotension, headache, dizziness and sedation. Clonidine is infrequently used due to adverse events.[68] Antiepileptic drugs, such as gabapentin and pregabalin, have been found to provide symptomatic relief.[71] The SSRIs, SNRIs and clonidine should not be used routinely as first-line therapy for VMS.[3] Paroxetine and fluoxetine are contraindicated in women taking tamoxifen.[8] There is no clear evidence that SSRIs and SNRIs improve low mood for women who have not been diagnosed with depression.[3]

Non-pharmacological Management

Non-pharmacological therapies include mind-body techniques, lifestyle changes, dietary management and supplements.[68] There is some evidence that lifestyle changes, such as weight loss and mindfulness-based stress reduction, may alleviate vasomotor symptoms.[68] Evidence is insufficient, negative or inconclusive for avoiding triggers, cooling techniques, exercise, relaxation and paced respiration.[68] Vaginal moisturisers, silicone-based lubricants or acidic gels can be used for vaginal dryness.[1,2]

Women with a history of affective disorders may be referred to a mental health care professional.[1] Cognitive behavioural therapy may be considered to improve low mood and anxiety associated with menopause.[3] Both cognitive behavioural therapy and clinical hypnosis have been found to reduce vasomotor symptoms.[67,68]

There is some evidence that the anaesthesia treatment stellate ganglion blockade may reduce VMS.[68] The stellate ganglion in the C6–T2 vertebral region is blocked by ultrasound-guided injection of local anaesthetic at the level of C6.[68] The mechanism of stellate ganglion blockade is unclear.

Isoflavones from soy foods and soy extracts are non-steroidal compounds that bind to oestrogen receptors.[68] There is some evidence that isoflavones can reduce VMS, and the S-equol derivatives of soy isoflavones are recommended with caution by the North American Menopause Society.[68] Soy preparations can vary in composition and the safety profile for individual preparations is not clear. Interactions with other drugs have been reported.[3] Women should be advised of this when considering soy products.

Complementary and Alternative Medicine

Women who do not receive adequate symptom relief from pharmacological and non-pharmacological treatments may look to complementary and alternative medicine (CAM). Indeed, CAM use among menopausal women is high.[74] The evidence for many of these is lacking, and the North American Menopause Society states that over-the-counter supplements and herbal therapies, acupuncture, yoga and chiropractic should not be recommended.[68] Black cohosh and other phytoestrogens should not be used by breast cancer survivors.[71] Women should be supported in their decision making about non-hormonal treatment of vasomotor symptoms, particularly as women may not feel fully informed about herbal products.[68]

Prognosis

Menopausal symptoms are usually self-limiting, but may persist for more than ten years.[20] Women taking HT should be reviewed after three months for any issues arising from commencement of therapy.[8] Annual review should include assessment of efficacy, dose and need for continued treatment, and benefits and risks should be re-evaluated.[8]

Ceasing HT gradually may reduce the chance of recurrence of the symptoms in the short term; however, stopping HT gradually or immediately does not influence symptoms long term.[3] For approximately 50% of women, ceasing HT may result in recurrence of vasomotor symptoms. Vaginal atrophy can persist and recur when treatment ceases.[8]

Age-related chronic diseases such as diabetes, cardiovascular disease, osteoporosis, cognitive decline and depression may appear after menopause.[75] Assessment of risks factors and screening can begin at menopause.[75] Lifestyle advice recommended for menopause (see 'Management') are also applicable for age-related chronic diseases. Although not recommended as a preventative strategy, HT has been found to decrease the risk of coronary heart disease and all-cause mortality.[75]

References

1. Robson S, Harvey J, Yazdani A, *et al.* (2014) Management of the menopause (C-Gyn 09). Royal Australian and New Zealand College of Obstetricians and Gynaecologists, Melbourne, Australia.
2. Stuenkel CA, Davis SR, Gompel A, *et al.* (2015) Treatment of symptoms of the menopause: An Endocrine Society Clinical Practice Guideline. *J Clin Endocrinol Metab* **100**(11): 3975–4011.

3. Sarri G, Davies M, Lumsden MA. (2015) Diagnosis and management of menopause: Summary of NICE guidance. *BMJ* **351**: h5746.
4. Gold EB, Crawford SL, Avis NE, *et al.* (2013) Factors related to age at natural menopause: Longitudinal analyses from SWAN. *Am J Epidemiol* **178**(1): 70–83.
5. Freedman RR, Roehrs TA. (2006) Effects of REM sleep and ambient temperature on hot flash-induced sleep disturbance. *Menopause* **13**(4): 576–583.
6. Williams RE, Kalilani L, DiBenedetti DB, *et al.* (2007) Healthcare seeking and treatment for menopausal symptoms in the United States. *Maturitas* **58**(4): 348–358.
7. Im EO, Seung Hee L, Chee W. (2010) Subethnic differences in the menopausal symptom experience of Asian American midlife women. *J Transcult Nurs* **21**(2): 123–133.
8. Neves ECM, Birkhauser M, Samsioe G, *et al.* (2015) EMAS position statement: The ten point guide to the integral management of menopausal health. *Maturitas* **81**(1): 88–92.
9. Mishra GD, Kuh D. (2012) Health symptoms during midlife in relation to menopausal transition: British prospective cohort study. *BMJ* **344**: e402.
10. Liu M, Wang Y, Li X, *et al.* (2013) A health survey of Beijing middle-aged registered nurses during menopause. *Maturitas* **74**(1): 84–88.
11. The National Institute of Health and Care Excellence (NICE) Guideline. (2015) Menopause: Diagnosis and management. Available from: https://www.nice.org.uk/guidance/ng23.
12. Woods NF, Mitchell ES. (2005) Symptoms during the perimenopause: Prevalence, severity, trajectory, and significance in women's lives. *Am J Med* **118**(Suppl 12B): 14–24.
13. Avis NE, Stellato R, Crawford S, *et al.* (2001) Is there a menopausal syndrome? Menopausal status and symptoms across racial/ethnic groups. *Soc Sci Med* **52**(3): 345–356.
14. Schneider HPG, Birkhauser M. (2017) Quality of life in climacteric women. *Climacteric* **20**(3): 187–194.
15. Harlow SD, Karvonen-Gutierrez C, Elliott MR, *et al.* (2017) It is not just menopause: Symptom clustering in the Study of Women's Health Across the Nation. *Womens Midlife Health* **3**.
16. Ang SB, How CH. (2013) Menopause: An important milestone in women's health. *Singapore Med J* **54**(2): 60–63.

17. Zheng W, Chow WH, Yang G, *et al.* (2005) The Shanghai Women's Health Study: Rationale, study design, and baseline characteristics. *Am J Epidemiol* **162**(11): 1123–1131.
18. Palacios S, Nappi RE, Bruyniks N, *et al.* (2018) The European Vulvovaginal Epidemiological Survey (EVES): Prevalence, symptoms and impact of vulvovaginal atrophy of menopause. *Climacteric* **21**(3): 286–291.
19. Whiteley J, DiBonaventura M, Wagner JS, *et al.* (2013) The impact of menopausal symptoms on quality of life, productivity, and economic outcomes. *J Womens Health (Larchmt)* **22**(11): 983–990.
20. Freeman EW. (2014) Hot flushes and the menopause: How long should they be expected to last? *Maturitas* **78**(3): 153–154.
21. Avis NE, Crawford SL, Greendale G, *et al.* (2015) Duration of menopausal vasomotor symptoms over the menopause transition. *JAMA Intern Med* **175**(4): 531–539.
22. Sun N, Xing J, Li L, *et al.* (2018) Impact of menopause on quality of life in community-based women in China: 1 year follow-up. *Arch Psychiatr Nurs* **32**(2): 224–228.
23. Avis NE, Ory M, Matthews KA, *et al.* (2003) Health-related quality of life in a multiethnic sample of middle-aged women: Study of Women's Health Across the Nation (SWAN). *Med Care* **41**(11): 1262–1276.
24. Utian WH. (2005) Psychosocial and socioeconomic burden of vasomotor symptoms in menopause: A comprehensive review. *Health Qual Life Outcomes* **3**: 47.
25. Dibonaventura MD, Chandran A, Hsu MA, *et al.* (2013) Burden of vasomotor symptoms in France, Germany, Italy, Spain, and the United Kingdom. *Int J Womens Health* **5**: 261–269.
26. Bobula JD. (2003) Vasomotor symptoms and quality of life (QoL) in postmenopausal women. *Value Health* **6**: 707.
27. Assaf AR, Bushmakin AG, Joyce N, *et al.* (2017) The relative burden of menopausal and postmenopausal symptoms versus other major conditions: A retrospective analysis of the medical expenditure panel survey data. *Am Health Drug Benefits* **10**(6): 311–321.
28. Sarrel P, Portman D, Lefebvre P, *et al.* (2015) Incremental direct and indirect costs of untreated vasomotor symptoms. *Menopause* **22**(3): 260–266.
29. Herber-Gast GC, Mishra GD, van der Schouw YT, *et al.* (2013) Risk factors for night sweats and hot flushes in midlife: Results from a prospective cohort study. *Menopause* **20**(9): 953–959.

30. Hall JE. (2015) Endocrinology of the menopause. *Endocrinol Metab Clin North Am* **44**(3): 485–496.
31. Hale GE, Robertson DM, Burger HG. (2014) The perimenopausal woman: Endocrinology and management. *J Steroid Biochem Mol Biol* **142**: 121–131.
32. Gosden RG, Faddy MJ. (1994) Ovarian aging, follicular depletion, and steroidogenesis. *Exp Gerontol* **29**(3–4): 265–274.
33. Burger HG, Hale GE, Robertson DM, *et al.* (2007) A review of hormonal changes during the menopausal transition: Focus on findings from the Melbourne Women's Midlife Health Project. *Hum Reprod Update* **13**(6): 559–565.
34. Klein NA, Houmard BS, Hansen KR, *et al.* (2004) Age-related analysis of inhibin A, inhibin B, and activin A relative to the intercycle monotropic follicle-stimulating hormone rise in normal ovulatory women. *J Clin Endocrinol Metab* **89**(6): 2977–2981.
35. Robertson DM, Hale GE, Fraser IS, *et al.* (2011) Changes in serum anti-mullerian hormone levels across the ovulatory menstrual cycle in late reproductive age. *Menopause* **18**(5): 521–524.
36. Landgren BM, Collins A, Csemiczky G, *et al.* (2004) Menopause transition: Annual changes in serum hormonal patterns over the menstrual cycle in women during a nine-year period prior to menopause. *J Clin Endocrinol Metab* **89**(6): 2763–2769.
37. Hale GE, Zhao X, Hughes CL, *et al.* (2007) Endocrine features of menstrual cycles in middle and late reproductive age and the menopausal transition classified according to the Staging of Reproductive Aging Workshop (STRAW) staging system. *J Clin Endocrinol Metab* **92**(8): 3060–3067.
38. Freedman RR. (2014) Menopausal hot flashes: Mechanisms, endocrinology, treatment. *J Steroid Biochem Mol Biol* **142**: 115–120.
39. Freedman RR. (1998) Biochemical, metabolic, and vascular mechanisms in menopausal hot flashes. *Fertil Steril* **70**(2): 332–337.
40. Freedman RR, Woodward S, Sabharwal SC. (1990) Alpha 2-adrenergic mechanism in menopausal hot flushes. *Obstet Gynecol* **76**(4): 573–578.
41. The North American Menopause Society. (2018) Changes in hormone levels. Available from: https://www.menopause.org/for-women/sexual-health-menopause-online/changes-at-midlife/changes-in-hormone-levels.
42. Robinson D, Toozs-Hobson P, Cardozo L. (2013) The effect of hormones on the lower urinary tract. *Menopause Int* **19**(4): 155–162.

43. Portman DJ, Gass ML. (2014) Genitourinary syndrome of menopause: New terminology for vulvovaginal atrophy from the International Society for the Study of Women's Sexual Health and The North American Menopause Society. *Climacteric* **17**(5): 557–563.
44. Naumova I, Castelo-Branco C. (2018) Current treatment options for postmenopausal vaginal atrophy. *Int J Womens Health* **10**: 387–395.
45. Goldstein I. (2010) Recognizing and treating urogenital atrophy in postmenopausal women. *J Womens Health (Larchmt)* **19**(3): 425–432.
46. Robinson GE. (2001) Psychotic and mood disorders associated with the perimenopausal period: Epidemiology, aetiology and management. *CNS Drugs* **15**(3): 175–184.
47. Gundlah C, Lu NZ, Bethea CL. (2002) Ovarian steroid regulation of monoamine oxidase-A and -B mRNAs in the macaque dorsal raphe and hypothalamic nuclei. *Psychopharmacology (Berl)* **160**(3): 271–282.
48. McEwen BS, Alves SE. (1999) Estrogen actions in the central nervous system. *Endocr Rev* **20**(3): 279–307.
49. Sherwin B. (1996) Menopause, early aging and elderly women. In: Jensvold M, Halbreich U, Hamilton J (eds), *Psychopharmacology and Women: Sex, Gender and Hormones.* American Psychiatric Press Inc., Washington, DC, pp. 225–237.
50. Pau KY, Hess DL, Kohama S, *et al.* (2000) Oestrogen upregulates noradrenaline release in the mediobasal hypothalamus and tyrosine hydroxylase gene expression in the brainstem of ovariectomized rhesus macaques. *J Neuroendocrinol* **12**(9): 899–909.
51. Caruso D, Masci I, Cipollone G, *et al.* (2019) Insomnia and depressive symptoms during the menopausal transition: Theoretical and therapeutic implications of a self-reinforcing feedback loop. *Maturitas* **123**: 78–81.
52. Parry BL, Fernando Martinez L, Maurer EL, *et al.* (2006) Sleep, rhythms and women's mood. Part II. Menopause. *Sleep Med Rev* **10**(3): 197–208.
53. Shanmugan S, Epperson CN. (2014) Estrogen and the prefrontal cortex: Towards a new understanding of estrogen's effects on executive functions in the menopause transition. *Hum Brain Mapp* **35**(3): 847–865.
54. Henderson VW, Popat RA. (2011) Effects of endogenous and exogenous estrogen exposures in midlife and late-life women on episodic memory and executive functions. *Neuroscience* **191**: 129–138.
55. Wilkinson HN, Hardman MJ. (2017) The role of estrogen in cutaneous ageing and repair. *Maturitas* **103**: 60–64.

56. Sharif-Alhoseini M, Rahimi-Movaghar V, Vaccaro A. (2012) Underlying causes of paresthesia. In: Imbelloni L, Gouveia M (eds), *Paresthesia.* InTech, Rijeka, Croatia.
57. Watt FE. (2018) Musculoskeletal pain and menopause. *Post Reprod Health* **24**(1): 34–43.
58. Roman-Blas JA, Castaneda S, Largo R, *et al.* (2009) Osteoarthritis associated with estrogen deficiency. *Arthritis Res Ther* **11**(5): 241.
59. Karsdal MA, Bay-Jensen AC, Henriksen K, *et al.* (2012) The pathogenesis of osteoarthritis involves bone, cartilage and synovial inflammation: May estrogen be a magic bullet? *Menopause Int* **18**(4): 139–146.
60. da Silva JA, Colville-Nash P, Spector TD, *et al.* (1993) Inflammation-induced cartilage degradation in female rodents: Protective role of sex hormones. *Arthritis Rheum* **36**(7): 1007–1013.
61. Santen RJ, Allred DC, Ardoin SP, *et al.* (2010) Postmenopausal hormone therapy: An Endocrine Society scientific statement. *J Clin Endocrinol Metab* **95**(7 Suppl 1): s1–s66.
62. Lugo L, Villalvilla A, Largo R, *et al.* (2014) Selective estrogen receptor modulators (SERMs): New alternatives for osteoarthritis? *Maturitas* **77**(4): 380–384.
63. Cirillo DJ, Wallace RB, Wu L, *et al.* (2006) Effect of hormone therapy on risk of hip and knee joint replacement in the Women's Health Initiative. *Arthritis Rheum* **54**(10): 3194–3204.
64. Lumsden MA, Davies M, Sarri G. (2016) Diagnosis and management of menopause: The National Institute of Health and Care Excellence (NICE) Guideline. *JAMA Intern Med* **176**(8): 1205–1206.
65. Casper RF. (2019) Clinical manifestations and diagnosis of menopause. Available from: https://www.uptodate.com/contents/clinical-manifestations-and-diagnosis-of-menopause.
66. Harlow SD, Gass M, Hall JE, *et al.* (2012) Executive summary of the Stages of Reproductive Aging Workshop +10: Addressing the unfinished agenda of staging reproductive aging. *Climacteric* **15**(2): 105–114.
67. The North American Menopause Society. (2017) The 2017 hormone therapy position statement of The North American Menopause Society. *Menopause* **24**(7): 728–753.
68. The North American Menopause Society. (2015) Nonhormonal management of menopause-associated vasomotor symptoms: 2015 position statement of The North American Menopause Society. *Menopause* **22**(11): 1155–1172; quiz 73–74.

69. Mintziori G, Lambrinoudaki I, Goulis DG, *et al.* (2015) EMAS position statement: Non-hormonal management of menopausal vasomotor symptoms. *Maturitas* **81**(3): 410–413.
70. Brockie J, Lambrinoudaki I, Ceausu I, *et al.* (2014) EMAS position statement: Menopause for medical students. *Maturitas* **78**(1): 67–69.
71. Cobin RH, Goodman NF. (2017) American Association of Clinical Endocrinologists and American College of Endocrinology Position Statement on Menopause: 2017 Update. *Endocr Pract* **23**(7): 869–880.
72. Baber RJ, Panay N, Fenton A. (2016) 2016 IMS Recommendations on women's midlife health and menopause hormone therapy. *Climacteric* **19**(2): 109–150.
73. Hammar ML, van de Weijer P, Franke HR, *et al.* (2007) Tibolone and low-dose continuous combined hormone treatment: Vaginal bleeding pattern, efficacy and tolerability. *BJOG* **114**(12): 1522–1529.
74. Posadzki P, Lee MS, Moon TW, *et al.* (2013) Prevalence of complementary and alternative medicine (CAM) use by menopausal women: A systematic review of surveys. *Maturitas* **75**(1): 34–43.
75. Lobo RA, Davis SR, De Villiers TJ, *et al.* (2014) Prevention of diseases after menopause. *Climacteric* **17**(5): 540–556.

2

Menopause in Chinese Medicine

OVERVIEW

Syndrome differentiation is used to treat menopause in Chinese medicine. Modern research suggests that the pathogenesis of menopause is mainly related to Kidney deficiency, as well as dysfunction of the Liver, Spleen, Heart and other organs. This chapter reviews the terminology, aetiology, pathogenesis and syndrome differentiation for menopausal syndrome from key Chinese medicine textbooks and guidelines. Treatments with Chinese herbal medicine, acupuncture and other therapies are described.

Introduction

Menopause is not classified as a syndrome in the World Health Organization's International Classification of Diseases (ICD-10).[1] Chinese medicine (CM) describes the collection, or grouping, of related symptoms as a 'syndrome' (*zheng* 证); this term can be found in several of the terms used for menopause in contemporary texts. Terms include *geng nian qi zong he zheng* 更年期综合征 (climacteric syndrome),[2] *jing duan qian hou zhu zheng* 经断前后诸证 (syndrome associated with the end of menstruation) and *jue jing qian hou zhu zheng* 绝经前后诸证 (signs and symptoms that are associated with the end of menstruation).[3,4] The term *geng nian qi zong he zheng* 更年期综合征 is typically used in conventional medicine, while the latter two terms are used in CM.

Jing duan qian hou zhu zheng 经断前后诸证 is a recent term, having first appeared in the CM gynaecology textbook *Zhong Yi Fu Ke Xue Jiang Yi* 中医妇科学讲义 in 1964.[5] Despite this, both CM terms appear to have roots in classical CM texts. *Jing duan* 经断, translated as 'cessation of menstruation', can be found in classical CM texts.[5] Other terms used to describe menopause in past eras include *zang zao* 脏躁, translated literally as 'restless organs' and often used to describe hysteria, and *bai he bing* 百合病, translated as 'lily disease'.[3,4] The term *bai he bing* 百合病 refers to the use of the herb *bai he* 百合, the bulb of the lily, in formulas that alleviated psychological symptoms commonly seen after childbirth and at the end of menstruation.

Scheid (2006)[6] posits that menopause was not considered a medical problem in classical texts, although symptoms common during menopause were described. This view was also expressed by Flaws,[7] who states that in classical texts the symptoms were the diagnosis. The description of menopause as a syndrome in contemporary CM texts is likely due to efforts in the 1960s to systematise CM to align with the biomedical model of disease.[5]

Aetiology and Pathogenesis

Menopause in CM is often described in terms of life cycles. The famous passage from *Huang Di Nei Jing Su Wen* 黄帝内经素问 describes the seven-year life cycles for women, which culminates in depletion of Kidneys, *tian gui* 天癸, and the *Ren* 任 and *Chong* 冲 vessels in the seventh seven-year cycle (age 49). This passage also describes decline from the fifth and sixth seven-year cycles: the decline of *Yangming* 陽明vessels, drying of the complexion and hair loss at age 35; and decline of the three *yang* vessels, dried out complexion and hair turning white at age 42 (Guo (1992), cited in Scheid (2007)).[5] The decline in the digestive function means less Blood is created and menses become irregular.[8] This highlights that the onset of menopause is preceded by decline of *qi*, Blood, *yin, yang, jing* 精 and *tian gui* 天癸.[7]

Kidney deficiency and exhaustion of *tian gui* 天癸 are the main causes of menopause, while imbalance of *yin* and *yang* are key in the pathogenesis.[3] The Kidney rules the reproductive functions, while *tian gui* 天癸 promotes the growth, development and reproduction functions. The *Ren* 任 (Conception) and *Chong* 冲 (Thoroughfare) vessels also play an important role in the regulation of menstruation. Weak constitution, multiparity, excessive coitus, imbalanced lifestyle, emotional instability and environmental factors can affect the balance of *yin* and *yang*, and can lead to menopause symptoms.[3,9]

During the menopausal transition, depletion of Kidney *qi*, exhaustion of *tian gui* 天癸, and deficiency of *Ren* 任 and *Chong* 冲 vessels[2–4,9] impair the ability of the body to adapt to the physiological changes. When menopause starts, Kidney *qi* and *tian gui* 天癸 will gradually decline, and the two vessels will deplete in their functions. The insufficiency of *jing* 精 and Blood, and exhausting reproductive function, will result in a lack of nourishment of the *zang fu* 脏腑 and an imbalance in *yin* and *yang*, resulting in menopause syndrome.

Constitutional *yin* deficiency or excessive blood loss caused by multiparity, combined with anxiety and insomnia, depletes Kidney *yin*. This results in an imbalance of *yin* and *yang* and disharmony between *ying* 營 and *wei* 衛, and the appearance of hot flushes.[3] Decline of Kidney *qi* results in decline of the *ming men* 命門 fire, which fails to warm the *zang fu* 脏腑. This results in aversion to cold with cold limbs and frequent urination at night. Deficient Kidney *yin* or *yang* will ultimately influence the other; for example, Kidney *yin* deficiency will lead to Kidney *yang* deficiency over time. With deficiency of both Kidney *yin* and *yang*, the *zang fu* 脏腑 will not be nourished or warmed, leading to sudden bouts of fever and cold.

Depletion of the Kidney can result in deficiency of the *Ren* 任 and *Chong* 冲 vessels. Menstruation becomes disordered and the symptoms may include hypomenorrhoea or menorrhagia. Depletion of the Kidney and insufficiency of *jing* 精 will result in a lack of nourishment of the Sea of Marrow (*sui hai* 髓海), bones and muscles, and leads to dizziness, tinnitus, and pain around the waist, back, knees and heels.[9]

Imbalance in Kidney *yin* and *yang* can affect other *zang fu* 脏腑.[2,3,10] For example, insufficiency of Kidney *jing* 精 will reduce nourishment of the Liver and bind Liver *qi*. Stagnation of Liver *qi* combined with Kidney deficiency can lead to emotional symptoms such as feeling irritable, excited, stressed or depressed. Constitutional deficiency of Kidney *jing* 精 will fail to support the Heart. Heart *yin* will become deficient and Heart fire will develop and disturb the *shen* 神; this can lead to palpitations, insomnia and excessive dreams. Sweat is considered the Blood of the Heart, so uncontrolled sweating can further weaken Heart *yin*.[8]

A breakdown in the relationship between organs can contribute to menopause syndrome. In addition, the imbalance between *yin* and *yang* in *zang fu* 脏腑 can be accompanied by other factors, such as *qi* stagnation, Blood stasis and phlegm dampness.

Syndrome Differentiation and Treatments

Kidney deficiency is the main pattern in menopausal syndrome, and the key to clinical differentiation is identifying *yin* or *yang* syndromes. The main syndromes in guidelines and textbooks were Kidney *yin* deficiency 肾阴虚, Kidney *yang* deficiency 肾阳虚 and Kidney *yin* and *yang* deficiency 肾阴阳两虚.[4,9] The relationship between the Kidney and other organs, such as the Heart and Liver, features in the pathogenesis of menopause. The syndromes Kidney deficiency and Liver stagnation 肾虚肝郁, and disharmony between the Heart and Kidney 心肾不交, were included in the *Guidelines for the Treatment of Common Gynecological Diseases* 中医妇科常见病诊疗指南 published in 2012 by the Chinese Medical Association,[2] and have been included in new editions of a key CM gynaecology textbook.[3,10] The five syndromes included in the *Guidelines for the Treatment of Common Gynecological Diseases* 中医妇科常见病诊疗指南 are consistent with recent clinical epidemiological studies.[11,12]

The principle of treatment is to regulate the *yin* and *yang* in the Kidneys, identify syndrome differentiation and administer clinical treatments accordingly. The main treatment methods include nourishing Kidney *yin*, warming the Kidney and supporting *yang*, tonifying the *yin* and *yang*, relieving the Liver and resolving stagnation, tonifying the Kidney and nourishing the Heart to calm the *shen* 神. Other therapies, such as acupuncture, moxibustion and ear acupuncture, can be used at the same time to complement the

Table 2.1 Summary of Chinese Herbal Medicines for Menopause Syndrome

Syndrome Differentiation	Treatment Principle	Formula
Kidney *yin* deficiency 肾阴虚	Nourish Kidney *yin* and subdue *yang*.	*Zuo gui wan* 左归丸 plus *Er zhi wan* 二至丸[2,3]
Kidney *yang* deficiency 肾阳虚	Warm the Kidney and support *yang*.	*You gui wan* 右归丸[2,3]
Kidney *yin* and *yang* deficiency 肾阴阳俱虚	Tonify both *yin* and *yang*.	*Er xian tang* 二仙汤[2,3]
Kidney deficiency with Liver stagnation 肾虚肝郁	Nourish Kidney *yin*, relieve the Liver and resolve stagnation.	*Yi guan jian* 一贯煎[3,13]
Heart and Kidney disharmony 心肾不交	Enrich *yin* and suppress fire, replenish the Kidney and calm the Heart.	Modified *Tian wang bu xin dan* 天王补心丹[2,3]

efficacy of herbal treatments. A summary of CM syndromes and treatments can be found in Table 2.1.

The following section describes the CHM formulas recommended in clinical guidelines, their herb ingredients and key actions of the herbs. The use of some herbs may be restricted in some countries. In addition, some herbs are restricted under the provisions of the Convention on International Trade in Endangered Species of Wild Fauna and Flora (CITES). Readers are advised to comply with relevant regulations.

Oral Chinese Herbal Medicine Treatment Based on Syndrome Differentiation

The following syndromes describe symptoms that occur during menopause, that is, both before and after the end of menstruation.

Kidney *Yin* Deficiency 肾阴虚

Clinical manifestations: Menopausal menstrual disorder, hypomenorrhoea or menorrhagia and flooding or spotting bright red coloured menstrual blood. Menstrual symptoms may be accompanied by dizziness and tinnitus, sweating with hot flush, 'five hearts hot' (heat in the palms, soles and chest), pain around the waist, knees and heels, itchy and dry skin, dry mouth, dry stools and decreased urine volume. The tongue will be red with little tongue coating and the pulse will be thin and rapid.

Treatment principle: Nourish Kidney *yin* and subdue *yang*.

Formulas: *Zuo gui wan* 左归丸 plus *Er zhi wan* 二至丸.[2,3]

Herbs in both formulas: *Shu di huang* 熟地黄, *shan yao* 山药, *gou qi* 枸杞, *shan zhu yu* 山茱萸, *chuan niu xi* 川牛膝, *gui ban jiao* 龟板胶, *lu jiao jiao* 鹿角胶, *tu si zi* 菟丝子, *han lian cao* 旱莲草 and *nü zhen zi* 女贞子.

Main actions of herbs: *Shu di huang* 熟地黄 and *gui ban jiao* 龟板胶 nourish the Kidney and replenish *jing* 精; *shan zhu yu* 山茱萸 and *gou qi* 枸杞 enrich the Kidney and nourish the Liver; *shan yao* 山药 replenishes the Spleen and tonifies *yin*; *lu jiao jiao* 鹿角胶 warms and replenishes Kidney *yang* and strongly tonifies *jing* 精 and marrow (*sui* 髓); *tu si zi* 菟丝子 and *chuan niu xi* 川牛膝 replenish the Liver and Kidney; *han lian cao* 旱莲草 and *nü zhen zi* 女贞子 tonify the Kidney *yin*.

Manufactured medicines: *Liu wei di huang wan* 六味地黄丸[2,3,13] enriches *yin* and tonifies the Kidney. *Kun bao wan* 坤宝丸[2,3] enriches the Liver and Kidney, calms and quiets the *shen* 神, nourishes the Blood and activates channels. *Geng nian an* 更年安[2,3,13] enriches *yin* and clears heat, relieves anxiety and quiets the *shen* 神.

Kidney *Yang* Deficiency 肾阳虚

Clinical manifestations: Menopausal menorrhagia with pale colour, sometimes flooding or spotting. The complexion will be dull and spiritless. Other symptoms include soreness and pain in the waist and knees, fear of cold with cold limbs or puffy face and swollen limbs, copious clear urine, frequent urination at night and thin loose stools. The tongue will be pale or enlarged with tooth marks on the margins and there will be a thin white tongue coat. The pulse will be weak, deep and thin.

Treatment principle: Warm the Kidney and support *yang*.

Formula: *You gui wan* 右归丸.[2,3]

Herbs: *Shu di huang* 熟地黄, *shan yao* 山药, *shan zhu yu* 山茱萸, *gou qi* 枸杞, *tu si zi* 菟丝子, *du zhong* 杜仲, *lu jiao jiao* 鹿角胶, *shu fu zi* 熟附子, *rou gui* 肉桂 and *dang gui* 当归.

Main actions of herbs: *Shu fu zi* 熟附子, *rou gui* 肉桂 and *lu jiao jiao* 鹿角胶 warm and tonify Kidney *yang*, and replenish *jing* 精 and marrow 髓; *shu di huang* 熟地黄, *gou qi* 枸杞, *shan zhu yu* 山茱萸 and *shan yao* 山药 enrich *yin* and nourish the Kidney, and enrich and nourish the Liver and Spleen; *tu si zi* 菟丝子 tonifies *yang* and nourishes *yin*; *du zhong* 杜仲 enriches and nourishes the Liver and Kidney and strengthens sinews and bones; and *dang gui* 当归 tonifies Blood and nourishes the Liver.

Manufactured medicines: *Long feng bao jiao nang* 龙凤宝胶囊 (capsule)[2,3,14] replenishes the Kidney, fortifies the Spleen, boosts *qi*, calms the *shen* 神 and sharpens the wits.

Kidney *Yin* and *Yang* Deficiency 肾阴阳俱虚

Clinical manifestations: Menopausal menstrual disorder and hypomenorrhoea or menorrhagia. Other symptoms include sudden bouts of fever and cold, sweating with hot flush, dizziness and tinnitus, forgetfulness, cold and pain in low back. The tongue will be pale with a thin tongue coat and the pulse will be deep and weak.

Treatment principle: Tonify both *yin* and *yang*.

Formula: *Er xian tang* 二仙汤.[2,3]

Herbs: *Xian mao* 仙茅, *xian ling pi* 仙灵脾, *dang gui* 当归, *ba ji tian* 巴戟天, *huang bai* 黄柏 and *zhi mu* 知母.

Main actions of herbs: *Xian mao* 仙茅, *xian ling pi* 仙灵脾 and *ba ji tian* 巴戟天 warm Kidney *yang* and enrich Kidney *jing* 精; *huang bai* 黄柏 and *zhi mu* 知母 drain Kidney fire and enrich Kidney *yin*; and *dang gui* 当归 warms and nourishes the Blood and regulates *Ren* 任 and *Chong* 冲 vessels.

Kidney Deficiency with Liver Stagnation 肾虚肝郁

Clinical manifestations: Sweating with hot flushes during menopause transition or hypomenorrhoea with red coloured menstrual blood. Menstrual changes may be accompanied by mood changes (irritability, excitability, stress or depression). Additional symptoms may include soreness and weakness in the waist and knees, dizziness and insomnia, distending pain in the breasts, rib pain, bitter taste in the mouth and dry throat. The tongue will be red with a thin white coating and the pulse will be fine and rapid.

Treatment principle: Nourish Kidney *yin*, relieve the Liver and resolve stagnation.

Formula: *Yi guan jian* 一贯煎.[3,13]

Herbs: *Sheng di huang* 生地黄, *bei sha shen* 北沙参, *mai dong* 麦冬, *dang gui* 当归, *gou qi zi* 枸杞子 and *chuan lian zi* 川楝子.

Main actions of herbs: *Sheng di huang* 生地黄 enriches *yin*, nourishes Blood and replenishes the Liver and Kidney; *dang gui* 当归 and *gou qi zi* 枸杞子 nourish the Blood, enrich *yin* and soften the Liver; *bei sha shen* 北沙参 and *mai dong* 麦冬 enrich and nourish the Lung and Stomach; and *chuan lian zi* 川楝子 relieves the Liver and discharges heat, corrects *qi* and relieves pain.

Heart and Kidney Disharmony 心肾不交

Clinical manifestations: Sweating with hot flushes during menopause transition, palpitations and hypomenorrhoea with red coloured menstrual blood. Other symptoms include soreness and weakness around the waist and knees, dizziness and tinnitus, vexation and agitation, insomnia and profuse dreaming at night, and mood changes. The tongue will be red with a thin white coating and the pulse will be thin and rapid.

Treatment principle: Enrich *yin* and suppress fire, replenish the Kidney and calm the Heart.

Formula: *Tian wang bu xin dan* 天王补心丹; replace *ren shen* 人参 and *zhu sha* 朱砂 with *tai zi shen* 太子参 and *sang shen* 桑葚.[2,3]

Herbs: *Suan zao ren* 酸枣仁, *bai zi ren* 柏子仁, *dang gui* 当归, *tian dong* 天冬, *mai dong* 麦冬, *sheng di huang* 生地黄, *tai zi shen* 太子参, *dan shen* 丹参, *xuan shen* 玄参, *fu ling* 茯苓, *wu wei zi* 五味子, *yuan zhi* 远志, *ji geng* 桔梗 and *sang shen* 桑葚.

Main actions of herbs: *Sheng di huang* 生地黄 and *sang shen* 桑葚 tonify the Heart and Kidney and nourish the Liver and Kidney; *tian dong* 天冬, *mai dong* 麦冬 and *xuan shen* 玄参 enrich *yin* and clear heat; *dan shen* 丹参 and *dang gui* 当归 nourish Heart Blood and promote Blood circulation; *tai zi shen* 太子参 and *fu ling* 茯苓 benefit the Heart *qi*; *bai zi ren* 柏子仁, *yuan zhi* 远志, *wu wei zi* 五味子 and *suan zao ren* 酸枣仁 constrain the Heart *qi*, sharpen the wits and calm the nerves; and *ji geng* 桔梗 guides the herbs.

Manufactured medicines: *Kun tai jiao nang* 坤泰胶囊 (capsule)[2,3,14] enriches *yin* and clears heat, calms the *shen* 神 and relieves anxiety. *Nü zhen ke li* 女珍颗粒 (granules)[2,3] nourishes the Kidney and calms the Heart.

Acupuncture Therapies

Several acupuncture therapies are recommended in clinical textbooks and guidelines. These include acupuncture, moxibustion and

Table 2.2 Summary of Acupuncture Therapies for Menopause

Intervention	Acupuncture Points/Body Area	Treatment Frequency
Acupuncture	Main points: KI3 *Taixi* 太溪, LR3 *Taichong* 太冲, CV4 *Guanyuan* 关元, HT7 *Shenmen* 神门, SP6 *Sanyinjiao* 三阴交, BL15 *Xinshu* 心俞, BL23 *Shenshu* 肾俞 and BL18 *Ganshu* 肝俞. For *yang* deficiency, add CV6 *Qihai* 气海, GV4 *Mingmen* 命门 and KI7 *Fuliu* 复溜. For *yin* deficiency, add KI2 *Rangu* 然谷, KI10 *Yingu* 阴谷 and KI7 *Fuliu* 复溜.	30 minutes treatment daily for six days, one rest day. Treat for four consecutive weeks (one course).
Moxibustion	Main points: GV4 *Mingmen* 命门, CV6 *Qihai* 气海 and CV4 *Guanyuan* 关元.	5–10 minutes per point, treat daily or on alternate days.
Ear acupuncture	TF2 *Zigong* (Uterus) 子宫, TF2 *Luanchao* (Ovary) 卵巢, CO18 *Neifenmi* (Endocrine) 内分泌, TF4 *Shenmen* 神门, AH6 *Jiaogan* (Sympathetic) 交感, AT4 *Pizhixia* (Subcortex) 皮质下, CO15 *Xin* (Heart) 心, CO12 *Gan* (Liver) 肝 and CO10 *Shen* (Kidney) 肾.	3–4 points daily or on alternate days, retain for 30–60 minutes.

ear acupuncture (Table 2.2). Acupuncture points are selected according to syndrome differentiation. Common acupuncture points include: CV4 *Guanyuan* 关元, CV6 *Qihai* 气海, GV4 *Mingmen* 命门, BL23 *Shenshu* 肾俞, LR3 *Taichong* 太冲, BL15 *Xinshu* 心俞, SP6 *Sanyinjiao* 三阴交 and BL18 *Ganshu* 肝俞. Their actions are described below:[15]

- CV4 *Guanyuan* 关元: Nourishes and tonifies the Kidneys and benefits *yuan qi* 元氣 and *jing* 精;
- CV6 *Qihai* 气海: Tonifies *qi* and the Kidneys, strengthens *yang*, regulates *qi* and harmonises Blood;

- GV4 *Mingmen* 命门: Tonifies the Kidneys and regulates the Governing Vessel;
- LR3 *Taichong* 太冲: Nourishes Liver Blood and *yin*, promotes free flow of *qi*, subdues Liver *yang* and regulates menstruation;
- SP6 *Sanyinjiao* 三阴交: Invigorates Blood, calms the *shen* 神, tonifies the Stomach and Spleen and resolves dampness;
- BL15 *Xinshu* 心俞: Tonifies the Heart and calms the *shen* 神, regulates Heart *qi* and clears Heart fire;
- BL18 *Ganshu* 肝俞: Regulates the Liver and free flow of Liver *qi*, nourishes Blood and cools fire;
- BL23 *Shenshu* 肾俞: Tonifies the Kidneys and Kidney *yin*, benefits *jing* 精, firms Kidney *qi*, and benefits and warms the uterus.

Acupuncture

Body acupuncture points should be selected according to syndrome differentiation. Commonly used acupuncture points include KI3 *Taixi* 太溪, LR3 *Taichong* 太冲, CV4 *Guanyuan* 关元, HT7 *Shenmen* 神门, SP6 *Sanyinjiao* 三阴交, BL15 *Xinshu* 心俞, BL23 *Shenshu* 肾俞 and BL18 *Ganshu* 肝俞.[2,3,13] A mild reinforcing and reducing technique should be used to stimulate the needles. Needles should be retained for 30 minutes and treatment provided daily for six days followed by a day of no treatment, for four weeks. This constitutes one course of treatment.[13] For cases of *yang* deficiency, acupuncture points CV6 *Qihai* 气海, GV4 *Mingmen* 命门 and KI7 *Fuliu* 复溜 can be added; for cases of *yin* deficiency add KI2 *Rangu* 然谷, KI10 *Yingu* 阴谷 and KI7 *Fuliu* 复溜.[3]

Moxibustion Therapy

Moxibustion is suitable for patients with *yang* deficiency. The main acupuncture points include GV4 *Mingmen* 命门, CV6 *Qihai* 气海 and CV4 *Guanyuan* 关元.[16] Moxibustion can be applied normally or as ginger moxibustion for five to ten minutes on each point; treat every day or every second day.[16]

Ear Acupuncture

Ear acupuncture may be used for menopausal syndrome.[9,17] The main ear points include TF2 *Zigong* (Uterus) 子宫, TF2 *Luanchao* (Ovary) 卵巢, CO18 *Neifenmi* (Endocrine) 内分泌, TF4 *Shenmen* 神门, AH6 *Jiaogan* (Sympathetic) 交感, AT4 *Pizhixia* (Subcortex) 皮质下, CO15 *Xin* (Heart) 心, CO12 *Gan* (Liver) 肝 and CO10 *Shen* (Kidney) 肾. Choose three or four points each time; treat every day or every second day, retaining the needles for 30–60 mins. Ear acupuncture can be used as auricular needle-embedding or auricular plaster therapy.[16]

Other Chinese Medicine Therapies

In addition to Chinese herbal medicine and acupuncture, CM-based psychotherapy can benefit menopause syndrome.[9,18] Chinese medicine psychotherapy is also called 'holistic CM treatment for psychosomatic diseases', which means combining CM-based psychotherapy with Chinese herbal medicine according to syndrome differentiation. The treatment principles of CM psychotherapy are based on the five-phase theory on emotional moods and the specific emotional characteristics of women in menopausal transition; the key principles are 'sorrow overcomes anger' and 'joy overcomes sorrow and anxiety'.[13] The combined treatments can provide long-term improvement in the mental and physical symptoms for women in menopausal transition.[19]

Other Management Strategies

Preventive health care advice and guidance for women during the menopausal transition are important health education activities. Health education should include information about the nature of common symptoms of menopause. Health education improves a women's readiness and adaption to the mental and physical changes they will experience during menopause and helps them to be better prepared for health care in older age.[3,10,20]

Lifestyle advice can relate to diet, physical activity and daily life. Women should be encouraged to eat a balanced diet low in calories, fat, salt and sugar, to have plenty of dietary fibre, and to use vitamins, calcium, iron and other trace element supplements when necessary.[10,18] Physical exercise that is appropriate for their abilities is recommended, but care should be taken to avoid injury to joints and/or the musculoskeletal system. Women should aim for 30 minutes of moderate intensity exercise at least three times per week, in combination with twice weekly strength training.[20] Moderate exercise should increase the heart rate to 150 beats per minute. Women should be encouraged to have a balanced daily routine with plenty of sleep, sexual abstinence, and cultivation of positive thoughts and emotions.[3]

A comprehensive annual physical examination is highly recommended for early detection and treatment of many high-risk diseases in menopausal women, such as cervical cancer, breast disorders, hypertension, hyperlipidaemia, diabetes, coronary heart disease, osteoporosis, depression and anxiety, and other related diseases.[3,20]

References

1. World Health Organization. (2016) *ICD-10: International Statistical Classification of Disease and Related Health Problems*, 10th revision, 2nd ed. World Health Organization, Geneva.
2. 中华中医药学会. (2012) 中医妇科常见病诊疗指南. 北京: 中国中医药出版社.
3. 罗颂平, 刘雁峰. (2017) 中医妇科学 ('十二五'普通高等教育本科国家级规划教材). 第3版. 北京: 人民卫生出版社.
4. 马宝璋. (2012) 中医妇科学 (普通高等教育'十一五'国家级规划教材). 北京: 中国中医药出版社.
5. Scheid V. (2007) Traditional Chinese medicine — What are we investigating? The case of menopause. *Complement Ther Med* **15**(1): 54–68.
6. Scheid V. (2006) Not very traditional, nor exactly Chinese, so what kind of medicine is it? TCM's discource on menopause and its implications for practice, teaching and research. *J Chin Med* **82**: 5–20.
7. Flaws B. (2006) *Menopause and Chinese Medicine*. Blue Poppy Press, Boulder, Colorado.

8. Wolfe HL. (1993) *Menopause: A Second Spring*, 3rd ed. Blue Poppy Press, Boulder, Colorado.
9. 罗颂平. (2008) 中医妇科学 (全国高等中医药院校规划教材). 第2版. 北京: 高等教育出版社.
10. 王小云 黄. (2018) 中西医结合妇产科学 (普通高等教育'十三五'规划教材). 第3版. 北京: 科学出版社.
11. 杜彩凤, 王天芳, 吴秀艳, *et al.* (2010) 基于专家咨询问卷调查的更年期综合征常见证候要素. *中西医结合学报* **8**(8): 757–761.
12. 朱玲桂. (2016) 围绝经期综合征中医证候分布规律及病机特点研究. 甘肃中医药大学.
13. 王小云, 黄健玲. (2013) 妇科专病中医临床诊治. 第3版. 北京: 人民卫生出版社.
14. 中华医学会妇产科学分会绝经学组. (2013) 绝经期管理与激素补充治疗临床应用指南. *中华妇产科杂志* **48**(10): 795–799.
15. Deadman P, Al-Khafaji M, Baker K. (2000) *A Manual of Acupuncture*. Journal of Chinese Medicine Publications, East Sussex, England.
16. 国家中医药管理局医政司. (2010) 22个专业95个病种中医诊疗方案. 北京: 国家中医药管理局.
17. 罗云坚, 张英哲. (2003) 常见病中西医结合诊疗常规. 广州: 广东科技出版社.
18. 罗云坚, 孙塑伦. (2007) 中医临床治疗特色与优势指南. 北京: 人民卫生出版社.
19. 杨洪艳, 王小云, 许, 等. (2011) 中医心身同治方案治疗绝经综合征抑郁症状的随机对照研究. *广东医学* **32**(16): 2209–2211.
20. 中华预防医学会妇女保健分会, 更年期保健学组. (2016) 更年期妇女保健指南 (2015年). *实用妇科内分泌杂志* **3**(2): 21–32.

3

Classical Chinese Medicine Literature

OVERVIEW

Classical Chinese medicine texts are an important source of information for symptoms related to menopause. This chapter reports the findings from a search of the *Zhong Hua Yi Dian* 中华医典, one of the largest digitalised collections of Chinese medical texts. Search terms were selected for the key symptoms of menopause and for two diagnoses commonly associated with menopause — *zang zao* 脏躁/脏燥 and *bai he bing* 百合病. The terms identified 291 citations that described treatment for symptoms consistent with menopause. Chinese herbal medicine was described in 288 citations and acupuncture was described in three citations. The symptoms, aetiology and treatments are discussed.

Introduction

Chinese medicine (CM) has a long history, with some of the earliest written records dating back to the Spring and Autumn (770–476 BC) and Warring States (474–221 BC) periods. In these passages concepts such as *yin* and *yang* are evident and therapeutic methods included the use of mugwort (*ai* 艾) for moxibustion, herbal decoctions and acupuncture.[1]

The end of reproductive years is described in the *Huang Di Nei Jing Su Wen* 黄帝内经素问 (c. 762 AD). The well-known passage describes the exhaustion of *tian gui* 天癸 occurring in the seventh seven-year life cycle. However, the end of menstruation is part of the normal physiological changes that occur during ageing and, as an event, does not require treatment. The symptoms that accompany menopause may have been bothersome to women and for this reason treatment may have been sought. Given the early reference to the end of reproductive years in key CM texts, it is likely that CM treatments have been used for symptoms of menopause for many centuries.

In order to obtain a sample of the classical and pre-modern medical literature, we conducted electronic searches of the *Zhong Hua Yi Dian* (ZHYD) 中华医典, *Encyclopaedia of Traditional Chinese Medicine*, a CD of more than 1,000 medical books.[2] This collection is the largest currently available and is representative of other large collections of classical and pre-modern CM literature.[3,4]

Search Terms

Contemporary terms used for menopause, such as *jing duan qian hou zhu zheng* 经断前后诸证, have their origins in classical texts. *Jing duan* 经断, the cessation of menstruation, can be found in classical texts;[5] however, this term is not exclusive to menopause. Similarly, other terms that describe changes in menstrual cycle, such as *yue jing xian qi* 月经先期 (early menstruation), *yue jing xian hou wu ding qi* 月经先后不定期 (irregular menstruation), *yue jing hou qi* 月经后期 (late menstruation) and *yue jing guo duo* 月经过多 (excessive menstruation or menorrhagia),[6] are not specific to menstrual changes in mid-life. Other contemporary terms, such as *nian lao xue beng* 年老血崩 (metrorrhagia) and *nian lao jing duan fu lai* 年老经断复来 (postmenopausal bleeding), are not present in classical literature.

Two terms that describe symptoms of menopause can be found throughout classical CM literature: *zang zao* 脏躁/脏燥 and *bai he bing* 百合病 (Luo (1998), cited in Scheid (2008)).[7] *Zang zao* (translated as 'restless organs') has been used as a gynaecology term since the late Han dynasty (after 220 AD).[6] This term has been linked with psychological symptoms, such as melancholy or depression, and in some cases has been used to describe psychological symptoms occurring before and after menopause.[8,9] Other symptoms associated with menopause include hot flushes (*chao re* 潮热), insomnia (*shi mian* 失眠 or *bu mian* 不眠), palpitations (*xin ji* 心悸) and dizziness (*xuan yun* 眩晕).[6] Again, these symptoms are not unique to menopause and, therefore, a search strategy was needed that identified these symptoms in women.

In order to identify examples of menopause in classical literature, search terms were identified through consulting a CM dictionary,[10] traditional medicine nomenclature,[11] and Chinese and integrative medicine gynaecology textbooks.[8,9,12–20] Trial searches were conducted in the ZHYD to test their relevance. Eighteen terms or combinations of terms were included in the final search, including two sets of characters for *zang zao* 脏躁/脏燥.

Two terms, *zang zao* 脏躁/脏燥 and *bai he bing* 百合病, were considered likely to identify relevant citations and, therefore, these terms were searched alone. Other terms for symptoms that were not unique to menopause were combined with *fu ren* 妇人 (woman) in order to increase the specificity of results. Terms used for menopausal symptoms included hot flushes (*chao re* 潮热), insomnia (*bu mei* 不寐, *wo bu an* 卧不安, *bu de mian* 不得眠, *bu ming* 不瞑 and *bu de wo* 不得卧), bone atrophy (*gu wei* 骨痿), palpitation (*xin ji* 心悸) and dizziness (*xuan yun* 眩晕).

Some psychological symptoms in women may be related to menopause. Terms for psychological symptoms included depressed (*yu* 郁), angry (*nu* 怒), worry (*you* 忧), scared (*kong* 恐), sadness (*bei* 悲) and frightened (*jing* 惊). Separate searches were conducted for these symptoms combined with *fu ren* 妇人 (woman) in a subset of gynaecology texts included in the ZHYD.

Procedures for Search, Data Coding and Data Analysis

Search terms were entered into both heading and text search fields of the ZHYD and the search results were downloaded into spreadsheets. Duplicate citations that were the same citation found by multiple search terms were excluded. A 'citation' was defined as a distinct passage of text referring to one or more of the search terms. Codes were allocated for types of citations, books, and the dynasties in which they were written according to the procedures described in

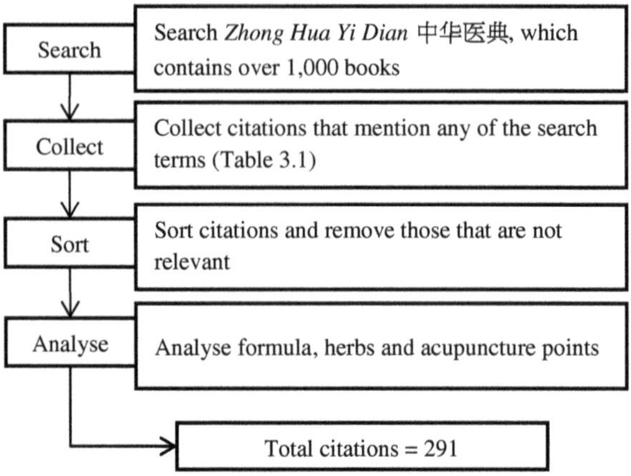

Fig. 3.1 Classical literature citations.

May *et al.* (2013).[4] Books written after 1949 were excluded. The process for searching, sorting and analysing information from classical literature is illustrated in Fig. 3.1.

The number of hits for each search term was recorded and summed to provide a total number of hits. Duplicate citations found by multiple search terms were removed from the dataset and the terms that identified the citation were recorded. Exclusion criteria were then applied to remove irrelevant citations. Citations were excluded if they were not related to menopause, were CM dictionary citations, or were pharmacopeia-style herb entries (for example, where menopause may have been listed as an indication with no additional information about menopause). Single acupuncture points were reviewed in a similar manner.

The remaining citations were reviewed to identify descriptions that were 'possibly' or 'most likely' related to menopause. Criteria were established to aid this judgment. Terms were grouped according to diagnosis (Group A) and symptoms (Groups B and C; Table 3.1). As terms in Groups A, B and C may be used for conditions other than menopause, additional criteria were added for menstruation (Group D), age (Group E) and symptoms accompanying dizziness, or palpitation (Group F).

Table 3.1 Term and Symptom Groups

Symptom Category	Descriptions	Possible Translation
Group A: Diagnosis 'most likely' to be menopause	A1: *Zang zao* 脏躁	Restless organs
	A2: *Zang zao* 脏燥	Restless organs
	A3: *Bai he bing* 百合病	Lily syndrome
Group B: Symptoms 'most likely' to relate to menopause	B1: *Chao re* 潮热 and *fu ren* 妇人	Hot flushes and women
	B2: Any emotional or sleep symptom below combined with *fu ren* 妇人:	Women and:
	Bei 悲	Sadness
	Yu 郁	Depressed
	Kong 恐	Fear
	Nu 怒	Angry
	Jing 惊	Frightened
	Bu de mian 不得眠, *bu de wo* 不得卧, *bu mei* 不寐, *wo bu an* 卧不安, *bu ming* 不瞑	Insomnia
Group C: Symptoms 'possibly' related to menopause	C1: *Xuan yun* 眩晕 and *fu ren* 妇人	Dizziness and women
	C2: *Xin ji* 心悸 and *fu ren* 妇人	Palpitations and women
	C3: *Gu wei* 骨痿 and *fu ren* 妇人	Bone atrophy and women
Group D: Terms related to amenorrhoea (*yue jing* 月经) in menopause	*Jing shui se shao* 经水涩少, *xue ku jing bi* 血枯经闭, *jing shui bi jue* 经水闭绝, *jing shui duan jue* 经水断绝, *jing duan* 经断, *tian gui jie* 天癸竭, *jing bi bu xing* 经闭不行 and *yue shui bu tong* 月水不通	Fewer menstrual periods and hypomenorrhoea, blood exhaustion and amenorrhoea, fewer menstrual periods and amenorrhoea, fewer menstrual periods and amenorrhoea, end of menstruation, exhaustion of *tian gui* 天癸, fewer menstrual periods and amenorrhoea, fewer menstrual periods and amenorrhoea

(*Continued*)

Table 3.1 (*Continued*)

Symptom Category	Descriptions	Possible Translation
Group E: Terms related to age (*nian ling* 年龄)	*Si shi ji qi yi shang nian liang* 四十及其以上年龄, *zhong nian yi hou* 中年以后, *niao lao* 年老, *lao fu* 老妇, *qi qi* 七七, *si xun wai* 四旬外 and *wu xun* 五旬	Age 40 and above, after middle age, old age, old woman, *seven seven* (referring to the seventh seven-year cycle), age 40 and above, age 50 and above
Group F: Symptoms combined with dizziness (*xuan yun* 眩晕) and/or palpitation (*xin ji* 心悸)	F1: *Ou tu* 呕吐, *er ming* 耳鸣, *er long* 耳聋 and *zhan li bu wen* 站立不稳	Vomit, tinnitus, deafness and astasia
	F2: *Ke chuan* 咳喘, *shui zhong* 水肿, *xiong men* 胸闷 and *xiong tong* 胸痛	Cough with asthma, oedema, chest tightness and chest pain
	F3: *Teng tong* 疼痛 and *gu zhe* 骨折	Pain and fracture

Citations were considered 'most likely' to be related to menopause when terms in Groups D or E were combined with terms in Group A, Group B1, Groups B1 and B2, or Group B1 and any term from Group C (Table 3.2). Citations were considered 'possibly' related to menopause where any term from Group A was described alone, when *chao re* 潮热 (Group B1) was used alone, when any of the emotional symptoms described in Group B2 were combined with terms in Groups D or E, and when any term from Group C was described in Groups D or E.

Citations which included any of the emotional symptoms from Group B2, or any symptoms from Group C alone, provided insufficient information to make a judgement about the likelihood of relating to menopause. These citations were excluded from the final dataset. Citations that described only symptoms from Groups D or E were excluded, as were citations with terms from C1 and F1, C2 and F2, and C2 and F3.

Table 3.2 Symptom Groups for Rating Citations

Likelihood of Relating to Menopause	Group Criteria
'Most likely' to be menopause	Any term from Group A plus any term from either Groups D or E
	Group B1 plus any term from either Groups D or E
	Any term from both Groups B1 and B2 plus any term from either Groups D or E
	Any term from both Groups B1 and C plus any term from either Groups D or E
'Possibly' related to menopause	Any term from Group A
	Group B1
	Any term from Group B2 plus any term from either Groups D or E
	Any term from Group C plus any term from either Groups D or E

Citations that only described menopause symptoms with no mention of treatment were excluded from analysis of treatments. Citations that described multiple treatments were considered as separate citations for the calculation of formulas, herbs or acupuncture points. Data are presented for the frequencies of identified formulas, herbs and acupuncture points for citations considered 'possibly' and 'most likely' related to menopause.

Search Results

After searches of both headings and text of the ZHYD were completed, 6,226 hits were found (Table 3.3). The selected search terms were productive, yielding over 100 hits for the majority of terms or combination of terms. Two combinations of terms produced fewer than 100 results: *Gu wei* 骨痿 and *fu ren* 妇人 (87 citations), and *bu ming* 不瞑 and *fu ren* 妇人 (8 citations). *Gu wei* 骨痿 can be translated as 'bone atrophy'. This may have referred to the loss of bone

Table 3.3 Hit Frequency by Search Term

Pinyin	Chinese Characters	Hit Frequency (*n*, %)
Xin ji and *fu ren*	心悸 and 妇人	1,441 (23.1)
Chao re and *fu ren*	潮热 and 妇人	622 (10.0)
Jing and *fu ren*	惊 and 妇人	475 (7.6)
Kong and *fu ren*	恐 and 妇人	463 (7.4)
Xuan yun and *fu ren*	眩晕 and 妇人	462 (7.4)
Yu and *fu ren*	郁 and 妇人	452 (7.3)
Nu and *fu ren*	怒 and 妇人	373 (6.0)
Bai he bing	百合病	327 (5.3)
Bu de wo and *fu ren*	不得卧 and 妇人	274 (4.4)
Bu mei and *fu ren*	不寐 and 妇人	238 (3.8)
You and *fu ren*	忧 and 妇人	194 (3.1)
Zang zao 2	脏燥	155 (2.5)
Wo bu an and *fu ren*	卧不安 and 妇人	151 (2.4)
Zang zao 1	脏躁	130 (2.1)
Bu de mian and *fu ren*	不得眠 and 妇人	129 (2.1)
Bei and *fu ren*	悲 and 妇人	113 (1.8)
Gu wei and *fu ren*	骨痿 and 妇人	87 (1.4)
Bu ming and *fu ren*	不瞑 and 妇人	8 (0.1)

mass and strength typically experienced by menopausal women. As only three citations from the 87 hits were ultimately included in the final dataset, it is difficult to know whether this is the case. Only eight citations were found for the combination of *bu ming* 不瞑 (insomnia) and *fu ren* 妇人. The number of citations for other terms referring to insomnia was much higher. For example, *bu mei* 不寐, *wo bu an* 卧不安, *bu de mian* 不得眠 and *bu de wo* 不得卧 all produced over 100 hits when combined with *fu ren* 妇人. This suggests that the term *bu ming* 不瞑 was used infrequently to describe insomnia in women.

The largest number of hits was found with the combination of *xin ji* 心悸 and *fu ren* 妇人, which identified 1,441 hits. This combination refers to palpitations in women. Although the initial number of hits was high, most of these hits were excluded after inclusion criteria were applied and only 11 citations describing treatment included in the final dataset.

Citations Related to Menopause

After exclusion of duplicates, irrelevant citations, and those with insufficient information to form a judgment, 196 citations were considered 'possibly' related to menopause. Thirty-six citations described menopause, menopausal symptoms, or the aetiology and pathogenesis of menopause without describing treatments. These citations were reviewed to identify the best examples of how menopause was conceptualised in past eras.

Fifty-four of the 196 included citations (27.6%) described two or more treatments. The greatest number of treatments described in any one citation was eight. Citations that included multiple treatments were separated for analysis of herbal formulas and acupuncture treatments. This process resulted in 291 treatment citations in the final dataset. The vast majority related to Chinese herbal medicine (CHM; 288 treatment citations), with three describing acupuncture treatment. The criteria described above were applied to the 291 treatment citations to identify those most likely to relate to menopause. Twenty-three treatment citations were identified, all of which described management of menopause symptoms with oral CHM.

Definitions of Menopause

Some of the best descriptions of menopause symptoms were also the earliest. Citations found by terms *zang zao* 1 脏躁 and *bai he bing* 百合病 were in the pre-Tang dynasty book *Jin Gui Yao Lue Fang Lun* 金匮要略方论 (commonly referred to as *Jin Gui Yao Lue* 金匮要略, c. 206 AD). A woman with *zang zao* 1 脏躁 was reported to 'feel sad and tend to cry with no apparent cause, yawn frequently, and should be treated with *Gan mai da zao tang* 甘麦大枣汤' (妇人脏躁悲伤欲哭, 象如神灵所作, 数欠伸者, 宜甘麦大枣汤). A later description of emotional symptoms in *Yin Chan Quan Shu* 胤产全书 (c. 1608) suggested *zang zao* 1 脏躁 could be due to Heart deficiency: 'Woman with Heart deficiency and palpitate with fear, and feel much sadness, which was named *zang zao* 1 脏躁, should be treated with *Dan zhu ru tang* 淡竹茹汤' (妇人心虚惊悸, 悲伤不止, 此名脏躁, 宜服此淡竹茹汤).

In *Jin Gui Yao Lue* 金匮要略, physical symptoms of *bai he bing* 百合病 were diverse: 'People with *bai he bing* 百合病 want to eat but cannot, are often silent, want to rest but cannot feel rested, want to walk but cannot, feel hot with no fever, feel cold without cold symptoms, have a bitter taste in the mouth and red urine. This cannot be treated with any other herbs or formula, if the patient takes [other] formula they will have severe vomiting or diarrhoea, like possessed by a devil, with a fast pulse. The patient will look normal to the doctor' (百合病者, 百脉一宗, 悉致其病也. 意欲食, 复不能食. 常默默, 欲卧不能卧. 欲行不能行. 饮食或有美时, 或有不用, 恶闻食臭. 时如寒无寒, 如热无热, 口苦, 小便赤. 诸药不能治, 得药则剧吐利, 如有神灵者. 身形如和, 其脉微数). This passage appears to suggest that *bai he* 百合 is the only treatment that can treat these symptoms.

Physical symptoms were diverse. Books from the Ming dynasty described the characteristic menopause symptom experienced by women: hot flushes. 'Steaming bone' hot flushes, a sensation of heat coming from the bones and moving to the exterior of the body, were described in *Wan Shi Nv Ke* 万氏女科 (c. 1549). 'Steaming bone' hot flushes occur with an empty pulse and can be treated with *Zeng sun ba wu chai hu tang* 增损八物柴胡汤 (妇人经闭不行, 骨蒸潮热, 脉虚者, 增损八物柴胡汤主之). The term 'steaming bone' typically refers to internal heat due to severe *yin* deficiency.

Another Ming dynasty book, *Nv Ke Zheng Zhi Zhun Sheng* 女科证治准绳 (c. 1607), depicted menstruation occurring every two or three months and hot flushes appearing in the afternoon when women are about 50 years old. This is due to Blood deficiency with heat, and these symptoms can be treated with *Xiao yao san* 逍遥散 with added *shan zhu yu* 山茱萸 (妇人年五十, 内热晡热, 经水两三月一至. 此血虚有热, 用逍遥散加山茱萸治之而愈).

Other menopausal symptoms found in classical citations included dizziness, sensations of cold, pain in the abdomen and legs, and palpitations. A case report in *Fu Ren Da Quan Liang Fang* 妇人大全良方

(c. 1237) describes a woman aged 44 or 45 years with a weak voice: 'If she walks weakly (slowly or with short steps), she will feel cold in her mouth, like a frost. She has three menstrual periods in 70 days, every time she walks she always feels cold in her mouth, feels dizzy and has cold feet, feeling like the cold and pain will go into her Heart' (一妇人, 年四十四, 五, 其证说话气短, 足弱, 行得数步则口若含霜. 七十日内三次经行, 遇行则口冷, 头目眩晕, 足冷则透心冷痛). The reference to cold sensations and weak voice suggests she has a deficiency of *qi* or *yang*. Deficiency of *wei qi* 衛氣 and the Sea of Blood underpinned symptoms of hot flushes and upset, dry mouth with preference for cold (food or drink), pain around the abdomen, chest, lower back and legs, cough with phlegm, palpitations and irregularity or the end of menstruation (妇人血海虚损, 荣卫不足, 多致潮热心烦, 口干喜冷, 腹胁刺痛, 腰腿疼, 痰多咳嗽, 惊惕怔忡, 经候不调, 或闭断不通; *Shi Yi De Xiao Fang* 世医得效方, c. 1345).

Descriptions of the Aetiology of Menopause

The aetiology and pathogenesis of menopausal symptoms were predominantly related to disorders of *qi* and Blood, and/or deficiency of *zang fu* 脏腑. Citations from *Pu Ji Fang* 普济方 (c. 1406) and *Shang Han Wen Yi Tiao Bian* 伤寒瘟疫条辨 (c. 1784) suggest that *bai he bing* 百合病 occurs in women who are unable to recover after a period of illness. In these women, both *zang* 脏 and *fu* 腑 organs are deficient, *rong* 荣 (Blood and nutritive fluids) and *wei* 卫 (*qi*) are both weak. *Bai he bing* 百合病 will develop (百合病, 脏腑俱虚, 荣卫耗弱, 不能平复, 变成斯疾也 — *Pu Ji Fang* 普济方; 百合病, 百脉一宗, 举身皆病, 无复经络传次, 故曰百合。大抵病后虚劳, 脏腑不调所致 — *Shang Han Wen Yi Tiao Bian* 伤寒瘟疫条辨).

The various causes and development of Blood exhaustion and amenorrhoea were detailed in *Han Dan Yi Gao* 邯郸遗稿 (c. 1617). Stomach *qi* deficiency prevents absorption of nutrition from food and drink, so that the body cannot produce *jin ye* 津液 (body fluids); this will lead to Blood deficiency (妇人血枯经闭, 有因胃气虚, 水谷难化, 津液不生, 而血虚不来者). *Qi* will be deficient in women who vomit blood during their youth, who have abnormally heavy menses, or have bleeding between menses (有因少时吐衄, 崩漏大脱血, 气亦不足者). 'Steaming bone' hot flushes consume *jin ye* 津液, the body will stop producing *jin ye* 津液 and the menses will cease (有因潮热骨蒸, 不生津液, 而经水闭绝者). Finally, in women with excessive sexual activity and multiple births, the body will become deficient and exhausted and menses will stop (有因房劳多产, 枯竭于内, 而经不通者). This description appears to describe the loss of *jing* 精 (essence).

Discussions of *zang zao* 脏躁/脏燥 naturally included references to the internal organs (*zang fu* 脏腑). Organ dryness, especially Lung dryness, was mentioned in several citations. A passage from *Jin Gui Yao Lue Xin Dian* 金匮要略心典 (c. 1729) connects organ dryness with Blood deficiency. When women have deficiency of Blood and *zang zao 2* 脏燥 (meaning organ dryness), internal fire will disturb the *shen* 神 and women will feel sad and want to cry, like possessed by the devil. This appears to be an excess disease, but is actually due to deficiency (此证沈氏所谓子宫血虚, 受风化热者是也. 血虚脏躁, 则内火扰而神不宁, 悲伤欲哭, 有如神灵, 而实为虚病). The consumption of *jin* 津 by excessive fire leads to Lungs losing their moisture and a feeling of upset and depression (脏燥者, 火盛烁津, 肺失其润, 心系了戾而然 — *Zhang Shi Yi Tong* 张氏医通, c. 1695).

A detailed passage from the Qing dynasty book *Su Ling Wei Yun* 素灵微蕴 (c. 1800) discusses the interrelationships in function and emotions of the *zang* 脏 organs in terms of the five phases (*wu xing* 五行). This citation offers two explanations for *zang zao* 脏躁. The first describes 'dry Metal' leading to 'cold Water' (燥金生其寒水). In this case Metal likely refers to the Lungs, and Water likely refers to the Kidney. In the generating (*sheng* 生) cycle of the five phases, Metal is the 'mother' of Water and provides nourishment when the body is in harmony. When Metal is dry, Water will not receive sufficient *qi*. The citation goes on to explain that when 'cold Water is too strong, it puts out the Fire' (水寒则火灭). This seems to suggest that cold Water is an excess condition, rather than a deficiency. For the Water to be in excess, the more likely case is that the 'child' (Water) has taken too much *qi* from the 'mother' (Metal). Metal dryness will manifest as sadness.

The second explanation describes imbalance of emotions in the five phases. In this case, the Wood and Fire are weak, allowing Metal and Water to become too strong. Women will feel fear and sadness (emotions associated with Metal and Water), but not happy or angry (emotions associated with Wood and Fire) (木火衰而金水旺, 故有悲恐而无喜怒, 水寒则火灭, 金燥则木伤故也).

Chinese Herbal Medicine

Among the 291 treatment citations, it was clear that CHM was the main treatment for symptoms of menopause. Two hundred and eighty-eight citations in 94 books described CHM. The book that provided the most citations was *Zhang Shi Yi Tong* 张氏医通 by Zhang Lu 张璐 (c. 1695); 15 citations were included from this book. Three other books provided ten or more citations: *Shang Han Zhi Zhi* 伤寒直指 (c. 1156; 14 citations), *Chi Shui Xuan Zhu* 赤水玄珠 (c. 1573; 11 citations) and *Ji Yin Gang Mu* 济阴纲目 (c. 1620; ten citations).

Frequency of Treatment Citations by Dynasty

The majority of included citations were from books published in the Ming and Qing dynasties (81.4%; Table 3.4). This most likely relates

Table 3.4 Dynastic Distribution of Treatment Citations

Dynasty	No. of Treatment Citations
Before Tang dynasty (before 618)	9
Tang and 5 dynasties (618–960)	7
Song and Jin dynasties (961–1271)	33
Yuan Dynasty (1272–1368)	6
Ming Dynasty (1369–1644)	62
Qing Dynasty (1645–1911)	171
Min Guo/Republic of China (1912–1949)	3
Total	**291**

to advances in book publication techniques during these eras. The earliest citations were found in the text *Jin Gui Yao Lue Fang Lun* 金匮要略方论 (c. 206 AD) by Zhang Zhongjing 张仲景. The term *bai he bing* 百合病 located two of the four citations in this book, and treatments included *Hua shi dai zhe tang* 滑石代赭汤 and *Bai he zhi mu tang* 百合知母汤. These citations are well known as being among the earliest references to menopause symptoms. The term *bai he bing* 百合病 has been used from the pre-Tang dynasties (before 618) to the Min Guo period (1912–1949).

The most recent citation was from the *Zhong Guo Nei Ke Yi Jian* 中国内科医鉴, published in the Min Guo period (1933). This citation was identified by *zang zao* 1 脏躁. This is not to say that this is a modern term; indeed, *zang zao* 1 脏躁' was found in books dating back to the pre-Tang dynasties. This term appeared to have a longer duration of use compared to *zang zao* 2 脏燥, which was limited to books from the Song and Jin, Qing, and Min Guo dynasties. *Zang zao* 2 脏燥 did not identify any citations related to menopause symptoms in books from the Ming dynasty. The reason for this is unclear but is more likely to relate to the criteria used to select citations rather than an absence of this term in books from the Ming dynasty.

Treatment with Chinese Herbal Medicine

As described, 288 of the 291 treatment citations used CHM for menopause symptoms. The majority of formulas were for oral administration (266 treatment citations), with topical treatments described in 22 citations. These citations were judged as either 'possible' cases of menopausal symptoms or cases 'most likely' to be related to menopause symptoms.

Most Frequent Formulas in 'Possible' Menopause Citations

Oral Chinese Herbal Medicine

Fifty-three different formulas for oral CHM use were described in the 266 citations. Many formulas were named after the herb ingredients.

For example, one of the most frequently used formulas was *Bai he zhi mu tang* 百合知母汤, with herbs *bai he* 百合 and *zhi mu* 知母 as the key ingredients. The majority of formulas were described by name (249 of 266 citations, 93.6%), while 17 citations described herb ingredients for unnamed formulas.

The most frequently cited formulas for oral use can be found in Table 3.5. *Gan mai da zao tang* 甘麦大枣汤 was the most common formula, found in 63 citations. The key actions of *Gan mai da zao tang* 甘麦大枣汤 are to nourish the Heart and calm the spirit.[6] The earliest use of this formula for menopause symptoms was in *Jin Gui Yao Lue Fang Lun* 金匮要略方论 in 206 AD. This book also described the second and third most frequently used formulas: *Bai he zhi mu tang* 百合知母汤 and *Hua shi dai zhe tang* 滑石代赭汤. The importance of the herb *bai he* 百合 for menopause-like symptoms is clear; the herb was included in the name of four of the ten most frequently described oral CHM formulas.

Two formulas with similar names and identical ingredients of the core formula were found in multiple citations: *Zeng jian ba wu chai hu tang* 增减八物柴胡汤 and *Zeng sun ba wu chai hu tang* 增损八物柴胡汤. The earliest citation of *Zeng jian ba wu chai hu tang* 增减八物柴胡汤 came from *Luo Shi Hui Yue Yi Jing* 罗氏会约医镜 (c. 1789). This book also described modifications of the formula, adding *di gu pi* 地骨皮, *gan jiang* 干姜, or both *mu dan pi* 牡丹皮 and *dan zhu ye* 淡竹叶. The earliest citation of the second formula, *Zeng sun ba wu chai hu tang* 增损八物柴胡汤, came from an earlier source. The text *Wan Shi Nv Ke* 万氏女科 (c. 1549) described the same core formula, as well as additions of *gu pi* 骨皮 or both *mu dan pi* 牡丹皮 and *dan zhu ye* 淡竹叶. These herb ingredients and modifications of this version of the formula are described in Table 3.5.

Topical Chinese Herbal Medicine

Topical application of CHM was described in 17 different books. The earliest use of topical CHM for menopause symptoms was from *Wai Tai Mi Yao* 外台秘要 (c. 752 AD) in the Tang and Five dynasties. This

Table 3.5 Most Frequent Oral Use Formulas in 'Possible' Menopause Citations

Formula Name	Herb Ingredients	No. of Citations (*n*)
Gan mai da zao tang 甘麦大枣汤	*Da zao* 大枣, *xiao mai* 小麦 and *gan cao* 甘草 (*Jin Gui Yao Lue Fang Lun* 金匮要略方论, c. 206 AD).	63
Bai he zhi mu tang 百合知母汤	*Bai he* 百合 and *zhi mu* 知母 (*Jin Gui Yao Lue Fang Lun* 金匮要略方论, c. 206 AD).	24
Hua shi dai zhe tang 滑石代赭汤	*Bai he* 百合, *hua shi* 滑石 and *zhe shi* 赭石 (*Jin Gui Yao Lue Fang Lun* 金匮要略方论, c. 206 AD).	22
Bai he di huang tang 百合地黄汤	*Bai he* 百合 and *di huang* 生地 (*Shang Han Zong Bing Lun* 伤寒总病论, c. 1100).	21
Bai he ji zi huang tang 百合鸡子黄汤	*Bai he* 百合 and *ji zi huang* 鸡子黄 (*Hua Tuo Shen Fang* 华佗神方, c. 682 AD).	18
Gua lou mu li san 栝蒌牡蛎散	*Gua lou gen* 栝蒌根 and *mu li* 牡蛎 (*Wai Tai Mi Yao* 外台秘要, c. 752 AD).	16
Bai he hua shi san 百合滑石散	*Bai he* 百合 and *hua shi* 滑石 (*Wai Tai Mi Yao* 外台秘要, c. 752 AD).	16
Zeng jian ba wu chai hu tang 增减八物柴胡汤/*Zeng sun ba wu chai hu tang* 增损八物柴胡汤	Core formula: *Ren shen* 人参, *fu ling* 茯苓, *bai shao* 白芍, *mai men dong* 麦门冬, *dang gui* 当归, *sheng di* 生地, *gan cao* 甘草, *zhi mu* 知母 and *chai hu* 柴胡. Variants include addition of (1) *gu pi* 骨皮 or (2) *mu dan pi* 牡丹皮 and *dan zhu ye* 淡竹叶 (*Wan Shi Nv Ke* 万氏女科, c. 1549).	7 (4/3)
Si wu tang jia jian 四物汤加减	*Chuan xiong* 川芎, *dang gui* 当归, *bai shao* 白芍, *shu di huang* 熟地黄 and *ze lan* 泽兰 (*Han Dan Yi Gao* 邯郸遗稿, c. 1617).	4

Note: The use of some herbs may be restricted in some countries. Readers are advised to comply with relevant regulations.

passage describes preparing *bai he* 百合 in water to wash the skin. The most recent citation was found in the Qing dynasty book *Jing Fang Li Shi* 经方例释 (c. 1884) and describes the same method of application.

Three named formulas and three unnamed formulas for topical use were described in 22 citations. All formulas used the herb *bai he* 百合. The three named formulas were *Bai he xi fang* 百合洗方 (17 citations), *Bai he xi tang* 百合洗汤 (one citation) and *Bai he tang* 百合汤 (one citation). Both *Bai he xi fang* 百合洗方 and *Bai he xi tang* 百合洗汤 were applied as a topical wash.

Most Frequent Herbs in 'Possible' Menopause Citations

A total of 112 different herbs were described in the 288 CHM treatment citations. The frequency of each herb was calculated separately for herbs described for oral use and those described for topical use. *Bai he* 百合 was the only herb described in topical CHM treatments and was also included in oral CHM formulas.

Not surprisingly, the most common herb was *bai he* 百合, found in 117 citations (Table 3.6). *Gan cao* 甘草 was the second most frequently used herb, found in 106 citations. This is most likely related to its action of harmonising the herbs in oral CHM formulas. The herbs *da zao* 大枣 (78 citations) and *xiao mai* 小麦 (70 citations) were also found to have high frequency of use. This is due to the finding that *Gan mai da zao tang* 甘麦大枣汤 was the most frequently described oral CHM formula. *Gan mai da zao tang* 甘麦大枣汤 includes the herbs *da zao* 大枣, *xiao mai* 小麦 and *gan cao* 甘草.

The number of herbs in formulas ranged from one to 22 and the median was three herbs. Many formulas used few herbs; 199 oral CHM formulas included three or fewer herbs. Again, this was likely to be due to the finding that *Gan mai da zao tang* 甘麦大枣汤, with its three herb ingredients, was the most frequently cited oral treatment for menopause symptoms. Ten citations prescribed the use of single herbs such as *bai he* 百合, *zhi mu* 知母 and *sheng di* 生地.

Table 3.6 Most Frequent Oral Use Herbs in 'Possible' Menopause Citations

Herb Name	Scientific Name	No. of Citations (*n*)
Bai he 百合	*Lilium* spp.	117
Gan cao 甘草	*Glycyrrhiza* spp.	106
Da zao 大枣	*Ziziphus jujuba* Mill.	78
Xiao mai 小麦	*Triticum aestivum* L.	70
Zhi mu 知母	*Anemarrhena asphodeloides* Bge.	43
Sheng di 生地	*Rehmannia glutinosa* Libosch.	41
Dang gui 当归	*Angelica sinensis* (Oliv.) Diels	40
Hua shi 滑石	Hydrated magnesium silicate	36
Fu ling 茯苓	*Poria cocos* (Schw.) Wolf	31
Ren shen 人参	*Panax ginseng* C. A. Mey.	29
Bai shao 白芍	*Paeonia lactiflora* Pall.	28
Chai hu 柴胡	*Bupleurum* spp.	23
Zhe shi 赭石	Ferric oxide	22
Mai men dong 麦门冬	*Ophiopogon japonicus* (Thunb.) Ker-Gawl.	21
Bai zhu 白术	*Atractylodes macrocephala* Koidz.	18
Ji zi huang 鸡子黄	Chicken egg yolk	18
Mu li 牡蛎	*Ostrea* spp.	17
Chuan xiong 川芎	*Ligusticum chuangxiong* Hort.	16
Gua lou gen 栝蒌根	*Tirchosanthes kirilowii* Maxim.	16
Shu di huang 熟地黄	*Rehmannia glutinosa* Libosch.	15

Note: The use of some herbs may be restricted in some countries. Readers are advised to comply with relevant regulations.

Most Frequent Formulas in 'Most Likely' Menopause Citations

Based on the available descriptions, 23 citations were considered 'most likely' to relate to menopause. All treatments described in these citations prescribed CHM for oral use. Eleven named and six unnamed formulas were described in the 23 citations considered most likely to relate to menopause. Given that the number of citations in the 'most likely' group was much smaller than the 'possible' group, it was not surprising to see little overlap in formulas used for menopause symptoms.

Three formulas were described in two or more citations and two of these were also among the most frequently used formulas found in possible menopause citations. The formulas *Zeng jian ba wu chai hu tang* 增减八物柴胡汤 and *Zeng sun ba wu chai hu tang* 增损八物柴胡汤 described the same core ingredients and similar modifications. These two formulas were merged for analysis and ingredients from the earliest citation are described in Table 3.7. The only other formula found in two or more citations was modified *Si wu tang* 四物汤.

One citation from the Ming dynasty book *Jiao Zhu Fu Ren Liang Fang* 校注妇人良方 (c. 1558) described using the combination of *Gui pi tang* 归脾汤 and *Liu wei di huang wang* 六味地黄丸 for menopause symptoms. The use of this combination of formulas suggests a view that both the Kidney and Spleen should be tonified for women with menopause symptoms.

Table 3.7 Most Frequent Formulas in 'Most Likely' Menopause Citations

Formula Name	Herb Ingredients	No. of Citations (*n*)
Zeng jian ba wu chai hu tang 增减八物柴胡汤/*Zeng sun ba wu chai hu tang* 增损八物柴胡汤	Core formula: *Ren shen* 人参, *fu ling* 茯苓, *gan cao* 甘草, *dang gui* 当归, *bai shao* 白芍, *sheng di* 生地, *mai men dong* 麦门冬, *zhi mu* 知母 and *chai hu* 柴胡. Variants include addition of: (1) *gu pi* 骨皮 or (2) *mu dan pi* 牡丹皮 and *dan zhu ye* 淡竹叶 (*Wan Shi Nv Ke* 万氏女科, c. 1549).	7 (4/3)
Si wu tang jia jian 四物汤加减	*Chuan xiong* 川芎, *dang gui* 当归, *bai shao* 白芍, *shu di huang* 熟地黄 and *ze lan* 泽兰 (*Han Dan Yi Gao* 邯郸遗稿 c. 1617).	2

Note: The use of some herbs may be restricted in some countries. Readers are advised to comply with relevant regulations.

Most Frequent Herbs in 'Most Likely' Menopause Citations

Sixty-one herbs were described among the 23 citations judged 'most likely' to be related to menopause. Formulas in the 'most likely' group were more complex compared to the 'possible' group. The number of herbs in each formula ranged from five to 18 and the median number of herbs was nine.

The high-frequency herbs in citations 'most likely' to be related to menopause differed somewhat to those found in the citations that were 'possibly' related to menopause (Table 3.8). *Dang gui* 当归 was

Table 3.8 Most Frequent Herbs in 'Most Likely' Menopause Citations

Herb Name	Scientific Name	No. of Citations (*n*)
Dang gui 当归	*Angelica sinensis* (Oliv.) Diels	21
Fu ling 茯苓	*Poria cocos* (Schw.) Wolf	14
Gan cao 甘草	*Glycyrrhiza* spp.	12
Chai hu 柴胡	*Bupleurum* spp.	11
Bai shao 白芍	*Paeonia lactiflora* Pall.	11
Ren shen 人参	*Panax ginseng* C. A. Mey.	10
Zhi mu 知母	*Anemarrhena asphodeloides* Bge.	9
Sheng di 生地	*Rehmannia glutinosa* Libosch.	7
Mai men dong 麦门冬	*Ophiopogon japonicus* (Thunb.) Ker-Gawl.	7
Bai zi ren 柏子仁	*Platycladus orientalis* (L.) Franco	6
Shi hu 石斛	*Dendrobium* spp.	6
Zi shi ying 紫石英	Calcium fluoride	6
Bie jia 鳖甲	*Trionyx sinensis* Wiegmann	6
Lu rong 鹿茸	*Cervus* spp.	6
Shu di huang 熟地黄	*Rehmannia glutinosa* Libosch.	5
Mu dan pi 牡丹皮	*Paeonia suffruticosa* Andr.	5
Bai zhu 白术	*Atractylodes macrocephala* Koidz.	5
Chuan xiong 川芎	*Ligusticum chuangxiong* Hort.	4
Niu xi 牛膝	*Achyranthes bidentata* Bl.	4

Note: The use of some herbs may be restricted in some countries. Readers are advised to comply with relevant regulations.

the most frequently used herb (21 citations), followed by *fu ling* 茯苓 (14 citations), *gan cao* 甘草 (12 citations), *chai hu* 柴胡 (11 citations) and *bai shao* 白芍 (11 citations). Notably, herbs *da zao* 大枣, *bai he* 百合 and *xiao mai* 小麦, which were among the most frequently used in 'possible' menopause citations, were absent from the list of high-frequency herbs in 'most likely' menopause citations. In fact, neither *bai he* 百合 nor *xiao mai* 小麦 was used in any formula among citations most likely to be menopause.

Discussion of Chinese Herbal Medicine for Menopause

The results of this systematic search of the classical CM literature showed that oral CHM was a common treatment for menopause-like symptoms. The formula with the highest frequency of use among citations 'possibly' related to menopause was *Gan mai da zao tang* 甘麦大枣汤. This formula is a well-known prescription for depression and emotional disturbances, with actions that nourish the Heart, calm the *shen* and tonify Spleen *qi*. Many of the citations described psychological symptoms of menopause (data not presented), so the high frequency for *Gan mai da zao tang* 甘麦大枣汤 was not surprising. Similarly, the presence of *da zao* 大枣, *xiao mai* 小麦 and *gan cao* 甘草 in the 20 most frequently used herbs was not surprising. These three herbs are the ingredients of *Gan mai da zao tang* 甘麦大枣汤 and the high frequency of this formula naturally influenced the frequency of herbs.

Despite being the most frequently cited formula in citations 'possibly' related to menopause, *Gan mai da zao tang* 甘麦大枣汤 was not found in citations 'most likely' to be related to menopause. This may be related to the criteria used to rate citations. Citations that described *Gan mai da zao tang* 甘麦大枣汤 as a treatment included diagnosis of either *zang zao* 脏躁/脏燥 (62 of 63 citations) or *bai he bing* 百合病 (one of 63 citations) and no other relevant symptoms. Furthermore, these citations did not mention the disease occurring in the context of amenorrhoea (*yue jing* 月经) or in relation to age (*nian ling* 年龄). This does not mean that *Gan mai da zao tang* 甘麦大枣汤 should not be used to treat emotional symptoms of menopause;

rather, the lack of information about cessation of menstruation and female age prevented these citations as being selected as the best examples of menopause.

The combination of *Gui pi tang* 归脾汤 and *Liu wei di huang wan* 六味地黄丸 was used in one citation judged 'most likely' to be menopause. *Gui pi tang* 归脾汤 strengthens the *qi* and Blood of the Spleen and Heart and may have been used to address the decline of *Yang Ming* vessels in the fifth seven-year cycle described in the *Huang Di Nei Jing Su Wen* 黄帝内经素问. *Liu wei di huang wan* 六味地黄丸 is a well-known formula to tonify the Kidney and nourish *yin*. *Liu wei di huang wan* 六味地黄丸 is a commercially available product that is recommended in gynaecology textbooks and guidelines (see Chapter 2).[8,21,22]

Aside from the formulas *Zeng jian ba wu chai hu tang* 增减八物柴胡汤 and *Zeng sun ba wu chai hu tang* 增损八物柴胡汤, the only other formula found in multiple citations judged most likely to be menopause was modified *Si wu tang* 四物汤. *Si wu tang* 四物汤 is often used for gynaecological and postpartum conditions due to its action of nourishing Blood, *Chong* 冲 (Thoroughfare) and *Ren* 任 (Conception) vessels.

Oral-use formulas in citations 'possibly' related to menopause involved fewer herb ingredients than those judged 'most likely' to be related to menopause (median three versus nine herbs, respectively). Topical-use formulas were simple, with all citations describing the application of a single herb: *bai he* 百合. *Bai he* 百合 was the most frequently used herb in 'possible' menopause citations yet was not found in citations 'most likely' to be menopause. Again, the lack of description of amenorrhoea or age is likely to be the reason for this finding.

Citations in which *bai he* 百合 was a formula ingredient were identified solely by the term *bai he bing* 百合病. The actions of *bai he* 百合 are to nourish Lung *yin*, clear the Heart and calm the *shen*.[23] This aligns with the descriptions of menopause symptoms being due to Lung dryness. The frequent use of *bai he* 百合 in both oral- and topical-use formulas highlights its importance in treating menopause symptoms.

Dang gui 当归 was the most frequently used herb in citations 'most likely' to relate to menopause. *Dang gui* 当归 tonifies Blood and nourishes the Liver,[23] and is used for gynaecological diseases. The importance of tonifying Blood and Spleen *qi* is demonstrated by the use of *fu ling* 茯苓, *gan cao* 甘草 and *bai shao* 白芍.

Acupuncture and Related Therapies

Acupuncture points were infrequently described in included citations. Three citations from the Ming dynasty (1369–1644) described treatment of menopause with acupuncture therapies, and all were considered to 'possibly' be related to menopause. Acupuncture therapies were not described in citations judged 'most likely' to relate to menopause. Two citations were found using the combination of *fu ren* 妇人 and *bei* 悲 and were from the books *Yi Xue Gang Mu* 医学纲目 (c. 1565) and *Zheng Zhi Zhun Sheng — Za Bing* 证治准绳 — 杂病 (c. 1602). Both citations described applying acupuncture to points on the Liver and Pericardium (*Jue Yin*) and Heart channels, although the points to be used were not named.

The third citation was found using *fu ren* 妇人 and *xin ji* 心悸. This citation, from the book *Yi Xue Gang Mu* 医学纲目 (c. 1565), described dizziness in an older woman, and acupuncture points BL12 *Fengmen* 风门, CV14 *Juque* 巨阙, ST40 *Fenglong* 丰隆 and GB21 *Jianjing* 肩井 were used. While BL12 *Fengmen* 风门 and GB21 *Jianjing* 肩井 are typically used to regulate *qi* and expel wind, the inclusion of CV14 *Juque* 巨阙 and ST40 *Fenglong* 丰隆 suggests organ dysfunction of the Lung, Heart and Stomach.[24]

Classical Literature in Perspective

The classical CM literature is a valuable source of information about the management of many health conditions in past eras. When health conditions have a clear name and/or unique identifiable features, for example the characteristic rash of herpes zoster (*she chuan chuang* 蛇串疮), information about the understanding and treatment can be located relatively easily. Identifying citations for conditions that have a diverse range of symptoms is more challenging. This review used a systematic approach to identify terms used for menopause symptoms and to search a representative sample of classical CM books.

The terms *zang zao* 脏躁/脏燥 and *bai he bing* 百合病 are the CM diagnoses frequently associated with symptoms of menopause. Together, these terms identified more than 600 citations, but did not identify citations judged 'most likely' to relate to menopause. Whilst both terms are used for menopause symptoms, commentators of classical CM literature agree that *zang zao* 脏躁/脏燥 describes a kind of nutritive *qi* deficiency, while *bai he bing* 百合病 refers to the presence of excess heat (Li (1989), cited in Scheid (2008)).[7] Nutritive (*ying*) *qi* 營氣 moves within the meridians and nourishes the organs and tissues. Lack of nourishment will result in impaired functions of the organs, leading to disease. While *zang zao* 脏躁/脏燥 may not have an exclusive connection with menopause symptoms, the pathogenesis is likely to be relevant when considering the diversity of symptoms women experience.

The suggestion that *bai he bing* 百合病 refers to excess heat appears to be at odds with the contemporary understanding of menopause symptoms as arising due to deficient heat (particularly in Kidney *yin* deficiency). However, when one examines the historical development of CM gynaecology, the reason for this becomes apparent. Scheid (2008) states that the prevailing view during the Eastern Han (pre-Tang) dynasty was that gynaecology and obstetrics diseases were a 'failure of regulation of *qi*, Blood and body fluids and their disturbance by outside factors like wind and cold.'[7, p. 495] During the Jin, Yuan and Ming dynasties there was a greater emphasis on organ systems in gynaecology books, although there was little discussion of the importance of the Kidneys in treating women.[7] Indeed, few of the citations identified by *bai he bing* 百合病 in this analysis mention the Kidneys in relation to menopause symptoms.

In the 1960s, the Chinese Ministry of Health sought to systematise CM education through the development of biomedical-style textbooks. The term for menopause syndrome, *jing duan qian hou zhu zheng* 经断前后诸证, was not present in the first edition of the

Lecture Notes for Chinese Medicine Gynaecology (*Zhong yi fu ke xue jiang yi* 中医妇科学讲义, 1960), but appeared in the second edition published in 1964.[5] It was at this time that menopause syndrome was defined as a problem relating to the Kidneys[5] and this view can be found in many contemporary textbooks and clinical guidelines published since the 1960s.

The majority of citations judged 'most likely' to be related to menopause were found by the combination of terms for hot flushes and women (*chao re* 潮热 and *fu ren* 妇人, 19 citations). Contemporary research shows vasomotor symptoms, hot flushes and night sweats are the most bothersome symptoms for women[25] and are the symptoms most often discussed with contemporary health care providers.[26] This may have also been the case in past eras in China.

Terms for other symptoms related to menopause, such as insomnia, palpitations and emotional symptoms, identified many more hits than *zang zao* 1 脏躁, *zang zao* 2 脏燥 and *bai he bing* 百合病. These symptoms are common to many health conditions and a significant number of citations were excluded when criteria relating to age and amenorrhoea were applied. Aside from hot flushes, terms for three other symptoms (searched with *fu ren* 妇人) identified citations 'most likely' to relate to menopause — *nu* 怒 (angry, two citations), *yu* 郁 (depressed, two citations) and *xuan yun* 眩晕 (dizziness, one citation). Irritability and depression are reported by many women during the menopause transition[27] and this appears to be the case for Chinese women in previous eras.

Descriptions of women with menopause symptoms highlighted many factors that contributed to symptom development. Stomach *qi* deficiency resulted in impaired production of *jin ye* 津液, leading to Blood deficiency. Chronic or prolonged illness consumed *jin ye* 津液, *qi* and Blood. Excessive sexual activity and multiple childbirths resulted in loss of *jing* 精. Some citations described a general deficiency of *zang* 脏 and *fu* 腑 organs which is consistent with ageing or with prolonged illness. Other syndromes described in multiple citations included Heart deficiency and Lung dryness. The diversity in descriptions of aetiology and CM syndromes was not surprising given the diversity in symptoms reported during menopause.

The earliest treatment citations were found in *Jin Gui Yao Lue Fang Lun* 金匮要略方论 (c. 206 AD) from the late Han dynasty. Passages from this book are well known as some of the earliest descriptions of menopause symptoms. Citations described treatment with *Gan mai da zao tang* 甘麦大枣汤, *Bai he zhi mu tang* 百合知母汤 and *Hua shi dai zhe tang* 滑石代赭汤. These formulas were not recommended in key textbooks and clinical guidelines included in Chapter 2, although some formulas have been found in other specialist textbooks. For example, *Gan mai da zao tang* 甘麦大枣汤 is prescribed with *Sheng mai san* 生脉散 in Bob Flaw's *Menopause and Chinese Medicine* (2006) for the CM syndrome dual deficiency of the Heart and Spleen.[6] Evidence from other sources confirms that this formula continues to be a mainstay of CHM treatment, with *Gan mai da zao tang* 甘麦大枣汤 ranked as the fourth most used herbal formula for menopause syndrome.[28] Whether other formulas that were popular for menopause symptoms in past eras are still used in contemporary CM practice remains unclear.

Oral CHM formulas were the predominant treatment choice for menopause symptoms. *Gan mai da zao tang* 甘麦大枣汤 was the most frequently used formula in citations 'possibly' related to menopause. Among possible menopause citations, five of the top nine oral CHM formulas used *bai he* 百合 as one of the key ingredients and *bai he* 百合 was included in all formulas for topical application. *Bai he* 百合 appears to have been an important herb in past eras.

However, *bai he* 百合 did not appear as a herb ingredient in CHM formulas described in Chapter 2, and it was not among the most frequently used single herbs for menopause symptoms in Taiwan.[28] There are several possible explanations for this. Firstly, when CM treatments were systematised in the 1960s, menopause syndrome was aligned with the syndrome of Kidney deficiency. The focus on the Kidney may have resulted in treatments addressing other organ dysfunction being overlooked. Secondly, it is possible that a shift in views of gynaecology and obstetrics diseases over time meant that *bai he* 百合 was no longer as important as in previous times. Thirdly, it is possible that the absence of *bai he* 百合 in books published after *Jing Fang Li Shi* 经方例释 and *Xue Zheng Lun* 血证论

(both published in 1884) is a result of the search terms used and criteria applied for citation selection; other terms or criteria may have found *bai he* 百合 as a herb ingredient for menopause symptoms in the late Qing and Min Guo periods.

Only two treatments in citations 'most likely' to be menopause were found in multiple citations: *Zeng jian ba wu chai hu tang* 增减八物柴胡汤/*Zeng sun ba wu chai hu tang* 增损八物柴胡汤 and modified *Si wu tang* 四物汤. There was no overlap in other formulas. This is likely due to the small number of citations meeting the criteria for 'most likely' cases of menopause. When considering the herbs that appeared frequently in 'most likely' cases of menopause, it was clear that formulas focused on tonifying Blood, with *dang gui* 当归 used in 21 of the 23 citations included in this group. *Dang gui* 当归 appears in several formulas described in Chapter 2: *You gui wan* 右归丸, *Er xian tang* 二仙汤, *Yi guan jian* 一贯煎 and *Tian wang bu xin dan* 天王补心丹.

Acupuncture was used less frequently than oral CHM for menopause symptoms. One citation described using the acupuncture points BL12 *Fengmen* 风门, CV14 *Juque* 巨阙, ST40 *Fenglong* 丰隆 and GB21 *Jianjing* 肩井. These acupuncture points were not found in clinical textbooks and guidelines included in Chapter 2. One acupuncture point on the Liver channel was recommended in clinical textbooks and guidelines for menopausal symptoms: LR3 *Taichong* 太冲. This point nourishes Liver Blood and *yin*, promotes the free flow of *qi* and regulates menstruation.[24] As the *yuan* point 原穴 on the Liver channel, LR3 *Taichong* 太冲 is commonly used in clinical practice. Whilst it is possible that this point was used for menopausal symptoms, we cannot be certain of its use in past eras.

This analysis of classical literature was designed to capture information about the treatment of menopause symptoms in past eras. Selection of search terms included the key symptoms reported by women and some physical signs, but it is possible that other terms were used for menopause symptoms in classical texts. It is unlikely that vaginal atrophy would have been discussed in classical texts and terms were not included to search for urinary symptoms. In addition to the challenge posed by a diverse range of symptoms, the absence of a name for menopause in classical texts may have limited the information obtained. The inclusion of additional terms may alter the findings in this analysis of classical texts.

Finally, criteria were developed to locate the best examples of menopause symptoms. It is possible that other citations exist that describe menopause without including references to amenorrhoea and age; such citations may have been excluded during the selection process. Different criteria for selecting citations may also produce different results.

References

1. Needham J, Lu G, Sivin N. (2000) *Science and Civilisation in China. Vol 5, Part VI: Medicine*. Cambridge University Press, UK.
2. Hu R, ed. (2000) *Encyclopedia of Traditional Chinese Medicine*. Hunan Electronic and Audio-Visual Publishing House, Changsha.
3. May B, Lu C, Xue C. (2012) Collections of traditional Chinese medical literature as resources for systematic searches. *J Altern Complement Med* **18**(12): 1101–1107.
4. May B, Lu Y, Lu C, *et al.* (2013) Systematic assessment of the representativeness of published collections of the traditional literature on Chinese medicine. *J Altern Complement Med* **19**(5): 403–409.
5. Scheid V. (2007) Traditional Chinese Medicine — What Are We Investigating?: The Case of Menopause. *Complement Ther Med* **15**(1): 54–68.
6. Flaws B. (2006) *Menopause and Chinese Medicine*. Blue Poppy Press, Boulder, Colorado.
7. Scheid V. (2008) Globalising Chinese medical understandings of menopause. *East Asian Sci Technol Soc* **2**(4): 485–506.
8. 罗颂平, 刘雁峰. (2017) 中医妇科学 ('十二五'普通高等教育本科国家级规划教材). 第3版. 北京: 人民卫生出版社.
9. 马宝璋. (2012) 中医妇科学 (普通高等教育'十一五'国家级规划教材). 北京: 中国中医药出版社.
10. 林昭庚. (2002) 中西医病名对照大词典. 人民卫生出版社; 北京.
11. World Health Organization. (2007) WHO International Standard Terminologies on Traditional Medicine in the Western Pacific Region. WHO Regional Office for the Western Pacific, Manila.

12. 刘敏如. (1988) 中医妇科学(高等中医院校教学参考丛书)(第2版). 人民卫生出版社; 北京.
13. 司徒仪. (2012) 中西医结合妇产科学(第2版). 科学出版社; 北京.
14. 尤昭玲. (2006) 中西医结合妇产科学(新世纪全国高等医药院校规划教材). 中国中医药出版社; 北京.
15. 张玉珍. (2002) 中医妇科学(普通高等教育'十五'国家级规划教材). 中国中医药出版社; 北京.
16. 欧阳惠卿. (2002) 中医妇科学(21世纪课程教材). 人民卫生出版社; 北京.
17. 王小云 黄. (2018) 中西医结合妇产科学 (普通高等教育'十三五'规划教材). 第3版. 科学出版社; 北京.
18. 罗颂平. (2008) 中医妇科学(全国高等中医药院校规划教材). 第2版. 高等教育出版社; 北京.
19. 连方, 齐聪. (2016) 中西医结合妇产科学(卫生部'十二五'规划教材). 人民卫生出版社; 北京.
20. 钱静, 湖波. (2013) 中医妇科学(全国高等医学院校中医药类系列教材). 科学出版社; 北京.
21. 中华中医药学会. (2012) 中医妇科常见病诊疗指南. 北京: 中国中医药出版社.
22. 王小云, 黄健玲. (2013) 妇科专病中医临床诊治. 第3版. 北京: 人民卫生出版社.
23. Bensky D, Clavey S, Stoger E. (2004) *Chinese Herbal Medicine Materia Medica*, 3rd ed. Eastland Press, Inc., Seattle, WA.
24. Deadman P, Al-Khafaji M, Baker K. (2000) *A Manual of Acupuncture.* Journal of Chinese Medicine Publications, East Sussex, UK.
25. Robson S, Harvey J, Yazdani A, *et al.* (2014) Management of the menopause (C-Gyn 09). Royal Australian and New Zealand College of Obstetricians and Gynaecologists, Melbourne, Australia.
26. Williams RE, Kalilani L, DiBenedetti DB, *et al.* (2007) Healthcare seeking and treatment for menopausal symptoms in the United States. *Maturitas* **58**(4): 348–358.
27. The National Institute of Health and Care Excellence (NICE) Guideline. (2015) Menopause: Diagnosis and management. Available from: https://www.nice.org.uk/guidance/ng23.
28. Chen HY, Lin YH, Wu JC, *et al.* (2011) Prescription patterns of Chinese herbal products for menopausal syndrome: Analysis of a nationwide prescription database. *J Ethnopharmacol* **137**(3): 1261–1266.

4

Methods for Evaluating Clinical Evidence

OVERVIEW

A comprehensive search of English and Chinese language biomedical databases was conducted to identify clinical studies of Chinese medicine interventions for menopause. Potentially relevant studies were screened against eligibility criteria. Characteristics of the studies are described and a review of findings conducted using standardised methods. This chapter describes the methods used to evaluate the efficacy and safety of Chinese medicine treatments for menopause.

Introduction

The use of Chinese medicine (CM) for menopause has been described in contemporary literature (Chapter 2) and in classical CM texts (Chapter 3). Many clinical studies and systematic reviews have been conducted to evaluate the efficacy, effectiveness and safety of CM treatments for menopause. The evidence from controlled clinical trials was analysed using meta-analysis where possible and details from non-controlled studies have been described. The findings of these analyses have been presented according to the type of intervention: Chinese herbal medicine (CHM; see Chapter 5), acupuncture and related therapies (see Chapter 7), other CM therapies (see Chapter 8) and combinations of CM therapies such as CHM plus acupuncture, or acupuncture plus *taichi* 太极 (see Chapter 9).

This chapter describes the methods used to evaluate evidence from clinical studies. References to clinical trials were obtained and assessed by an expert group. Evidence from randomised controlled trials (RCTs), non-randomised controlled clinical trials (CCTs) and non-controlled studies were evaluated separately. The same approach was used to evaluate RCTs and CCTs, which was to describe the characteristics of the studies and CM treatments and to conduct meta-analysis using the approach outlined below. This approach was not suitable for non-controlled studies. Instead, a summary is provided of the characteristics of the studies, CM treatments and any adverse events reported.

References to included studies are indicated by a letter followed by a number. Studies of CHM are indicated by an 'H', for example H1; studies of acupuncture and related therapies indicated by an 'A', for example A1; studies of other CM therapies indicated by an 'O', for example O1; and studies of combinations of CM therapies (see Table 4.1) indicated by a 'C', for example C1.

Search Strategy

A comprehensive search was conducted in English and Chinese language databases guided by the methods of the Cochrane Handbook for Systematic Reviews of Interventions.[1] English language databases included PubMed, Excerpta Medica Database (Embase), Cumulative Index of Nursing and Allied Health Literature (CINAHL), the Cochrane Central Register of Controlled Trials (CENTRAL), including the Cochrane Library, and Allied and Complementary Medicine Database (AMED). Chinese language databases included China BioMedical Literature (CBM), China National Knowledge Infrastructure (CNKI), Chongqing VIP (CQVIP) and Wanfang. Databases were searched from inception to April 2018. No restrictions were applied. Search terms were mapped to controlled vocabulary (where applicable), in addition to being searched as keywords.

To conduct a comprehensive search of the literature, searches were run according to the study design (reviews, controlled trials and non-controlled studies). This was done for each of the three intervention types (CHM, acupuncture and related therapies and other CM therapies) resulting in nine searches in each of the nine databases:

1. CHM reviews;
2. CHM controlled trials (randomised and non-randomised);

3. CHM non-controlled studies;
4. Acupuncture and related therapies reviews;
5. Acupuncture and related therapies controlled trials (randomised and non-randomised);
6. Acupuncture and related therapies non-controlled studies;
7. Other CM therapies reviews;
8. Other CM therapies controlled trials (randomised and non-randomised);
9. Other CM therapies non-controlled studies.

Studies of combination CM therapies were identified through the above searches. In addition to electronic databases, reference lists of systematic reviews and included studies were searched for additional publications. Clinical trial registries were searched to identify clinical trials that were ongoing or completed and, where required, trial investigators were contacted to obtain data. The searched trial registries were the Australian New Zealand Clinical Trial Registry (ANZCTR), the Chinese Clinical Trial Registry (ChiCTR), the European Union Clinical Trials Register (EU-CTR) and the United States of America National Institutes of Health register (ClinicalTrials.gov).

If required, trial investigators were contacted to obtain further information. Trial investigators were contacted by email or telephone and were followed up after two weeks if no reply was received. Where no response was received after one month, any unknown information was marked as not available.

Inclusion Criteria

Studies that met the inclusion criteria for participants, interventions, comparators and outcome measures were included. Criteria were as follows:

- Participants: Premenopausal, perimenopausal or postmenopausal women with spontaneous menopause or bilateral oophorectomy (surgical menopause);
- Interventions: CHM, acupuncture and related therapies, other CM therapies, or combinations of CM therapies (see Table 4.1);

Table 4.1 Chinese Medicine Interventions Included in Clinical Evidence Evaluation

Category	Intervention
Chinese herbal medicines (CHM)	Oral or topical
Acupuncture and related therapies	Acupuncture, acupressure, ear acupressure, electroacupuncture, laser acupuncture, moxibustion and point percussion therapy
Other Chinese medicine therapies	*Qigong* therapy 气功, Chinese medicine psychological intervention, *tuina* 推拿 (Chinese massage) and *taichi* therapy太極.
Combination Chinese medicine	Combination therapies are defined as two or more Chinese medicine interventions from different categories administered together (e.g., CHM plus acupuncture or CHM plus *qigong* 气功).

- Comparators: No treatment/waitlist control, placebo/sham or interventions recommended in clinical practice guidelines for menopause;
- Outcome measures: Studies reported at least one of the pre-specified outcome measures (Table 4.2).

Clinical practice guidelines of the following organisations were reviewed to identify treatments recommended for menopausal symptoms: The American Association of Clinical Endocrinologists (AACE)/ American College of Endocrinology (ACE),[2] The Royal Australian and New Zealand College of Obstetricians and Gynaecologists,[3] The North American Menopause Society,[4,5] The Endocrine Society[6] and the European Menopause and Androgen Society.[7] Guidelines were largely consistent in recommendations.

Treatments included patient education, hormone therapy, non-hormonal pharmacotherapy, and non-hormonal and non-pharmacological interventions. Patient education included information and advice for self-management of symptoms, stress reduction, diet and exercise advice, alcohol and caffeine intake, and weight management. Hormone therapy included systemic or vaginal oestrogen therapy, oestrogen plus progestogen therapy and bazedoxifene. Non-hormonal pharmacotherapy included selective serotonin reuptake inhibitors (SSRIs, for example paroxetine, escitalopram and citalopram), serotonin and noradrenaline (norepinephrine) reuptake inhibitors (SNRIs, for example venlafaxine and desvenlafaxine), tibolone, pregabalin, gabapentin, clonidine and ospemifene. Non-hormonal and non-pharmacological interventions included vaginal moisturisers, vaginal lubricants, cognitive behavioural therapy, clinical hypnosis, mindfulness-based stress reduction, black cohosh, isoflavones and

Table 4.2 Pre-specified Outcomes

Outcome Categories	Outcome Measures	Scoring
Vasomotor symptoms	1. Hot flush frequency and/or severity	1. Various, lower is better
	2. Night sweats frequency and/or severity	2. Various, lower is better
Genitourinary symptoms	1. VMI[8]	1. 0–4 points, lower is better
	2. Vaginal pH	2. 0–14, see text
	3. VHI[9]	3. 0–25 points, higher is better
	4. SQF[10]	4. 0–100 points, higher is better
Musculoskeletal symptoms	1. VAS	1. 0–10 cm, lower is better*
	2. Likert scale	2. Variable, lower is better*
Sleep quality	1. PSQI[11]	1. 0–21 points, lower is better
	2. ISI[12]	2. 0–28 points, lower is better
	3. AIS[13]	3. 0–24 points, lower is better
	4. Spiegel Sleep Questionnaire[14]	4. See text
	5. SDRS[15]	5. 0–40 points, lower is better
	6. SRSS[16]	6. 10–50 points, lower is better
Psychological symptoms	1. Zung SDS[17]	1. 20–80 points, lower is better
	2. Zung SAS[18]	2. 20–80 points, lower is better
	3. HAM-D[19]	3. 0–50 points, lower is better
	4. HAM-A[20]	4. 0–56 points, lower is better
	5. CES-D[21]	5. 0–60 points, lower is better
	6. BDI[22]	6. 0–63 points, lower is better

(*Continued*)

Table 4.2 (*Continued*)

Outcome Categories	Outcome Measures	Scoring
Global symptom scales	1. Kupperman Index[23]	1. 0–51 points, lower is better
	2. GCS[24]	2. 0–63 points, lower is better
HRQoL	1. MRS[25]	1. 0–44 points, lower is better
	2. MENQOL[26]	2. Variable for domains, lower is better
	3. HFRDI[27]	3. 0–100 points, lower is better
	4. WHQ[28]	4. 0–1 for each domain, lower is better
	5. SF-36[29]	5. 0–100 points per domain, higher is better
Adverse events	Number and type of adverse events	

*Lower scores for VAS and Likert scales typically indicated better outcomes.
Abbreviations: AIS, Athens Insomnia Scale; BDI, Beck Depression Inventory; CES-D, Center for Epidemiologic Studies Depression Scale; GCS, Greene Climacteric Scale; HAM-A, Hamilton Rating Scale for Anxiety; HAM-D, Hamilton Rating Scale for Depression; HFRDI, Hot Flash Related Daily Interference Scale; HRQoL, health-related quality of life; ISI, Insomnia Severity Index; MENQOL, Menopause-specific Quality of Life Questionnaire; MRS, Menopause Rating Scale; PSQI, Pittsburgh Sleep Quality Index; SAS, Self-rating Anxiety Scale; SDRS, Sleep Dysfunction Rating Scale; SDS, Self-rating Depression Scale; SF-36, Medical Outcome Study 36-Item Short-form Health Survey; SQF, Sexual Quotient-Female version; SRSS, Self-rating Sleep Scale; VAS, visual analogue scale; VHI, Vaginal Health Index; VMI, Vaginal Maturation Index; WHQ, Women's Health Questionnaire.

stellate ganglion block. Studies that combined a CM therapy with a guideline-recommended treatment were included if the same guideline-recommended treatment was used as the comparator.

Exclusion Criteria

Studies were not eligible if:

- Only males were included (male andropause);
- Participants included women with premature ovarian insufficiency, chemically induced menopause, menopausal symptoms in women with breast or ovarian cancer, menopausal symptoms in women with endometriosis, and women with menstrual disorders in menopause such as abnormal uterine bleeding;

- Treatment focused on cardiovascular disease or osteoporosis in premenopausal, perimenopausal or postmenopausal women;
- The intervention was an over-the-counter Western herbal treatment. Examples include black cohosh (*Cimicifuga racemosa, Actaea racemosa*), soy isoflavones, phytoestrogens, evening primrose oil (*Oenothera biennis*), St John's wort (*Hypericum perforatum*), hop extract (*Humulus lupulus*), red clover (*Trifolium pratense*) and grape seed extract (*Vitis vinifera*);
- The comparator was a custom-compounded bioidentical hormone.

Outcomes

Outcomes were pre-specified and related to the common signs and symptoms reported in menopause. Outcomes were grouped into the following categories: vasomotor symptoms, genitourinary symptoms, sleep quality, psychological symptoms, musculoskeletal symptoms, global symptom scales and health-related quality of life (see Table 4.2). In addition, the nature and quantity of adverse events were collected.

Vasomotor Symptoms

The two key vasomotor symptoms are hot flushes and night sweats. These are patient-reported and are typically measured daily or weekly. Frequency and/or severity of hot flushes and night sweats may be measured. Severity is typically measured on a visual analogue scale (VAS) or a Likert scale. Objective physiological measures, such as sternal skin conductance, are less frequently used.

Genitourinary Symptoms

Vulvovaginal Atrophy

Vulvovaginal atrophy is common in menopausal women. There is no 'gold-standard' tool to measure vulvovaginal symptoms.[30] Both objective and subjective outcome measures were included. Objective measurements include vaginal cytology and/or measurement of vaginal pH, while subjective assessments include individual or composite symptom scores and physical examination.[31] The Vaginal Maturation Index is based on vaginal cytology, and is a ratio of parabasal, intermediate and superficial cell types.[8]

Subjective measurements vary in terms of components and scoring. A typical example of physician-assessed vaginal health is the Vaginal Health Index (VHI).[9] The VHI measures five aspects of vaginal health: moisture, fluid volume, elasticity, epithelial integrity and pH. Each item is scored from one (poorest) to five (best), and a total score can be derived from the sum of item scores. Other investigator-developed outcomes for vulvovaginal atrophy were included where the criteria were clearly described. Some global symptom scales also included assessment of genitourinary symptoms; these have been described below (see 'Global Symptom Scales').

Vaginal pH can be an indicator of menopausal status. Vaginal pH in the range of 3.8 to 4.2 is considered normal in premenopausal women.[32] Caillouette *et al.* (1997)[33] report that a pH of greater than 4.5 is associated with a low oestrogen level typical of menopause, in the absence of vaginitis.

Urinary Tract Dysfunction

Dysfunction of the urinary tract can include dysuria, change in urinary frequency or urgency, and impaired continence. Symptoms may be assessed individually using a VAS or Likert scale. Some global symptom scales include items related to urinary tract dysfunction (see 'Global Symptom Scales').

Sexual Dysfunction

Sexual dysfunction may be assessed as an individual symptom, or as part of global symptom scales. Various scales exist for assessing sexual dysfunction. The Sexual Quotient-Female (SQF) version includes ten items scored from zero to five.[10] The sum of scores for the ten items is multiplied by two to calculate a total score out of 100, where higher scores mean greater sexual performance/satisfaction.

Musculoskeletal Symptoms

Assessment of musculoskeletal symptoms, such as arthralgia and myalgia, are commonly made using a VAS or Likert scale. Some studies reported changes in musculoskeletal symptoms as part of the Kupperman Index (see 'Global Symptom Scales').

Sleep Quality

Objective assessment of sleep can be determined using polysomnography. However, the practicalities of using polysomnography are limited by cost, access and resources.[34] As such, subjective assessment is more common in research. The Pittsburgh Sleep Quality Index (PSQI)[11] is one of the most frequently used outcome tools to assess sleep quality and patterns of sleep. The PSQI includes seven domains: subjective sleep quality, sleep latency, sleep duration, habitual sleep efficiency, sleep disturbances, use of sleep medication and daytime dysfunction in the previous month. Each question is scored on a four-point scale and a total score is calculated from the sum of individual items. A lower score indicates better sleep quality.

The Insomnia Severity Index[12] assesses the severity of difficulties with sleep onset and sleep maintenance, satisfaction with sleep pattern, the degree to which it affects daily functioning, impairment due to sleep problems and degree of stress from sleep problems. Each of the seven items is scored from zero to four and the sum of all seven items determines the total score. Sleep quality is also included as a subscale of the Women's Health Questionnaire;[28] see 'Global Symptom Scales' for more information.

The Athens Insomnia Scale includes eight items relating to sleep induction, nighttime awakenings, final awakening, sleep quality and total sleep duration.[13] Items are scored from zero to three and higher scores indicate poorer sleep. Item scores are summed to calculate a total score. According to Leger *et al.* (2006),[35] the Spiegel Sleep Questionnaire assesses sleep initiation, sleep quality, duration of sleep, nighttime awakenings, dreams and feeling refreshed on waking. Each of the six items is scored from zero to five, with higher scores indicating poorer sleep. The original reference for the Spiegel Sleep Questionnaire does not report this scoring and is somewhat ambiguous in the description of items.[14] No additional information was able to be identified on validation and standardised scoring of this outcome.

Two Chinese outcome measures are often used to assess sleep: The Sleep Dysfunction Rating Scale (SDRS)[15] and the Self-rating Sleep Scale (SRSS).[16] The SDRS includes ten items scored from zero to four, where a lower score indicates better sleep quality. The sum of item scores provides a total score in the range of zero to 40 points. The SRSS is a ten-item scale scored from one to five, where higher scores indicate worse sleep. Scores are summed to provide a total score between 10 and 50.

Psychological Symptoms

Many validated questionnaires exist for measuring psychological symptoms. Frequently used outcome tools in clinical practice and research include Zung's Self-rating Depression Scale (SDS),[17] Zung's Self-rating Anxiety Scale (SAS),[18] the Hamilton Rating Scale for Depression (HAM-D)[19] and the Hamilton Rating Scale for Anxiety (HAM-A).[20]

The SDS includes 20 items related to depressive symptoms, with each item scored from one to four points. The total score is calculated from the sum of individual item scores. An index score can be calculated by dividing the total score by the maximum possible score of 80 and multiplying by 100 (index score ranges from 0.25 to 1.0). The SAS also includes 20 items and scoring is the same as for the SDS. For both scales, higher scores indicate greater severity.

The HAM-D, also known as HRSD or HDRS, is a clinician-rated measure of depressive symptoms in adults. It includes 21 items, with the first 17 used for scoring. The four unscored items relate to other factors that may be related to depression, such as paranoia, obsessive and compulsive symptoms, but which are not necessarily indicators of severity.[36] Eight items are rated on a five-point scale from zero to four and nine items are scored from zero to two. Higher scores indicate greater severity of depression. The HAM-A is a 14-item clinician-rated questionnaire that measures anxiety symptoms. Like the HAM-D, items are scored from zero to four. Scores are summed to produce an overall score, with higher scores indicating greater levels of anxiety.

The Center for Epidemiologic Studies Depression Scale (CES-D)[21] is a 20-item scale, with each item rated from zero to three. Item scores are summed to provide a total score ranging from zero to 60. Higher scores indicate greater depressive symptoms. The Beck Depression Inventory (BDI)[22] is another common scale for assessing depression severity. The BDI includes 21 items scored zero to three, with higher scores indicating worse severity of symptoms. A total score is calculated by summing scores for each item. Various versions of this scale exist and the BDI-II is the most recent version. Other measures of psychological symptoms were included where a description of assessment criteria was provided. Furthermore, psychological symptoms are included in global symptom scales; see below.

Global Symptom Scales

Several widely used and validated scales exist for providing a global assessment of symptoms. The Kupperman Index (also known as the Kupperman Index Score, Kupperman Menopause Index and Blatt-Kupperman Menopausal Index)[23] measures the severity of 11 symptoms: vasomotor, paraesthesia, insomnia, nervousness, melancholia, vertigo, weakness/fatigue, arthralgia and myalgia, headaches, palpitation and formication (a tactile hallucination where a physical sensation is felt where there is no physical cause; a type of paraesthesia). Symptoms are scored by the clinician from zero (no symptoms) to three (severe symptoms). Severity is multiplied by a conversion factor and the scores for each symptom summed to produce a total score. Results are typically presented as the total score or may be reported for each symptom. The Chinese version of the Kupperman Index typically includes two extra items relating to urinary tract infections and dyspareunia.

The Greene Climacteric Scale[24] measures 'bother' from menopause symptoms. Twenty-one items are scored from zero (not at all) to three (extremely). Scores for all 21 items are summed to provide a total summary score. The first 20 items are used to calculate summary scores for the domains 'psychological', 'physical' and 'vasomotor'. The final question, relating to loss of interest in sex, is used for the total score only.

Health-related Quality of Life

As menopause is known to have a significant impact on a woman's quality of life, health-related quality of life is an important outcome. Several menopause-specific and generic wellbeing scales were included. The Menopause Rating Scale (MRS)[25] is a patient-completed assessment of the impact of menopause on health-related quality of life. Eleven items are scored from zero (no complaints) to four (very severe symptoms). Items are grouped into three dimensions (subscales): psychological, somatic and urogenital. Results can be reported for individual dimensions or summed to provide a total composite score.

The Menopause-specific Quality of Life questionnaire (MENQOL, also abbreviated to MSQOL)[26] was designed to measure health-related quality of life in the period after menopause. Twenty-nine items relating to symptoms are grouped into four domains: vasomotor, physical, psychosocial and sexual. Each symptom is rated as either present or not present and, if present, is scored from zero (not bothersome) to six (extremely bothersome). The score for each item is the sum of not present (scored as 1) or present (scored as 2), plus the symptom rating score. Thus, the score range for one symptom is one to eight. Domain means are calculated by dividing the sum of domain scores by the number of items in the domain.

The Hot Flash Related Daily Interference Scale (HFRDI)[27] measures the impact of hot flushes on quality of life in the previous week. Nine questions relate to the impact of hot flushes on specific activities of work, social activities, leisure, sleep, mood, concentration, relations with others, sexuality and enjoyment of life, while the final question is a global assessment. Items are scored from zero (do not interfere) to ten (completely interfere) and the total score is calculated by summing the scores for all items. The Hot Flash Interference (HFI) questionnaire was developed from the HFRDI, and uses three items to measure the degree to which hot flushes interfere with mood, sleep and concentration.[37]

The Women's Health Questionnaire (WHQ) was developed to assess the physical and emotional symptoms experienced by women in the menopausal years.[28] The WHQ includes 36 items grouped into nine domains: depressed mood, somatic symptoms, anxiety/fears, vasomotor symptoms, sleep problems, sexual behaviour, menstrual symptoms, memory/concentration and attractiveness. Items are scored by the patient on a four-point scale (yes definitely, yes sometimes, no not much, no not at all) and are reduced to binary options of zero or one. Scores for nine subscales are calculated by summing the scores for each item and dividing by the number of items.

The Medical Outcome Study 36-Item Short-form Health Survey (SF-36)[29] includes 36 items relating to eight domains: physical functioning, role functioning due to health problems, role functioning due to emotional problems, bodily pain, general health perceptions, vitality, social function and mental health. Scores for each domain are weighted and converted to range from zero to 100, where higher scores indicate better outcomes.

Risk of Bias Assessment

Risk of bias was assessed for RCTs using the Cochrane Collaboration's tool.[1] In clinical trials, bias can be categorised as selection bias, performance bias, detection bias, attrition bias and reporting bias. Each domain is assessed to determine whether the bias is at 'low', 'high' or 'unclear' risk. 'Low' risk of bias indicates that bias is unlikely, 'high' risk indicates plausible bias that seriously weakens confidence in the results and 'unclear' bias indicates lack of information or uncertainty over potential bias and raises some doubt about the results. Risk of bias assessment was verified by two people and disagreement was resolved by discussion or consultation with a third person.

Risk of bias is categorised using the following six domains:

- Sequence generation: The method used to generate the allocation sequence is given in sufficient detail to allow an assessment of whether it should produce comparable groups. 'Low' risk of bias refers to the use of appropriate methods, such as a random-number table or computer random generator. 'High' risk of bias includes studies that describe a non-random sequence generation such as odd or even date of birth or date of admission.
- Allocation concealment: The method used to conceal the allocation sequence is given in enough detail to determine whether intervention allocations could have been foreseen before, or during, enrolment. Examples of 'low' risk of bias include central randomisation or sealed envelopes, and examples of 'high' risk of bias includes open random sequence.
- Blinding of participants and personnel: Measures used to describe whether the study participants and personnel are blind to the intervention received. In addition, information relating to whether the blinding was effective is also assessed. Studies that ensure blinding of participants and personnel are at 'low' risk of bias. If the study is not blind, or incompletely blind, it is at 'high' risk of bias.
- Blinding of outcome assessors: Measures used to describe whether the outcome assessors are blind to knowledge of which intervention a participant received. In addition, information relating to whether the blinding was effective is also assessed. Studies that ensure blinding of outcome assessors are at 'low' risk of bias. If the study is not blind, or incompletely blind, it is at 'high' risk of bias.
- Incomplete outcome data: Completeness of outcome data for each main outcome, including drop-outs, exclusions from the analysis with numbers missing in each group and reasons for drop-out or exclusions. Studies with 'low' risk of bias would include all

outcome data or if there is missing data, it is unlikely to relate to the true outcome or is balanced between groups. Studies at 'high' risk of bias would have unexplained missing data.

- Selective reporting: The study protocol is available and the pre-specified outcomes are included in the report. Studies with a published protocol which include all pre-specified outcomes in their report would be at 'low' risk of bias. Studies at 'high' risk of bias would not include all pre-specified outcomes or the outcome data may be reported incompletely.

Statistical Analyses

Frequency of CM syndromes, CHM formulas, herbs and acupuncture points reported in included studies are presented using descriptive statistics. Chinese medicine syndromes reported in two or more studies were presented. The ten most frequently reported CHM formulas and 20 most frequently reported herbs are presented when used in at least two studies, although for CHM formulas this was not always possible. The top ten acupuncture points used in two or more studies are presented, or as available. Where data were limited, reports of single CM syndromes or acupuncture points are provided as a guide for the reader.

Definitions of statistical tests and results are described in the glossary. Dichotomous data are reported as a risk ratio (RR) with 95% confidence interval (CI) and continuous data are reported as mean difference (MD) or standardised mean difference (SMD) with 95% CI. For dichotomous data, when the RR is greater than one and the upper and lower values of the 95% CI are both greater than one, this indicates we can be 95% certain that there is a difference between the groups and that the true effect lies within these CIs. The same is true for values less than one. In such cases, we say there is a 'significant difference' between the groups. For continuous data, when the MD is greater than zero and both the upper and lower values of the 95% CI are greater than zero, we say there is a 'significant difference' between the groups. The same is true on the negative side of the scale.[1] For all analyses, RR or MD/SMD and 95% CI were reported, together with a formal test for heterogeneity using the I^2 statistic. An I^2 score greater than 50% was considered to indicate substantial heterogeneity.[1]

Sensitivity analyses were undertaken to explore potential sources of heterogeneity, based on 'low' risk of bias for one of the risk of bias domains of sequence generation. Where possible and appropriate, planned subgroup analyses included ethnicity, menopause status, duration of treatment, CM syndromes, CM formula and comparator type. Available case analysis with a random effects model was used in all analyses. The random effects model was used to take into account the clinical heterogeneity likely to be encountered within and between included studies, and the variation in treatment effects between included studies.

Assessment Using Grading of Recommendations Assessment, Development and Evaluation

The Grading of Recommendations Assessment, Development and Evaluation (GRADE) approach was used.[38,39] The GRADE approach summarises and rates the strength and quality ('certainty') of evidence in systematic reviews using a structured process for presenting evidence summaries. The results are presented in summary of findings tables. The results provide an important overview for menopause outcomes.

A panel of experts was established to evaluate the certainty of evidence. The panel included the systematic review team, CM practitioners, integrative medicine experts, research methodologists and conventional medicine physicians. The experts were asked to rate the clinical importance of key interventions from CHM, acupuncture therapies and other CM therapies, as well as comparators and outcomes. Results were collated and, based on the rating scores and subsequent discussion, a consensus on the content for the summary of findings tables was achieved.

The certainty of evidence for each outcome was rated according to five factors outlined in the GRADE approach. The certainty of evidence may be rated based on:

- Limitations in study design (risk of bias);
- Inconsistency of results (unexplained heterogeneity);
- Indirectness of evidence (interventions, populations and outcomes important to the patients with the condition);
- Imprecision (uncertainty about the results);
- Publication bias (selective publication of studies).

These five factors are additive and a reduction in one factor, or more than one factor, will reduce the certainty of the evidence for that outcome. The GRADE approach also includes methods for assessing observational studies. The GRADE summaries in this book only include RCTs.

Treatment recommendations can also be assessed using the GRADE approach, but due to the diverse nature of CM practice, treatment recommendations were not included with the summary of findings. Therefore, the reader should interpret the evidence with reference to the local practice environment. It should also be noted that the GRADE approach requires judgements about the strength and quality of evidence and some subjective assessment. However, the experience of the panel members suggests the judgements are reliable and transparent representations of the certainty of evidence.

The GRADE levels of evidence are grouped into four categories:

1. 'High' certainty: We are very confident that the true effect lies close to that of the estimate of the effect.
2. 'Moderate' certainty: We are moderately confident in the effect estimate. The true effect is likely to be close to the estimate of the effect, but there is a possibility that it is substantially different.
3. 'Low' certainty: Our confidence in the effect estimate is limited. The true effect may be substantially different from the estimate of the effect.

4. 'Very low' certainty: We have very little confidence in the effect estimate. The true effect is likely to be substantially different from the estimate of effect.

References

1. Higgins JPT, Green S, eds. (2011) Cochrane Handbook for Systematic Reviews of Interventions Version 5.1.0 The Cochrane Collaboration. Available from: www.cochrane-handbook.org2011.
2. Cobin RH, Goodman NF. (2017) American Association of Clinical Endocrinologists and American College of Endocrinology position statement on menopause 2017 update. *Endocr Pract* **23**(7): 869–880.
3. Royal Australian and New Zealand College of Obstetricians and Gynaecologists. (2014) (C-Gyn 9) Management of the menopause.
4. The North American Menopause Society. (2015) Nonhormonal management of menopause-associated vasomotor symptoms: 2015 position statement of The North American Menopause Society. *Menopause* **22**(11): 1155–1172; quiz 73–74.
5. The North American Menopause Society. (2017) The 2017 hormone therapy position statement of The North American Menopause Society. *Menopause* **24**(7): 728–753.
6. Stuenkel CA, Davis SR, Gompel A, *et al.* (2015) Treatment of symptoms of the menopause: An Endocrine Society Clinical Practice Guideline. *J Clin Endocrinol Metab* **100**(11): 3975–4011.
7. Mintziori G, Lambrinoudaki I, Goulis DG, *et al.* (2015) EMAS position statement: Non-hormonal management of menopausal vasomotor symptoms. *Maturitas* **81**(3): 410–413.
8. McEndree B. (1999) Clinical application of the vaginal maturation index. *Nurse Pract* **24**(9): 48, 51–52, 55–56.
9. Bachmann G, Notelovitz M, Gonzalez S, *et al.* (1991) Vaginal dryness in menopausal women: Clinical characteristics and nonhormonal treatment. *Clin Pract Sex* **9**: 25–32.
10. Abdo C. (2006) Development and validation of female sexual quotient: A questionnaire to assess female sexual function. *Revista Brasileira de Medicina* **63**(9): 477–482.
11. Buysse DJ, Reynolds CF III, Monk TH, *et al.* (1989) The Pittsburgh Sleep Quality Index: A new instrument for psychiatric practice and research. *Psychiatry Res* **28**(2): 193–213.

12. Bastien CH, Vallieres A, Morin CM. (2001) Validation of the Insomnia Severity Index as an outcome measure for insomnia research. *Sleep Med* **2**(4): 297–307.
13. Soldatos CR, Dikeos DG, Paparrigopoulos TJ. (2000) Athens Insomnia Scale: Validation of an instrument based on ICD-10 criteria. *J Psychosom Res* **48**(6): 555–560.
14. Spiegel R. (1981) *Sleep and Sleepiness in Advanced Age*. M.T.P. Press, Lancaster, UK.
15. 肖卫东, 刘平, 马弘, *et al.* (2007) 睡眠障碍评定量表的信度和效度分析. 中国心理卫生杂志 **21**(1): 41–42, 51.
16. 李建明. (2012) 睡眠状况自评量表 (SRSS) 简介. 中国健康心理学杂志 **20**(12): 1851.
17. Zung WW. (1965) A self-rating depression scale. *Arch Gen Psychiatry* **12**: 63–70.
18. Zung WW. (1971) A rating instrument for anxiety disorders. *Psychosomatics* **12**(6): 371–379.
19. Hamilton M. (1960) A rating scale for depression. *J Neurol Neurosurg Psychiatry* **23**: 56–62.
20. Hamilton M. (1959) The assessment of anxiety states by rating. *Br J Med Psychol* **32**(1): 50–55.
21. Radloff L. (1977) The CES-D Scale: A self-report depression scale for research in the general population. *Appl Psychol Meas* **1**(3): 385–401.
22. Beck AT, Ward CH, Mendelson M, *et al.* (1961) An inventory for measuring depression. *Arch Gen Psychiatry* **4**: 561–571.
23. Kupperman HS, Wetchler BB, Blatt MH. (1959) Contemporary therapy of the menopausal syndrome. *J Am Med Assoc* **171**: 1627–1637.
24. Greene JG. (1976) A factor analytic study of climacteric symptoms. *J Psychosom Res* **20**(5): 425–430.
25. Heinemann LA, Potthoff P, Schneider HP. (2003) International versions of the Menopause Rating Scale (MRS). *Health Qual Life Outcomes* **1**: 28.
26. Hilditch JR, Lewis J, Peter A, *et al.* (2008) A menopause-specific quality of life questionnaire: Development and psychometric properties. *Maturitas* **61**(1–2): 107–121.
27. Carpenter JS. (2001) The Hot Flash Related Daily Interference Scale: A tool for assessing the impact of hot flashes on quality of life following breast cancer. *J Pain Symptom Manage* **22**(6): 979–989.
28. Hunter M. (1992) The Women's Health Questionnaire: A measure of mid-aged women's perceptions of their emotional and physical health. *Psychol Health* **7**: 45–54.

29. Ware JJ, Sherbourne C. (1992) The MOS 36-item Short-Form Health Survey (SF-36). I. Conceptual framework and item selection. *Med Care* **30**: 473–483.
30. Erekson EA, Yip SO, Wedderburn TS, *et al.* (2013) The Vulvovaginal Symptoms Questionnaire: A questionnaire for measuring vulvovaginal symptoms in postmenopausal women. *Menopause* **20**(9): 973–979.
31. Weber MA, Limpens J, Roovers JP. (2015) Assessment of vaginal atrophy: A review. *Int Urogynecol J* **26**(1): 15–28.
32. Goldstein I. (2010) Recognizing and treating urogenital atrophy in postmenopausal women. *J Womens Health (Larchmt)* **19**(3): 425–432.
33. Caillouette JC, Sharp CF, Jr., Zimmerman GJ, *et al.* (1997) Vaginal pH as a marker for bacterial pathogens and menopausal status. *Am J Obstet Gynecol* **176**(6): 1270–1275; discussion 5–7.
34. Van de Water A, Holmes A, Hurley D. (2011) Objective measurements of sleep for non-laboratory settings as alternatives to polysomnography: A systematic review. *J Sleep Res* **20**: 183–200.
35. Leger D, Massuel MA, Metlaine A. (2006) Professional correlates of insomnia. *Sleep* **29**(2): 171–8.
36. Sharp R. (2015) The Hamilton Rating Scale for Depression. *Occup Med (Lond)* **65**(4): 340.
37. Carpenter JS, Bakoyannis G, Otte JL, *et al.* (2017) Validity, cut-points, and minimally important differences for two hot flash-related daily interference scales. *Menopause* **24**(8): 877–85.
38. Schünemann H, Higgins J, Vist G, *et al.* (2019) Chapter 14: Completing 'Summary of findings' tables and grading the certainty of the evidence. In: Higgins JPT, Thomas J, Chandler J, *et al.* (eds), Cochrane Handbook for Systematic Reviews of Interventions version 6.0. Available from: www.training.cochrane.org/handbook.
39. Schünemann H, Brozek J, Guyatt G, Oxman A, eds. (2013) GRADE handbook for grading quality of evidence and strength of recommendations. The Grade Working Group. Available from: www.guidelinedevelopment.org/handbook.

5

Clinical Evidence for Chinese Herbal Medicine

OVERVIEW

Clinical studies have tested Chinese herbal medicines and published the results in scientific journals. This chapter presents the Chinese medicine syndromes described, treatments tested, and efficacy and safety of Chinese herbal medicine in a selection of 282 clinical studies. Oral Chinese herbal medicine was the main treatment test, with some benefits seen in improving vasomotor, sleep and psychological symptoms, as well as improvements in global symptom severity.

Introduction

Chinese herbal medicine (CHM) is a common Chinese medicine (CM) treatment for menopause symptoms. Contemporary clinical guidelines and textbooks describe the formulas that can be used according to CM syndrome differentiation (Chapter 2). Analysis of the classical CM texts show that CHM was the main approach used for the management of menopause symptoms (Chapter 3). Many clinical studies have evaluated the potential role for CHM for women experiencing the menopausal transition. Studies have been published in English and Chinese. This chapter reviews the clinical evidence from randomised controlled trials (RCTs), controlled clinical trials (CCTs) and non-controlled studies using systematic review and meta-analysis techniques. Findings have been grouped according to the route of administration, with studies of oral CHM presented first, followed by studies of topical CHM and finally studies that evaluated the combination of oral and topical CHM. Studies are indicated by the letter 'H' followed by a number, and the references for studies can be found at the end of the chapter.

Previous Systematic Reviews

The efficacy of CHM for menopause symptoms has been evaluated in many previous systematic reviews. Eight systematic reviews published in English language journals[1–8] and seven systematic reviews published in Chinese language journals[9–15] were identified. Several reviews evaluated CHM used alone or in combination with pharmacotherapy, while others focused on a specific formula or herb. Key findings from these systematic reviews are summarised.

A Cochrane systematic review of CHM for menopausal symptoms included 22 RCTs,[7] most of which were conducted in China. Meta-analyses showed no benefit of CHM over placebo or hormone therapy (HT) on hot flushes and no benefit of CHM over HT on menopause symptoms. Results from single studies showed no benefit of CHM on health-related quality of life (HRQoL). There was inconclusive evidence on safety of CHM. Based on 'very low' to 'moderate' quality evidence, the authors concluded that the evidence was insufficient to state that CHM is any more or less effective than either placebo or HT.

Two systematic reviews have shown the combination of CHM with pharmacotherapy to be more effective than pharmacotherapy alone in reducing Kupperman Index (KI) score.[11,14] Three reviews found CHM to be more effective than pharmacotherapy in improving sleep quality, with reduced scores on the Pittsburgh Sleep Quality Index (PSQI).[9,10,13] These three reviews also found fewer adverse events (AEs) among women who received CHM. Meta-analysis in one review by Zhang *et al.* (2017)[8] found CHM improved clinical efficacy and reduced depressive symptoms compared to controls, but the quality of studies was limited.

Three systematic reviews provided a narrative synthesis of the evidence,[3–5] as authors considered meta-analysis was not appropriate given heterogeneity in interventions and outcome measures. Taylor-Swanson *et al.* (2015)[3] reported improvements in hot flushes in three of the four CHM studies, improvement in pain in two studies, and improvement in mood and sleep in one study. In 13 high-quality RCTs, results of studies which described CM syndrome differentiation reported better outcomes than studies that did not describe CM syndromes.[4] Chinese herbal medicine was considered to be safe, but not without side effects. A second review by the same authors[5] found CHM to be effective in all nine trials published in Chinese, and in nine of the 14 trials published in non-Chinese journals. Side effects were mild and infrequent.

Three systematic reviews evaluated the efficacy and safety of the manufactured product *Kun tai jiao nang* 坤泰胶囊 (*Kun tai* capsules).[6,12,15] One review of 17 RCTs showed no benefit of *Kun tai* capsules on KI, global symptom improvement (effective rate) or hormone levels.[6] Fewer AEs were seen with *Kun tai* capsules compared to HT. Two meta-analyses reported *Kun tai jiao nang* 坤泰胶囊 was superior to HT in terms of KI score, with low frequency of AEs.[12,15] However, the general methodological quality of the included trials was 'low'.

The formula *Er xian tang* 二仙汤 was examined in a review by Chen *et al.* (2008).[1] Five RCTs were included and comparators included HT, diazepam, oryzanol (a rice bran oil), vitamins and CHM. The low quality of the studies, as well as the use of CHM as a comparator, limited conclusions. Finally, one review focused on ginseng (*ren shen* 人参) in ten placebo-controlled RCTs.[2] Meta-analysis showed ginseng may be beneficial for sexual symptoms, while no such benefit was found for hot flushes. Results from individual studies showed ginseng improved menopause symptoms, depression, wellbeing and general health. Few AEs were attributed to ginseng.

Identification of Clinical Studies

After searching in nine biomedical databases, results for 49,278 potentially relevant citations were exported to reference management software for further screening and evaluation (Fig. 5.1). More

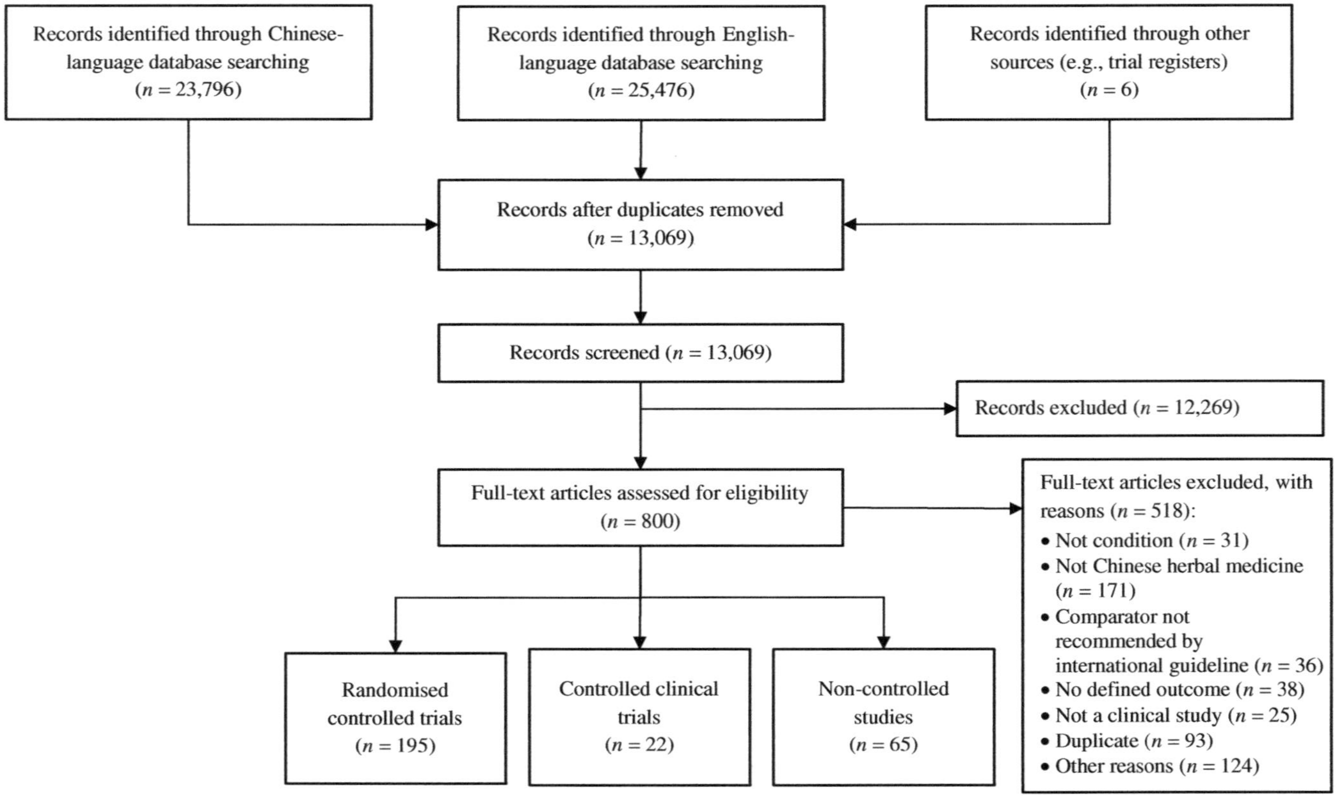

Fig. 5.1 Flowchart of study selection process: Chinese herbal medicine.

than 36,000 duplicates were removed and more than 12,000 citations were excluded after reading the titles and abstracts. The full-text article was retrieved for 800 citations. After reading the full-text articles, 518 were not relevant and were excluded from review in this chapter. Of the 282 studies (reported in 283 publications), 195 were RCTs, 22 were CCTs and 65 were non-controlled studies.

Oral Chinese Herbal Medicine

The vast majority of studies evaluated orally administered CHM. Of these, 191 studies were RCTs (H1–H185, H277–H282), 21 were CCTs (H186–H206) and 65 were non-controlled studies (H207–H271). The findings from evaluation of these studies are presented.

Randomised Controlled Trials of Oral Chinese Herbal Medicine

Oral CHM was tested in 191 RCTs (H1–H185, H277–H279, H280–H282) involving 17,599 women. The majority of studies were conducted in mainland China (156 studies), with other studies conducted in Iran (ten studies), Australia (three studies), Brazil (three studies), Korea (three studies), Hong Kong or Macau (two studies), Taiwan (two studies), Ukraine (two studies), the United States (two studies), Finland (one study), India (one study), Israel (one study), Japan (one study), the Netherlands (one study), Switzerland (one study) and Thailand (one study). Eight studies (H25, H35, H36, H120, H163, H182, H184, H185) were three-armed trials and three studies (H24, H127, H179) included four arms. Some included multiple control arms, for example HT and no treatment. Other studies included multiple treatment arms for different CM therapies. Studies that included a treatment arm of other CM therapies are described in Chapters 7, 8 and 9. Study settings included hospital inpatient and outpatient departments, community clinics and university or research institutes.

Many studies focused on menopausal women with comorbidities such as depression, anxiety, insomnia, vaginal atrophy, sexual dysfunction, or combinations of symptoms. Most studies described women as perimenopausal (154 studies). Studies including postmenopausal women were generally conducted in countries other than China (25 studies) and five studies involved perimenopausal and postmenopausal women. One study included only women who had undergone ovariectomy; women in this study were younger than women in other studies. Thirty-five studies reported inclusion criterion relating to follicle-stimulating hormone (FSH) levels and 27 described criteria relating to amenorrhoea.

Forty-six studies used CM syndrome differentiation as a study inclusion criterion and 44 considered syndromes when providing treatment. Syndromes involved *yin* and/or *yang* deficiency and *qi* stagnation. The most common syndrome was Kidney *yin* deficiency, reported in 11 studies. Other syndromes included Kidney deficiency with Liver stagnation (eight studies), *yin* deficiency with fire/heat (six studies), (Kidney) *yang* deficiency (five studies), Liver and Kidney *yin* deficiency (four studies), Liver *qi* stagnation (four studies), (Kidney) *yin* and *yang* both deficient (three studies), Heart and Kidney not communicating (three studies), Kidney deficiency and Blood stasis (three studies), Liver *yin* deficiency with Liver *yang* hyperactivity (two studies), Heart and Spleen both deficient (two studies), hyperactivity of Liver *yang* (two studies) and Liver stagnation with fire (two studies).

One hundred and forty studies evaluated oral CHM alone and 53 evaluated oral CHM used in combination with HT, antidepressants, benzodiazepines, sedatives or psychological therapy. Several studies tested multiple formulas, either in combination or individually when prescribed for specific syndromes. One hundred and twenty-nine different formulas were named in the included RCTs. Eleven studies were described as investigator developed; these were excluded from formula frequency analysis. The most frequently tested oral CHM was a commercial product, *Kun tai jiao nang* 坤泰胶囊, which was tested in ten studies (Table 5.1). This formula is prescribed for menopause symptoms. Formulas were used for general symptoms of menopause or for specific symptoms. For example, *Suan zao ren tang* 酸枣仁汤 is often prescribed for sleep problems, while *Gan mai da zao tang* 甘

Table 5.1 Frequently Reported Oral Formulas in Randomised Controlled Trials

Most Common Formulas	No. of Studies	Ingredients
Kun tai jiao nang 坤泰胶囊	10	*Shu di* 熟地, *huang lian* 黄连, *e jiao* 阿胶, *huang qin* 黄芩, *fu ling* 茯苓 and *bai shao* 白芍 (H1–H10)
Xiao yao wan/san 逍遥丸/散	9	*Chai hu* 柴胡, *bai shao* 白芍, *dang gui* 当归, *fu ling* 茯苓, *bai zhu* 白术, *gan cao* 甘草, *jiang* 姜 and *bo he* 薄荷
Er xian tang 二仙汤	8	*Xian mao* 仙茅, *xian ling pi* 仙灵脾, *ba ji tian* 巴戟天, *dang gui* 当归, *huang bai* 黄柏 and *zhi mu* 知母
Suan zao ren tang 酸枣仁汤	8	*Suan zao ren* 酸枣仁, *gan cao* 甘草, *zhi mu* 知母, *fu ling* 茯苓 and *chuan xiong* 川芎
Gan mai da zao tang 甘麦大枣汤	6	*Gan cao* 甘草, *da zao* 大枣 and *xiao mai* 小麦
Liu wei di huang wan 六味地黄丸	6	*Shu di* 熟地, *shan yao* 山药, *shan yu rou* 山萸肉, *fu ling* 茯苓, *ze xie* 泽泻 and *mu dan pi* 牡丹皮
Shu gan jie yu jiao nang 疏肝解郁胶囊	5	*Guan ye jin si tao* 贯叶金丝桃 and *ci wu jia* 刺五加 (H11–H15)
Zi shui qing gan yin 滋水清肝饮	4	*Shu di* 熟地, *dang gui* 当归, *bai shao* 白芍, *suan zao ren* 酸枣仁, *shan yu rou* 山萸肉, *fu ling* 茯苓, *shan yao* 山药, *chai hu* 柴胡, *shan zhi zi* 山栀子, *mu dan pi* 牡丹皮 and *ze xie* 泽泻

Notes: (1) Ingredients are referenced to the original studies where possible. If herb ingredients varied across studies, the herb ingredients were sourced from *Zhong Yi Fang Ji Da Ci Dian* 中医方剂大辞典.
(2) The use of some herbs may be restricted in some countries. Readers are advised to comply with relevant regulations.

麦大枣汤 is prescribed for psychological symptoms such as depression or anxiety.

There was diversity in herb ingredients among the studies with 176 different herbs described. The most frequently used herb was *fu ling* 茯苓, used 73 times (Table 5.2). Other common herbs were *bai shao* 白芍, *shu di huang* 熟地黄, *gan cao* 甘草 and *dang gui* 当归.

Table 5.2 Frequently Reported Orally Used Herbs in Randomised Controlled Trials

Most Common Herbs	Scientific Name	Frequency of Use
Fu ling 茯苓	*Poria cocos* (Schw.) Wolf	73
Bai shao 白芍	*Paeonia lactiflora* Pall.	69
Shu di huang 熟地黄	*Rehmannia glutinosa* Libosch.	69
Gan cao 甘草	*Glycyrrhiza* spp.	65
Dang gui 当归	*Angelica sinensis* (Oliv.) Diels	64
Suan zao ren 酸枣仁	*Ziziphus jujuba* Mill. var. spinosa (Bunge) Hu ex H. F. Chou	60
Chai hu 柴胡	*Bupleurum* spp.	57
Shan zhu yu 山茱萸	*Cornus officinalis* Sieb. et Zucc.	41
Shan yao 山药	*Dioscorea opposita* Thunb.	39
Zhi mu 知母	*Anemarrhena asphodeloides* Bge.	37
Sheng di huang 生地黄	*Rehmannia glutinosa* Libosch.	35
Yin yang huo 淫羊藿	*Epimedium* spp.	33
Mu dan pi 牡丹皮	*Paeonia suffruticosa* Andr.	32
Mu li 牡蛎	*Ostrea* spp.	32
Long gu 龙骨	Fossilised bones	28
Yu jin 郁金	*Curcuma* spp.	28
Huang lian 黄连	*Coptis* spp.	27
Chuan xiong 川芎	*Ligusticum chuangxiong* Hort.	26
Huang qin 黄芩	*Scutellaria baicalensis* Georgi	26
Nü zhen zi 女贞子	*Ligustrum lucidum* Ait.	26

Note: The use of some herbs may be restricted in some countries. Readers are advised to comply with relevant regulations.

Comparators included no treatment, placebo, HT, benzodiazepines, sedatives, psychological therapy and stellate ganglion block. Treatment ranged from 12 days to three years and the median duration of treatment was eight weeks. Seventeen studies conducted follow-up assessments after treatment ceased, which ranged from two weeks to three months.

Table 5.3 Risk of Bias of Randomised Controlled Trials: Oral Chinese Herbal Medicine

Risk of Bias Domain	Low Risk *n* (%)	Unclear Risk *n* (%)	High Risk *n* (%)
Sequence generation	71 (37.2)	112 (58.6)	8 (4.2)
Allocation concealment	22 (11.5)	166 (86.9)	3 (1.6)
Blinding of participants	38 (19.9)	4 (2.1)	149 (78.0)
Blinding of personnel	35 (18.3)	7 (3.7)	149 (78.0)
Blinding of outcome assessors	20 (10.5)	170 (89.0)	1 (52.4)
Incomplete outcome data	178 (93.2)	11 (5.8)	2 (1.0)
Selective outcome reporting	9 (4.7)	175 (91.6)	7 (3.6)

Risk of Bias

None of the studies were free from bias (Table 5.3). Over one third (37.2%) of studies posed 'low' risk for sequence generation as appropriate methods were used to allocate participants to groups. Eight studies (4.2%) used inappropriate methods and were judged to pose 'high' risk of bias. Over 85% of studies did not provide information about how group allocation was concealed, and these were judged as 'unclear' risk of bias. Over three quarters of studies were judged 'high' risk of bias for blinding of participants and personnel as the studies were considered unblinded. Blinding of participants and personnel was attempted in close to 20% of studies; these were judged 'low' risk of bias. Few studies explicitly stated that outcome assessors were blind to group allocation and 89% of studies were judged as 'unclear' risk. Many studies obtained outcome data for all participants or used statistical methods to account for missing data; 93.2% of studies were considered 'low' risk for the domain incomplete outcome data. While nine studies had published protocols or registered the study with trial registers, over 90% did not and were judged 'unclear' risk. Two studies, for which a trial registration or published trial protocol was identified, did not report all pre-specified outcomes; four studies with no identified trial protocol or registration reported outcomes in multiple publications, and one paper reported results for only one centre in a multi-centre trial. All seven studies were judged 'high' risk for selective outcome reporting.

Outcomes

Included studies reported outcomes for the broad range of menopause symptoms. Studies published in English reported outcomes for vasomotor, vaginal, urinary and sexual symptoms. Both English- and Chinese-language publications reported on sleep and psychological symptoms, global assessment of symptoms, HRQoL and safety.

Global assessment of symptoms was reported in 96 studies and the original or modified version of the KI (mKI)[16] was the most common outcome measure used (81 studies). Ninety-one studies reported on safety of oral CHM. Sixty-six studies assessed psychological symptoms; the Hamilton Rating Scale for Depression (HAM-D)[17] was the most frequently reported outcome (43 studies). Of the 48 studies that assessed sleep symptoms, 41 used the PSQI[18] to assess symptoms.

Twenty-three studies assessed the impact of oral CHM on HRQoL. The Menopause-specific Quality of Life questionnaire (MENQOL)[19] was used in 12 of the 23 studies. Fifteen studies reported vasomotor symptoms, with the frequency and/or severity of hot flushes reported in 14 of these studies. Outcomes less frequently reported included vaginal symptoms (four studies), urinary symptoms (one study) and sexual symptoms (four studies). None of the studies that tested oral CHM measured outcomes relating to musculoskeletal symptoms.

The findings from analysis of included studies are presented according to the specific outcome measures (see Chapter 4 for descriptions and scoring ranges for each outcome). Several studies reported results in a way that did not permit re-analysis and these data were excluded from the results presented in this section.

Vasomotor Symptoms

Results from 14 studies (H16–H29) that tested the effect of oral CHM on vasomotor symptoms were analysed. All studies compared oral

CHM with placebo except one that compared oral CHM with HT (H21).

Oral Chinese herbal medicine versus placebo

Hot flush severity was measured daily, weekly and monthly, and was reported as end-of-treatment scores or as change from baseline scores. Considering the diversity in approaches, it was considered inappropriate to pool results for analysis. Analysis of results is presented according to these factors.

Five studies (H19, H22, H23, H27, H29) involving 474 women measured daily frequency of hot flushes. Women who received oral CHM reported 2.3 fewer hot flushes at the end of treatment than women who received placebo (mean difference [MD] −2.33 flushes [95% confidence intervals −4.02, −0.65], $I^2 = 98\%$). Subgroup analysis according to menopausal status showed no significant benefit of oral CHM over placebo (Table 5.4). The overall positive finding appeared to have been influenced by one double-blind study (112 participants; H19) that showed a large effect in favour of oral CHM (MD −8.60 flushes [−10.53, −6.67]). When this study was removed from analysis, the magnitude of the effect was more modest (MD −1.07 flushes [−2.67, 0.52], $I^2 = 98\%$) and was not statistically different to placebo.

Furthermore, there was considerable statistical heterogeneity in the included studies which limits confidence in the results. Additional sensitivity analysis (with studies assessed as 'low' risk of bias for sequence generation) and subgroup analyses (according to treatment duration dichotomised at eight weeks) were conducted to identify possible causes of statistical heterogeneity. Meta-analysis of studies assessed as 'low' risk for sequence generation produced a result that was more homogeneous (200 women, MD 0.35 flushes [−0.26, 0.95], $I^2 = 43\%$; H27, H29), but showed no difference between oral CHM and placebo.

When hot flush frequency was assessed at follow-up, the result appeared to favour oral CHM over placebo (MD −1.04 [−1.97, −0.11], $I^2 = 94\%$). A small benefit was seen in perimenopausal

Table 5.4 Oral Chinese Herbal Medicine versus Placebo: Daily Hot Flush Frequency

Measurement Time (Menopausal Status)	No. of Studies (Participants)	Effect Size (MD [95% CI], I²)	Included Studies
End of treatment: all women	5 (474)	−2.33 [−4.02, −0.65]*, 98%	H19, H22, H23, H27, H29
Subgroup: perimenopausal	2 (220)	−4.36 [−12.59, 3.87], 98%	H19, H29
Subgroup: postmenopausal	3 (254)	−1.34 [−3.24, 0.55], 99%	H22, H23, H27
Follow-up: all women	3 (270)	−1.04 [−1.97, −0.11]*, 94%	H22, H23, H29
Subgroup: perimenopausal	1 (108)	−0.70 [−0.97, −0.43]*, NA	H29
Subgroup: postmenopausal	2 (162)	−1.33 [−3.81, 1.15], 97%	H22, H23

*Statistically significant, see Chapter 4.
Abbreviations: CI, confidence interval; MD, mean difference; NA, not applicable.

women, while no benefit was seen in analysis of studies that included postmenopausal women (Table 5.4). Again, statistical heterogeneity was considerable and limited certainty about the results.

Daily severity of hot flushes was measured in six studies (H22–H24, H27–H29). Four studies (H22, H23, H28, H29) reported severity at the end of treatment calculated using a variety of methods and two studies (H24, H27) reported change score from baseline to end of treatment. These two groups were kept separate for analysis.

Analysis of hot flush severity was conducted using standardised mean difference (SMD) to account for differences in the method for calculating severity. The overall analysis showed a borderline benefit of oral CHM over placebo in reducing hot flush severity at the end of treatment (334 women, SMD −1.00 [−1.99, −0.02], $p = 0.05$, $I^2 = 94\%$). However, when results were analysed according to menopausal status, the treatment effect disappeared and no difference was

Table 5.5 Oral Chinese Herbal Medicine versus Placebo: Daily Hot Flush Severity

Measurement Time (Menopausal Status)	No. of Studies (Participants)	Effect Size (SMD [95% CI], I^2)	Included Studies
End of treatment: all women	4 (334)	−1.00 [−1.99, −0.02]*, 94%	H22, H23, H28, H29
Subgroup: perimenopausal	2 (176)	−0.26 [−0.56, 0.04], 0%	H28, H29
Subgroup: postmenopausal	2 (162)	−1.81 [−4.09, 0.47], 97%	H22, H23
Follow-up: all women	3 (270)	−0.82 [−2.04, 0.41], 95%	H22, H23, H29
Subgroup: perimenopausal	1 (108)	−0.47 [−0.85, −0.09]*, NA	H29
Subgroup: postmenopausal	2 (162)	−1.01 [−3.41, 1.40], 94%	H22, H23

*Statistically significant, see Chapter 4.
Abbreviations: CI, confidence interval; NA, not applicable; SMD, standardised mean difference.

seen between the two groups (Table 5.5). Given the considerable statistical heterogeneity detected, it remains unclear whether oral CHM is more beneficial than placebo. Sensitivity analysis including two studies that used appropriate methods of group allocation eliminated heterogeneity but found no benefit of oral CHM over placebo (172 women, SMD −0.26 [−0.56, 0.04], I^2 = 0%; H28, H29). Statistical heterogeneity remained high in subgroup analyses according to treatment duration.

The potential benefit seen at the end of treatment diminished before follow-up assessment, with no difference in daily hot flush severity between oral CHM and placebo (SMD −0.82 [−2.04, 0.41], I^2 = 95%). The amount of statistical heterogeneity was considerable in the overall analysis (I^2 = 95%) and in the subgroup for postmenopausal women (I^2 = 94%), limiting confidence in the results.

Analysis of change score results in postmenopausal women showed oral CHM was no better than placebo in reducing severity of daily hot flushes, either at the end of treatment (111 participants, MD −2.50 points [−22.73, 17.73], I^2 = 19%; H24, H27) or at follow-up (19 participants, MD −0.24 points [−1.15, 0.66], H24).

One study (H19) measured weekly hot flushes in 112 perimenopausal women. A weighted weekly score was calculated by multiplying the number of mild flushes by one, the number of moderate flushes by two and the number of severe flushes by three. The weighted weekly score was calculated as the sum of scores. Extract of *Rheum rhaponticum* (*shi yong da huang* 食用大黄) resulted in a lower weekly score at the end of treatment than placebo (MD −113.70 points [−139.83, −87.57]).

The change in weekly hot flush frequency and severity was measured in 19 postmenopausal women (H24). Severity of hot flushes was calculated by multiplying the number of hot flushes by severity (mild = 1, moderate = 2, severe = 3) and change from baseline to end of treatment was measured. There was no difference between groups in the change in weekly hot flush frequency at the end of treatment (MD −18.60 flushes [−50.67, 13.47]), or at the 12-week follow-up (MD −15.40 flushes [−45.66, 14.86]). Similarly, no difference was seen between groups in weekly hot flush severity at the end of treatment (MD −34.40 [−96.59, 27.79]) or follow-up (MD −17.00 [−77.45, 43.45]).

The frequency of mild, moderate and severe hot flushes was reported per month by Haines *et al.* (H17). *Dang gui bu xue tang* 当归补血汤 was not statistically different to placebo in reducing monthly hot flush frequency for mild flushes (84 participants, MD −3.80 flushes [−11.25, 3.65]), moderate flushes (MD −5.10 flushes [−15.58, 5.38]), or severe flushes (MD 0.60 flushes [−0.23, 1.43]).

Two studies measured the effect of oral CHM on night sweats. Modified *Qing'e fang* 青蛾方 was no more effective than placebo in terms of daily night sweat frequency in 64 perimenopausal women (MD 0.07 night sweats [−0.19, 0.33]; H28). *Dang gui bu xue tang* 当归补血汤 was no more effective than placebo in reducing monthly night sweat frequency in 84 women (MD 1.30 [−1.76, 4.36]; H17).

One study (H16) used a composite measure of hot flushes and night sweats in 55 postmenopausal women. An unspecified CHM formula was not statistically different to placebo, in terms of the percentage change at the end of treatment (MD −10.53% [−55.29, 34.23]).

Oral Chinese herbal medicine versus hormone therapy

Fifty-two postmenopausal women participated in the study by Menati *et al.* (H21). The change in hot flush frequency and severity was evaluated at the end of treatment, although no details were provided of how these were assessed. Oral CHM (licorice extract) was not statistically different to the combination of conjugated equine estrogens (CEE) and medroxyprogesterone in the frequency of flushes (MD 0.58 flushes [−0.92, 2.08]). Hormone therapy was more effective than licorice extract in reducing the severity of flushes (MD 1.12 [0.05, 2.19]).

Vaginal Symptoms

Four studies (H30–H33) reported a diverse range of vaginal symptoms and signs, with all comparing oral CHM to placebo. The Vaginal Maturation Index is a ratio of parabasal, intermediate and superficial cell types of the vaginal epithelium. The percentage of each cell type was reported in 159 women in three studies (H30–H32). Analysis showed mixed results (Table 5.6). Meta-analysis showed oral CHM was not different to placebo in parabasal/basal cell count (MD −8.36 [−33.09, 16.38], I^2 = 86%), intermediate cell count (MD −1.11 [−21.78, 19.56], I^2 = 83%) or superficial cell count (MD 8.42 [−1.67, 18.51], I^2 = 85%). However, subgroup analysis showed differing results. One study (H31) that included both perimenopausal and postmenopausal women showed a statistically significant decrease in parabasal and intermediate cells and an increase in superficial cells. This suggests an increase in the effect of oestrogen on the vaginal mucosa in the group who received oral CHM. In a subgroup of two studies that included only postmenopausal women, no statistical difference was seen between groups in the the proportion of parabasal, intermediate and superficial cells.

Table 5.6 Oral Chinese Herbal Medicine versus Placebo: Vaginal Maturation Index

Outcome	No. of Studies (Participants)	Effect Size (MD [95% CI], I^2)	Included Studies
Parabasal/basal cells, %	3 (159)	−8.36 [−33.09, 16.38], 86%	H30–H32
Subgroup: all women	1 (69)	−2.50 [−3.17, −1.83]*, NA	H31
Subgroup: postmenopausal	2 (90)	−9.59 [−61.58, 42.40], 87%	H30, H32
Intermediate cells, %	3 (159)	−1.11 [−21.78, 19.56], 83%	H30–H32
Subgroup: all women	1 (69)	−9.00 [−11.12, −6.88]*, NA	H31
Subgroup: postmenopausal	2 (90)	3.71 [−29.77, 37.19], 71%	H30, H32
Superficial cells, %	3 (159)	8.42 [−1.67, 18.51], 85%	H30–H32
Subgroup: all women	1 (69)	11.50 [6.83, 16.17]*, NA	H31
Subgroup: postmenopausal	2 (90)	6.92 [−11.10, 24.94], 90%	H30, H32

*Statistically significant, see Chapter 4.
Abbreviations: CI, confidence interval; MD, mean difference; NA, not applicable.

Meta-analysis was also possible with two studies (H32, H30) that reported vaginal pH and the Vaginal Health Index (VHI).[20] The VHI is a physician-assessed measure of five aspects of vaginal health: moisture, fluid volume, elasticity, epithelial integrity and pH. Each item is scored from one (poorest) to five (best) and a total score can be derived from the sum of item scores. Meta-analysis included 197 postmenopausal women. There was a non-significant trend for the VHI score to be higher at the end of treatment in the oral CHM group compared to the placebo group (MD 1.43 points [0.00, 2.86], $p = 0.05$, $I^2 = 52\%$). There was no difference between the two groups in vaginal pH at the end of treatment (MD −0.49 points [−1.51, 0.54], I^2 = 86%).

Scores for individual items of the VHI were reported by Manonai *et al.* (H30). Results favoured placebo for fluid volume (MD 0.56 points [0.05, 1.07]) and pH score (MD 1.19 points [0.80, 1.58]), while no difference was seen between groups for moisture (MD 0.32 points [−0.17, 0.81]), elasticity (MD 0.20 points [−0.15, 0.55]) and epithelial integrity (MD 0.20 points [−0.15, 0.55]). This study also reported the maturation value for vaginal cytology, which was calculated by multiplying the number of each type of cells by a point value (0 for parabasal, 0.5 for intermediate and 1.0 for superficial) and adding the scores for each cell type. The total score was greater in the placebo group (MD 25.30 [13.51, 37.09]), indicating an increase in the effect of oestrogen on vaginal mucosa.

Various other vaginal outcomes were reported. There was no difference between the herb *guo ye ge* 裹叶葛 and placebo in dyspareunia scores at the end of treatment (81 postmenopausal women, MD −0.12 points [−0.66, 0.42]; H30), but the karyopyknotic index was greater among those who received placebo in this study (MD 16.40 [7.55, 25.25]). Larmo *et al.* (H32) found that postmenopausal women who received sea buckthorn (*sha ji* 沙棘) were less likely to report improvements in vaginal dryness (116 women, risk ratio [RR] 0.64 [0.44, 0.93]), while there was no difference between groups in the number of women who reported improvement in burning symptoms (RR 0.93 [0.63, 1.36]) or itching (RR 0.81 [0.53, 1.24]). The change in vaginal moisture from baseline to end of treatment was not statistically different in women who received *sha ji* 沙棘 and those who received placebo (MD 0.10, [−0.38, 0.58]). Finally, this study reported vaginal dryness, which was not statistically different between the two groups (MD −0.37 points, [−0.96, 0.22]).

Urinary Symptoms

One study (H30) involving 81 postmenopausal women assessed urinary symptoms. *Pueraria mirifica* (*guo ye ge* 裹叶葛) was compared with placebo. Symptoms of urinary frequency, urge incontinence, stress incontinence and frequent cystitis were scored from zero to three, where higher scores indicated worse symptoms. There was no statistical difference between groups at the end of treatment for any of the symptoms: urinary frequency (MD −0.13 points [−0.59, 0.33]), urge incontinence (MD 0.19 points [−0.29, 0.67]), stress incontinence (MD 0.03 points [−0.44, 0.50]) or frequent cystitis (MD 0.37 points [0.00, 0.74]). Oral CHM did not appear to improve urinary symptoms in postmenopausal women.

Sexual Symptoms

One study (H34) evaluated the actions of a single herb, *Tribulus terrestris* (*ji li* 蒺藜), on sexual symptoms in 60 postmenopausal women. The Sexual Quotient-Female version (SQF)[21] was used, which includes ten items scored from zero to five. The sum of scores for the ten items is multiplied by two to calculate a total score out of 100, where higher scores mean greater sexual performance/satisfaction. The total score at the end of treatment was 14.3 points higher in women who received *ji li* 蒺藜 than in women who received placebo ([5.32, 23.28]). Women who received *ji li* 蒺藜 also scored higher than women who received placebo on the domains for desire (MD 2.60 points [0.98, 4.22]), foreplay (MD 0.90 points, [0.25, 1.55]), arousal (MD 1.50 points, [0.30, 2.70]) and comfort (MD 1.50 points, [0.40, 2.60]). There was no difference between *ji li* 蒺藜 and placebo on the orgasm domain (MD 0.70 points [−0.59, 1.99]).

Pittsburgh Sleep Quality Index

Thirty-eight studies assessed the effect of CHM on sleep using the PSQI.[18] Scores range from zero to 21, with lower scores indicating better sleep. Three studies (H35–H37) compared oral CHM with placebo, 22 studies (H1, H38–H58) compared oral CHM with pharmacotherapy and 13 studies (H11, H12, H59–H69) tested the combination of oral CHM plus pharmacotherapy against pharmacotherapy alone.

Table 5.7 Oral Chinese Herbal Medicine versus Placebo: Pittsburgh Sleep Quality Index

Menopausal Status	No. of Studies (Participants)	Effect Size (MD [95% CI], I^2)	Included Studies
End of treatment: all women	3 (290)	−3.20 [−6.26, −0.14]*, 96%	H35–H37
Subgroup: all women	1 (86)	−5.56 [−6.59, −4.53]*, NA	H35
Subgroup: postmenopausal	2 (204)	−1.99 [−4.62, 0.64], 91%	H36, H37

*Statistically significant, see Chapter 4.
Abbreviations: CI, confidence interval; MD, mean difference; NA, not applicable.

Oral Chinese herbal medicine versus placebo

Three studies (H35–H37) that compared oral CHM with placebo evaluated impact on sleep using the PSQI. These studies included 290 women. Meta-analysis showed the PSQI scores to be 3.20 points lower, indicating better sleep quality, in women who received oral CHM ([−6.26, −0.14], I^2 = 96%; Table 5.7). In subgroup analysis a statistically significant result was seen in one study that included women of all menopausal stages, but no benefit was seen in postmenopausal women. Statistical heterogeneity was high in the overall meta-analysis and was not reduced in subgroup analysis for menopausal stage (Table 5.7). The significance of this result remains unclear.

Oral Chinese herbal medicine versus pharmacotherapy

The effect of oral CHM on sleep quality was assessed in 22 studies (H1, H38–H58) and 2,171 perimenopausal women. Meta-analysis showed oral CHM resulted in a score 2.33 points lower on the PSQI than pharmacotherapy ([−2.85, −1.80], I^2 = 93%; Table 5.8). Subgroup analysis was conducted to examine potential contributors to statistical heterogeneity. Six studies assessed as 'low' risk of bias for sequence generation showed a more modest reduction in score of 1.80 points with oral CHM and appeared to be more homogeneous

Table 5.8 Oral Chinese Herbal Medicine versus Pharmacotherapy: Pittsburgh Sleep Quality Index

Assessment	No. of Studies (Participants)	Effect Size (MD [95% CI], I^2)	Included Studies
End of treatment	22 (2,171)	−2.33 [−2.85, −1.80]*, 93%	H1, H38–H58
Subgroup: 'low' risk of bias SG	6 (515)	−1.80 [−2.16, −1.43]*, 13%	H38, H43, H46, H51, H52, H58
Subgroup: treatment duration ≤8 w	18 (1,833)	−2.37 [−3.03, −1.72]*, 94%	H1, H39–H44, H47–H56, H58
Subgroup: treatment >8 w	4 (338)	−1.72 [−2.18, −1.26]*, 0%	H38, H45, H46, H57

*Statistically significant, see Chapter 4.
Abbreviations: CI, confidence interval; MD, mean difference; SG, sequence generation; w, weeks.

([−2.16, −1.43], I^2 = 13%). Studies that provided treatment for over eight weeks showed similar results to studies at 'low' risk of bias (MD −1.72 points [−2.18, −1.26], I^2 = 0%). Additional subgroup analysis of studies where women had insomnia/sleep disorders produced a similar improvement to the total pool (15 studies, 1,542 women, MD −2.27 points [−2.93, −1.61], I^2 = 95%; H1, H38, H39, H41, H43–H45, H47–H49, H51, H52, H54–H56), while no difference was seen between groups in studies where comorbid insomnia was not reported (seven studies, 629 women, MD −0.68 points [−2.04, 0.68], I^2 = 87%; H40, H42, H46, H50, H53, H57, H58). Statistical heterogeneity remained 'high' in these analyses. The best estimate of the effect of oral CHM appears to come from studies at 'low' risk of bias for sequence generation and those where treatment was provided for more than eight weeks; a reduction of approximately 1.80 points appears to be more likely.

Oral Chinese herbal medicine plus pharmacotherapy versus pharmacotherapy alone

Thirteen studies (H11, H12, H59–H69) that used oral CHM as integrative medicine measured sleep quality using the PSQI. When

Table 5.9 Oral Chinese Herbal Medicine plus Pharmacotherapy versus Pharmacotherapy: Pittsburgh Sleep Quality Index

Assessment	No. of Studies (Participants)	Effect Size (MD [95% CI], I^2)	Included Studies
End of treatment	13 (1,249)	−1.55 [−2.80, −0.30]*, 97%	H11, H12, H59–H69
Subgroup: 'low' risk of bias SG	6 (544)	−0.27 [−2.50, 1.97], 98%	H12, H59, H60, H66, H67, H69
Subgroup: treatment duration ≤8 w	11 (1,052)	−1.85 [−3.25, −0.46]*, 98%	H11, H12, H60–H65, H67–H69
Subgroup: treatment >8 w	2 (197)	0.17 [−4.75, 5.09], 98%	H59, H66

*Statistically significant, see Chapter 4.

Abbreviations: CI, confidence interval; MD, mean difference; SG, sequence generation; w, weeks.

results for all 13 studies were combined for analysis, PSQI scores were 1.55 points lower in perimenopausal women who received oral CHM plus pharmacotherapy than in women who received pharmacotherapy alone (1,249 women, [−2.80, −0.30], I^2 = 97%; Table 5.9). However, considerable statistical heterogeneity lowers our confidence in the result.

Subgroup analyses were conducted to identify potential reasons for heterogeneity. In studies judged 'low' risk of bias for sequence generation, oral CHM plus pharmacotherapy was as effective as pharmacotherapy used alone (MD −0.27 points [−2.50, 1.97], I^2 = 98%). The result favoured oral CHM plus pharmacotherapy when treatment was provided for eight weeks or less (MD −1.85 points [−3.25, −0.46], I^2 = 98%), but showed no difference between groups in two studies that provided treatment for longer than eight weeks (MD 0.17 points [−4.75, 5.09], I^2 = 98%). Further subgroup analysis according to comorbid insomnia/sleep disorder (ten studies, 962 women, MD −1.91 points [−2.75, −1.06], I^2 = 91%: H11, H12, H59–H64, H67, H68) and no comorbid insomnia/sleep disorder (three studies, 287 women, MD −0.44 points [−4.68, 3.81], I^2 = 99%; H65, H66, H69) failed to identify the source of heterogeneity.

Thus, our confidence in the effects of oral CHM as integrative medicine on PSQI is limited.

Athens Insomnia Scale

The Athens Insomnia Scale (AIS)[22] was used to measure sleep quality in two studies (H70, H71). In 140 perimenopausal women, women who received oral CHM scored 2.16 points lower, indicating improved sleep, compared to women who received pharmacotherapy alone ([−2.82, −1.51], $I^2 = 27\%$).

Sleep Dysfunction Rating Scale

The Sleep Dysfunction Rating Scale (SDRS) is a subjective measure of sleep quality.[23] The SDRS includes ten items scored from zero to four; the sum of item scores provides a total score in the range of zero to 40 points. A lower score indicates better sleep quality. The SDRS was reported in one study of 73 perimenopausal women (H72). Women who received oral CHM scored 4.29 points lower than women who received diazepam ([−5.85, −2.73]).

Self-rating Scale of Sleep

Two studies (H52, H73) involving 160 perimenopausal women evaluated sleep using the Self-rating Scale of Sleep (SRSS).[24] The SRSS includes ten items scored from one to five, where higher scores indicate worse sleep. Scores are summed to provide a total score in the range 10 to 50. Meta-analysis showed women who received oral CHM scored 1.95 points lower on the SRSS than women who received benzodiazepines alone or with vitamin E and oryzanol (a rice bran oil) ([−2.73, −1.17], $I^2 = 0\%$).

Spiegel Sleep Questionnaire

The Spiegel Sleep Questionnaire[25] was used to measure sleep quality in three studies (H74–H76) with 236 perimenopausal women. The studies described scoring for ten items in five grades (scored 0, 1, 3, 5, 7), where a higher score means worse sleep. The score at the end of treatment was not statistically different between women who received oral CHM and women who received pharmacotherapy (MD −0.82 points [−2.62, 0.98], I^2 = 68%). The small number of included studies prevented examination of potential causes of statistical heterogeneity, and our confidence in the result is limited.

Zung's Self-rating Depression Scale

Five studies examined the role of oral CHM in improving depressive symptoms using Zung's Self-rating Depression Scale (SDS).[26] The SDS includes 20 items scored from one to four and the sum for each item provides a total score. An index score can be calculated by dividing the total score by the maximum score (80) and multiplying by 100; however, this method was not used in the included studies. Meta-analysis was conducted separately for studies that compared oral CHM with pharmacotherapy (H46, H77) and studies that compared oral CHM plus pharmacotherapy with pharmacotherapy alone (H11, H78, H79).

Oral Chinese herbal medicine versus pharmacotherapy

Two studies (H46, H77) with 212 perimenopausal women tested oral CHM. Meta-analysis showed oral CHM was as effective as pharmacotherapy in improving depressive symptoms (MD −0.83 points [−4.16, 2.50], I^2 = 79%), although statistical heterogeneity limits confidence in the results.

Oral Chinese herbal medicine plus pharmacotherapy versus pharmacotherapy alone

The combination of oral CHM and pharmacotherapy was tested in three studies (H11, H78, H79). Analysis of 282 perimenopausal women showed no benefit of adding oral CHM to pharmacotherapy in improving SDS scores (MD −3.64 point, [−7.37, 0.09], I^2 = 87%).

Subgroup analysis to explore reasons for statistical heterogeneity was not conducted due to the small number of included studies.

Zung's Self-rating Anxiety Scale

Four studies measured anxiety using Zung's Self-rating Anxiety Scale (SAS).[27] Two studies (H46, H77) compared oral CHM with pharmacotherapy and two studies (H11, H79) tested oral CHM as integrative medicine with pharmacotherapy.

Oral Chinese herbal medicine versus pharmacotherapy

Two studies (H46, H77), which included 212 perimenopausal women, measured anxiety symptoms using the SAS. When used alone, oral CHM was as effective as pharmacotherapy for anxiety symptoms (MD −1.83 points [−8.85, 5.20], $I^2 = 93\%$). Statistical heterogeneity was unable to be explored due to the small number of included studies and results should be interpreted in light of this.

Oral Chinese herbal medicine plus pharmacotherapy versus pharmacotherapy alone

Two hundred and twenty perimenopausal women were included in the two studies that assessed anxiety using the SAS (H11, H79). Anxiety was reduced in women who received the combination of oral CHM and pharmacotherapy compared to those who received pharmacotherapy alone (MD −8.17 points [−9.65, −6.70], $I^2 = 0\%$).

Beck Depression Inventory

The Beck Depression Inventory (BDI)[28] was used in one study (H36) to evaluate depressive symptom severity. The BDI includes 21 items scored zero to three, with higher scores indicating worse severity of symptoms. One hundred and four postmenopausal women were randomised to receive bitter orange capsules (*dai dai hua* 玳玳花) or placebo. Women who received *dai dai hua* 玳玳花 reported lower scores on the BDI compared to placebo (MD −2.30 points [−3.91, −0.69]).

Hamilton Rating Scale for Depression

Forty-three studies measured depressive symptoms using the HAM-D.[17] The HAM-D includes 21 items, with the first 17 contributing to the score. The total score ranges from zero to 50 points and lower scores indicate better outcomes. One study (H80) compared oral CHM with placebo, 20 studies (H14, H15, H40, H42, H47, H81–H95) compared oral CHM with pharmacotherapy and 22 studies (H12, H13, H69, H78, H96–H113) compared the combination of oral CHM plus pharmacotherapy with pharmacotherapy alone. Results are presented according to comparisons.

Oral Chinese herbal medicine versus placebo

One study (H80) of 56 postmenopausal women used the HAM-D to measure depressive symptoms. Women who received placebo achieved lower scores at the end of treatment compared to women who received saffron (*Crocus sativus, xi hong hua* 西红花) (MD 2.71 points [0.82, 4.60]).

Oral Chinese herbal medicine versus pharmacotherapy

Twenty studies (H14, H15, H40, H42, H47, H81–H95) that compared oral CHM to pharmacotherapy assessed depressive symptoms with the HAM-D. At the end of treatment, HAM-D scores were 2.10 points lower in those who received oral CHM compared to pharmacotherapy alone (1,591 participants, [−3.08, −1.11], $I^2 = 93\%$) (Table 5.10). Considerable statistical heterogeneity was identified, which was examined through subgroup and sensitivity analyses. Sensitivity analysis with studies assessed as 'low' risk of bias for sequence generation also showed oral CHM to produce lower HAM-D scores than pharmacotherapy alone,

Table 5.10 Oral Chinese Herbal Medicine versus Pharmacotherapy: Hamilton Rating Scale for Depression

Assessment	No. of Studies (Participants)	Effect Size (MD [95% CI], I^2)	Included Studies
End of treatment	20 (1,591)	−2.10 [−3.08, −1.11]*, 93%	H14, H15, H40, H42, H47, H81–H95
Subgroup: 'low' risk of bias SG	6 (379)	−2.25 [−4.48, −0.02]*, 82%	H81, H84, H85, H87, H92, H95
Subgroup: treatment duration ≤8 w	16 (1,354)	−2.23 [−3.30, −1.16]*, 94%	H14, H15, H40, H42, H47, H81–H90, H93
Subgroup: Treatment >8 w	4 (237)	−1.66 [−5.02, 1.71], 86%	H91, H92, H94, H95

*Statistically significant, see Chapter 4.
Abbreviations: CI, confidence interval; MD, mean difference; SG, sequence generation; w, weeks.

but statistical heterogeneity remained 'high' (Table 5.10). As 19 of the 20 studies included in the meta-analysis involved perimenopausal women, it was not surprising that the result for this group also showed high heterogeneity (1,525 women, MD −2.22 points [−3.23, −1.21], I^2 = 93%; H14, H15, H40, H42, H47, H81–H95).

Statistical heterogeneity persisted in subgroup analyses for treatment duration (Table 5.10). In this subgroup analysis, treatment provided for eight weeks or less produced a result that favoured oral CHM, while treatment for more than eight weeks showed similar results in both groups. Subgroup analyses failed to demonstrate sources of statistical heterogeneity. Characteristics of women were largely consistent, so it seems unlikely that heterogeneity is due to the population. It is possible that heterogeneity is a result of the different formulas and herbal ingredients.

Oral Chinese herbal medicine plus pharmacotherapy versus pharmacotherapy alone

Twenty-two studies (H12, H13, H69, H78, H96–H113) involving 1,754 perimenopausal women tested the combination of oral CHM

Table 5.11 Oral Chinese Herbal Medicine plus Pharmacotherapy versus Pharmacotherapy Alone: Hamilton Rating Scale for Depression

Assessment	No. of Studies (Participants)	Effect Size (MD [95% CI], I^2)	Included Studies
End of treatment	22 (1,754)	−2.64 [−4.31, −0.97]*, 98%	H12, H13, H69, H78, H96–H113
Subgroup: 'low' risk of bias SG	8 (629)	−1.10 [−4.61, 2.40], 99%	H12, H69, H96–H98, H102, H105, H111
Subgroup: treatment duration ≤8 w	19 (1,523)	−2.59 [−4.44, −0.74]*, 98%	H12, H13, H69, H78, H96–H98, H100–H105, H108–H113
Subgroup: treatment >8 w	2 (160)	−3.87 [−5.42, 2.32]*, 0%	H106, H107

*Statistically significant, see Chapter 4.
Abbreviations: CI, confidence interval; MD, mean difference; SG, sequence generation; w, weeks.

plus pharmacotherapy with pharmacotherapy alone and reported HAM-D scores at the end of treatment. The addition of oral CHM to pharmacotherapy appeared to improve outcomes; the mean HAM-D score at the end of treatment was 2.64 points lower with oral CHM plus pharmacotherapy than with pharmacotherapy alone ([−4.31, −0.97], I^2 = 98%; Table 5.11). Similar to the finding for oral CHM versus pharmacotherapy, considerable statistical heterogeneity was detected and examined through subgroup analysis.

When studies judged to pose 'low' risk for sequence generation were analysed, statistical heterogeneity remained, yet the treatment effect diminished such that no difference was seen between groups (Table 5.11). Eighteen of the 22 studies included perimenopausal women with comorbid insomnia. Meta-analysis of these studies also showed high levels of statistical heterogeneity (1,332 women, MD −2.56 points [−4.58, −0.53], I^2 = 98%; H69, H78, H96–H100, H102–H106, H108–H113). Studies where the intervention was provided for more than eight weeks were homogeneous (MD −3.87 points [−5.42, −2.32], I^2 = 0%), but only two studies were included in this meta-analysis. While many of the subgroup analyses showed a positive benefit of adding oral CHM to conventional pharmacological treatment, the unexplained heterogeneity limits our confidence in the results.

Hamilton Rating Scale for Anxiety

Sixteen RCTs measured anxiety using the Hamilton Rating Scale for Anxiety (HAM-A)[29] in perimenopausal women. The HAM-A consists of 14 items scored zero to four that are summed to produce a total score in the range of zero to 56. Higher scores indicate greater levels of anxiety. Seven studies (H14, H47, H58, H114–H117) compared oral CHM with pharmacotherapy and nine studies (H12, H61, H62, H67, H97, H104, H110, H118, H119) tested oral CHM as integrative medicine with pharmacotherapy.

Oral Chinese herbal medicine versus pharmacotherapy

Seven studies (H14, H47, H58, H114–H117) that compared oral CHM with pharmacotherapy measured anxiety using HAM-A in perimenopausal women. Women who received oral CHM scored 2.10 points lower on the HAM-A than women who received pharmacotherapy ([−2.71, −1.49], I^2 = 79%; Table 5.12). Statistical

Table 5.12 Oral Chinese Herbal Medicine versus Pharmacotherapy: Hamilton Rating Scale for Anxiety

Assessment	No. of Studies (Participants)	Effect Size (MD [95% CI], I^2)	Included Studies
End of treatment	7 (623)	−2.10 [−2.71, −1.49]*, 79%	H14, H47, H58, H114–H117
Subgroup: 'low' risk of bias SG	2 (140)	−2.27 [−3.09, −1.46]*, 0%	H58, H115
Subgroup: treatment duration ≤8 w	6 (537)	−2.36 [−2.77, −1.95]*, 38%	H14, H47, H58, H115–H117
Subgroup: treatment >8 w	1 (86)	−0.92 [−1.47, −0.37]*, NA	H114

*Statistically significant, see Chapter 4.

Abbreviations: CI, confidence interval; MD, mean difference; NA, not applicable; SG, sequence generation; w, weeks.

heterogeneity remained 'high' in subgroup analyses for studies that included women with a diagnosis of anxiety (three studies, 314 women, MD −2.35 points [−3.01, −1.69], $I^2 = 74\%$; H115, H116, H117). Studies of women who had not been diagnosed with anxiety showed a smaller treatment effect, but similar levels of statistical heterogeneity (four studies, 309 women, MD −1.86 points [−2.34, −1.38], $I^2 = 76\%$; H14, H47, H58, H114). Subgroup analysis showed lower heterogeneity in studies assessed as 'low' risk of bias for sequence generation and when the treatment duration was eight weeks or less (Table 5.12).

Oral Chinese herbal medicine plus pharmacotherapy versus pharmacotherapy alone

Nine studies (H12, H61, H62, H67, H97, H104, H110, H118, H119) measured anxiety using HAM-A in perimenopausal women. All studies provided treatment for up to eight weeks. There was no benefit of adding oral CHM to antidepressant/sedative therapy compared to using antidepressants/sedatives alone (780 women, MD −3.21 points [−6.83, 0.41], $I^2 = 99\%$; Table 5.13). Studies assessed

Table 5.13 Oral Chinese Herbal Medicine plus Pharmacotherapy versus Pharmacotherapy Alone: Hamilton Rating Scale for Anxiety

Assessment	No. of Studies (Participants)	Effect Size (MD [95% CI], I^2)	Included Studies
End of treatment	9 (780)	−3.21 [−6.83, 0.41], 99%	H12, H61, H62, H67, H97, H104, H110, H118, H119
Subgroup: 'low' risk of bias SG	3 (226)	−5.44 [−8.62, −2.26]*, 95%	H12, H67, H97
Subgroup: treatment duration ≤8 w	9 (780)	−3.21 [−6.83, 0.41], 99%	H12, H61, H62, H67, H97, H104, H110, H118, H119

*Statistically significant, see Chapter 4.

Abbreviations: CI, confidence interval; MD, mean difference, SG, sequence generation; w, weeks.

as 'low' risk of bias for sequence generation showed similar values for statistical heterogeneity. Planned subgroup analysis did not identify potential causes of heterogeneity, as all studies included perimenopausal women, provided treatment for up to eight weeks and used antidepressants/sedatives as the comparator. Thus, we can be confident that these factors are unlikely to be contributing to statistical heterogeneity. Given that the cause of heterogeneity was not able to be determined, confidence in the effect of oral CHM as integrative medicine to antidepressants/sedatives is limited.

Symptom Checklist-90 Item

One three-arm study by Qian *et al.* (H120) used a modified version of the Symptom Checklist (SCL)-90 item questionnaire[30] in perimenopausal women. The SCL-90 measures a broad range of psychological problems and includes dimensions for somatisation, obsessive-compulsive disorder, interpersonal sensitivity, depression, anxiety, hostility, phobic anxiety, paranoid ideation and psychoticism. The level of distress for each symptom is scored from zero (no distress) to four (extreme distress). Dimension scores can be calculated as the mean score of items for each dimension, and a global severity index is calculated as the average score of the 90 items. The study by Qian *et al.* (2010) reported the sum of dimension scores as a total score, which differs from the standard scoring approach. Combined use of *Kun bao wan* 坤宝丸 and modified *Xiao yao wan* 逍遥丸 was equally as effective as psychological treatment in 108 women (MD 0.18 points [−2.64, 3.00]). *Kun bao wan* 坤宝丸 and modified *Xiao yao wan* 逍遥丸 used in combination with psychological treatment resulted in a lower score, indicating an improvement in psychological symptoms (111 women, MD −4.00 points [−6.77, −1.23]).

Kupperman Index

The Kupperman Index[16] was the most common outcome reported among included studies. Data were able to be analysed for 79 of the

81 studies that reported KI. Studies published in English tended to use the original 11-item version, while studies originating from China frequently used an mKI to include two additional items: dyspareunia and urinary tract infections. In many studies, these two items were simply added to the questionnaires, while other studies replaced one or more of the original 11 items with items for dyspareunia, urinary tract infections or other symptoms. Lower scores indicate better outcomes. Meta-analysis was conducted using SMD, with subgroup analysis conducted for use of KI or mKI.

The KI/mKI was used in nine studies (H31, H33, H121–H127) that compared oral CHM with placebo, 48 studies (H1, H5, H6, H7, H10, H46, H48, H51, H82, H83, H88, H94, H128–H163) that compared oral CHM with pharmacotherapy and 22 studies (H2–H4, H60, H66, H97, H98, H102, H104, H106, H109, H113, H164–H173) that compared oral CHM plus pharmacotherapy with pharmacotherapy alone.

Oral Chinese herbal medicine versus placebo

Nine studies (H31, H33, H121–H127) that compared oral CHM with placebo used both KI and mKI to assess menopause symptoms. Meta-analysis of all nine studies showed oral CHM to be superior to placebo (SMD −1.43 [−2.08, −0.78], I^2 = 93%; Table 5.14). Subgroup analysis was conducted for menopausal status, instrument used, treatment duration and in studies judged 'low' risk of bias for sequence generation. One study that included only postmenopausal women showed no benefit of oral CHM over placebo (MD −1.78 points [−6.85, 3.29]; H125), whilst studies of perimenopausal women (four studies, 273 women, SMD −1.35 [−2.16, −0.55], I^2 = 88%; H121–H124) and both perimenopausal and postmenopausal women (three studies, 169 women, SMD −1.57 [−2.56, −0.58], I^2 = 87%; H31, H33, H126) showed oral CHM to be superior, albeit with considerable statistical heterogeneity.

Results for studies that used the KI showed oral CHM to be no different to placebo at the end of treatment (Table 5.14), while studies

Table 5.14 Oral Chinese Herbal Medicine versus Placebo: Kupperman Index Total Score

Assessment	No. of Studies (Participants)	Effect Size (SMD# [95% CI], I^2)	Included Studies
End of treatment	9 (729)	−1.43 [−2.08, −0.78]*, 93%	H31, H33, H121–H127
Subgroup: KI	3 (200)	MD −5.52 [−12.65, 1.61], 92%	H33, H121, H125
Subgoup: mKI	6 (529)	−1.76 [−2.43, −1.08]*, 89%	H31, H122–H124, H126, H127
Subgroup: 'low' risk of bias SG	6 (544)	−1.36 [−2.26, −0.47]*, 95%	H31, H33, H121, H122, H125, H127
Subgroup: treatment duration ≤8 w	4 (249)	−0.95 [−1.63, −0.27]*, 83%	H121–H123, H126
Subgroup: treatment duration >8 w	5 (480)	−1.82 [−2.79, −0.85]*, 94%	H31, H33, H124, H125, H127

*Statistically significant, see Chapter 4.
#Analysis using SMD unless otherwise specified.
Abbreviations: CI, confidence interval; KI, Kupperman Index; MD, mean difference; mKI, modified Kupperman Index; SG, sequence generation; SMD, standardised mean difference; w, weeks.

that used mKI produced a result that favoured oral CHM. Benefits of oral CHM over placebo were seen in studies judged 'low' risk of bias for sequence generation and when treatment was provided for eight weeks or less, or more than eight weeks. Statistical heterogeneity persisted through all subgroup analyses, which lowers confidence in the result.

One study (H126) conducted follow-up assessment using mKI six weeks after the end of treatment. Among the 36 perimenopausal and postmenopausal women who participated in the study, women who received *Schisandra chinensis* (*wu wei zi* 五味子) had scores 5.27 points lower than women who received placebo ([−9.42, −1.12]).

Results for individual items of the KI were reported in four studies (H31, H33, H125, H126) that compared oral CHM with placebo. Meta-analysis was possible for ten items (Table 5.15). Benefits were

Table 5.15 Oral Chinese Herbal Medicine versus Placebo: Kupperman Index Item Scores

Assessment	No. of Studies (Participants)	Effect Size (SMD [95% CI], I^2)	Included Studies
Vasomotor	4 (238)	−1.42 [−2.54, −0.30]*, 94%	H31, H33, H125, H126
Insomnia	3 (166)	−1.25 [−2.53, 0.03], 92%	H31, H33, H126
Nervousness	2 (100)	−0.68 [−1.27, −0.08]*, 51%	H33, H126
Melancholia	3 (166)	−0.29 [−0.68, 0.09], 35%	H31, H33, H126
Vertigo	3 (166)	−0.97 [−2.14, 0.19], 92%	H31, H33, H126
Weakness	2 (130)	−1.77 [−3.03, −0.52]*, 89%	H31, H33
Arthralgia	3 (166)	−0.92 [−1.73, −0.12]*, 83%	H31, H33, H126
Headache	2 (100)	−0.44 [−0.93, 0.05], 31%	H33, H126
Palpitations	3 (166)	−0.97 [−2.32, 0.38], 94%	H31, H33, H126
Formication	2 (130)	−0.40 [−0.75, −0.05]*, 1%	H31, H33

*Statistically significant, see Chapter 4.
Abbreviations: CI, confidence interval; SMD, standardised mean difference.

found for oral CHM over placebo for the items vasomotor (SMD −1.42 [−2.54, −0.30], I^2 = 94%), nervousness (SMD −0.68 [−1.27, −0.08], I^2 = 51%), weakness (SMD −1.77 [−3.03, −0.52], I^2 = 89%), arthralgia (SMD −0.92 [−1.73, −0.12], I^2 = 83%) and formication (SMD −0.40 [−0.75, −0.05], I^2 = 1%). No benefit was seen for oral CHM over placebo for items insomnia, melancholia, vertigo, headache and palpitations (Table 5.15).

One study (H33) reported scores for paraesthesia at the end of treatment. Scores for this item were 0.54 points lower in women who received oral CHM compared to placebo ([−0.96, −0.12]). Two studies reported individual item scores for mKI: sweating, tinnitus, irritability, concentration and vaginal dryness. At the end of treatment, women who received oral CHM scored lower for items relating to tinnitus (66 women, MD −0.49 points [−0.63, −0.35]; H31) and irritability (66 women, MD −1.52 points [−1.86, −1.18]; H31). No difference was seen between oral CHM and placebo for items relating to sweating (36 women, MD −0.89 [−2.10, 0.32];

H126), concentration (36 women, MD 0.16 [−0.50, 0.82]; H126) and vaginal dryness (36 women, MD −0.06 [−0.73, 0.61]; H126). Change in vaginal dryness was greater with oral CHM than with placebo in one study of 64 women (MD −0.69 points [−1.16, −0.22]; H33).

One study (H126) reported results for individual mKI item scores at a follow-up assessment that was conducted six weeks after treatment ceased. Results for 36 perimenopausal and postmenopausal women found those who received *Schisandra chinensis* (*wu wei zi* 五味子) reported better scores than women who received placebo for the items vasomotor (MD −1.70 points [−3.06, −0.34]), palpitations (MD −0.56 [−1.04, −0.08]) and sweating (MD −1.18 points [−2.17, −0.19]). No difference between groups was seen in scores for insomnia (MD −1.06 points [−2.31, 0.19]), nervousness (MD −0.56 points [−1.52, 0.40]), melancholia (MD −0.27 points [−0.86, 0.32]), vertigo (MD −0.09 points [−0.46, 0.28]), arthralgia (MD −0.11 points [−0.56, 0.34]), headache (MD −0.39 points [−0.90, 0.12]), concentration (MD 0.35 points [−0.16, 0.86]) and vaginal dryness (MD −0.23 points [−0.85, 0.39]).

Oral Chinese herbal medicine versus pharmacotherapy

Forty-eight studies (H1, H5–H7, H10, H46, H48, H51, H82, H83, H88, H94, H128–H163) that compared oral CHM with pharmacotherapy examined their effect on menopause symptoms using the KI/mKI. Analysis involved 4,195 women and showed oral CHM produced a greater improvement in symptoms than pharmacotherapy (SMD −0.50 [−0.73, −0.27], I^2 = 92%; Table 5.16). Subgroup analyses were conducted for several factors to identify possible reasons for the considerable amount of statistical heterogeneity seen. Forty-five of the 48 studies included perimenopausal women, so it was not surprising that the results of the analysis of this group of studies reflected the total pool (4,395 women, SMD −0.51 [−0.75, −0.26], I^2 = 93%; H1, H5–H7, H10, H46, H48, H51, H82, H83, H88, H94, H129–H136, H138–H162).

Table 5.16 Oral Chinese Herbal Medicine versus Pharmacotherapy: Kupperman Index Total Score

Assessment	No. of Studies (Participants)	Effect Size (SMD# [95% CI], I^2)	Included Studies
End of treatment	48 (4,195)	−0.50 [−0.73, −0.27]*, 92%	H1, H5–H7, H10, H46, H48, H51, H82, H83, H88, H94, H128–H163
Subgroup: KI	14 (1,101)	MD −2.58 [−3.72, −1.44]*, 87%	H5, H6, H48, H51, H88, H128, H138, H139, H144–H146, H148, H159, H162
Subgoup: mKI	34 (3,094)	−0.37 [−0.65, −0.09]*, 93%	H1, H7, H10, H46, H82, H83, H94, H129–H137, H140–H143, H147, H149 H158, H160, H161, H163
Subgroup: 'low' risk of bias SG	13 (924)	−0.10 [−0.38, 0.18], 78%	H6, H46, H51, H131, H136, H142, H144, H146, H148, H150, H156, H159, H163
Subgroup: treatment duration ≤8 w	17 (1,608)	−0.80 [−1.30, −0.30]*, 95%	H1, H48, H51, H82, H83, H88, H128–H130, H133, H140, H142, H146, H151, H157, H158, H163
Subgroup: treatment duration >8 w	31 (2,587)	−0.29 [−0.50, −0.08]*, 84%	H5–H7, H10, H46, H94, H131, H132, H134–H139, H141, H143–H145, H147–H150, H152–H156, H159–H162

*Statistically significant, see Chapter 4.
#Analysis using SMD unless otherwise specified.
Abbreviations: CI, confidence interval; KI, Kupperman Index; MD, mean difference; mKI, modified Kupperman Index; SG, sequence generation; SMD, standardised mean difference; w, weeks.

Results for subgroups using the KI or mKI to assess symptoms resulted in a treatment effect favouring oral CHM, with considerable statistical heterogeneity (Table 5.16). A smaller subset of studies judged as 'low' risk of bias for sequence generation showed no benefit of oral CHM over pharmacotherapy, with substantial heterogeneity. Duration of treatment did not appear to contribute to statistical heterogeneity, which remained 'high' in both groups.

Follow-up assessment at four weeks was conducted in two studies (H131, H143). Scores for the mKI were lower at follow-up among women who received oral CHM compared to pharmacotherapy (172 women, SMD −0.99 [−1.78, −0.20], $I^2 = 83\%$).

Two studies (H82, H137) involving 104 women reported scores for individual items of the mKI. Oral CHM was more beneficial than pharmacotherapy in improving vasomotor symptoms (MD −2.02 points [−3.82, −0.22], $I^2 = 58\%$) and insomnia (MD −1.12 points [−2.13, −0.12], $I^2 = 52\%$). Oral CHM was not statistically different to pharmacotherapy for the items paraesthesia, nervousness, melancholia, vertigo, weakness, arthralgia, headache, palpitations, formication, dyspareunia and urinary tract infection (Table 5.17).

Oral Chinese herbal medicine plus pharmacotherapy versus pharmacotherapy alone

Oral Chinese herbal medicine was combined with pharmacotherapy in 22 studies (H2–H4, H60, H66, H97, H98, H102, H104, H106, H109, H113, H164–H173) with over 2,500 perimenopausal women. The combination of oral CHM with pharmacotherapy was more effective in improving menopause symptoms than pharmacotherapy alone (SMD −1.39 [−1.90, −0.87], $I^2 = 97\%$; Table 5.18), although statistical heterogeneity lowers confidence in the results. Subgroup analyses were conducted with studies using the original KI or mKI, for studies assessed as 'low' risk of bias and according to treatment duration.

Results favoured the combination of oral CHM plus pharmacotherapy regardless of whether the KI or mKI was used; however,

Table 5.17 Oral Chinese Herbal Medicine versus Pharmacotherapy: Modified Kupperman Index Item Scores

Assessment	No. of Studies (Participants)	Effect Size (MD [95% CI], I^2)	Included Studies
Vasomotor	2 (104)	−2.02 [−3.82, −0.22]*, 58%	H82, H137
Paraesthesia	2 (104)	−0.21 [−0.58, 0.16], 0%	H82, H137
Insomnia	2 (104)	−1.12 [−2.13, −0.12]*, 52%	H82, H137
Nervousness	2 (104)	−0.35 [−0.86, 0.16], 0%	H82, H137
Melancholia	2 (104)	−0.29 [−0.96, 0.37], 77%	H82, H137
Vertigo	2 (104)	0.08 [−0.18, 0.35], 24%	H82, H137
Weakness	2 (104)	−0.14 [−0.34, 0.05], 0%	H82, H137
Arthralgia	2 (104)	−0.16 [−0.45, 0.13], 0%	H82, H137
Headache	2 (104)	−0.10 [−0.37, 0.17], 0%	H82, H137
Palpitations	2 (104)	−0.03 [−0.62, 0.55], 71%	H82, H137
Formication	2 (104)	0.08 [−0.13, 0.29], 0%	H82, H137
Dyspareunia	2 (104)	0.04 [−0.27, 0.36], 0%	H82, H137
Urinary tract infection	2 (104)	−0.24 [−0.70, 0.21], 3%	H82, H137

*Statistically significant, see Chapter 4.
Abbreviations: CI, confidence interval; MD, mean difference.

statistical heterogeneity remained high (Table 5.18). Analysis of studies judged as 'low' risk of bias for sequence generation produced results that were similar to the overall pool of studies. The magnitude of the effect appeared smaller in studies that provided treatment for more than eight weeks; however, this was not statistically different to studies that provided treatment for eight weeks or less. The cause of statistical heterogeneity was not identified through these subgroup analyses and the reason for heterogeneity remains unclear.

Individual scores for mKI items were reported in two studies (H4, H170), although one study reported only some items (Table 5.19). Meta-analysis showed favourable results for oral CHM plus pharmacotherapy over pharmacotherapy alone for vasomotor symptoms (MD −0.71 points [−1.24, −0.18], I^2 = 93%), while no benefit was seen for melancholia (MD −0.14 points [−0.36, 0.09], I^2 = 88%),

Table 5.18 Oral Chinese Herbal Medicine plus Pharmacotherapy versus Pharmacotherapy Alone: Kupperman Index Total Score

Assessment	No. of Studies (Participants)	Effect size SMD# [95% CI], I^2%	Included Studies
End of treatment	22 (2,541)	−1.39 [−1.90, −0.87]*, 97%	H2–H4, H60, H66, H97, H98, H102, H104, H106, H109, H113, H164–H173
Subgroup: KI	11 (1,486)	MD −4.42 [−6.32, −2.51]*, 96%	H2, H60, H66, H97, H98, H102, H113, H165, H167, H172, H173
Subgoup: mKI	11 (1,055)	−1.60 [−2.60, −0.60]*, 98%	H3, H4, H104, H106, H109, H164, H166, H168–H171
Subgroup: 'low' risk of bias SG	10 (1,261)	−1.67 [−2.51, −0.82]*, 98%	H2, H4, H60, H66, H97, H98, H102, H166, H169, H173
Subgroup: treatment duration ≤8 w	12 (1,219)	−1.85 [−2.80, −0.90]*, 98%	H60, H97, H98, H102, H104, H109, H113, H164, H166, H167, H169, H170
Subgroup: treatment duration >8 w	10 (1,322)	−0.84 [−1.25, −0.43]*, 92%	H2–H4, H66, H106, H165, H168, H171–H173

*Statistically significant, see Chapter 4.
#Analysis using SMD unless otherwise specified.
Abbreviations: CI, confidence interval; KI, Kupperman Index; MD, mean difference; mKI, modified Kupperman Index; SG, sequence generation; SMD, standardised mean difference; w, weeks.

vertigo (MD −0.09 points [−0.20, 0.01], I^2 = 64%) and palpitations (MD 0.05 points [−0.08, 0.17], I^2 = 92%).

Results from a single study showed that the combination of oral CHM and pharmacotherapy produced greater improvements in arthralgia (MD −0.11 points [−0.18, −0.04]) and dyspareunia (MD −0.70 points, [−0.82, −0.58]). No benefit of adding oral CHM to pharmacotherapy was shown for the mKI items paraesthesia, insomnia, nervousness, weakness, headache and formication (Table 5.19).

Table 5.19 Oral Chinese Herbal Medicine plus Pharmacotherapy versus Pharmacotherapy: Modified Kupperman Index Item Scores

Assessment	No. of Studies (Participants)	Effect Size (MD [95% CI], I^2)	Included Studies
Vasomotor	2 (178)	−0.71 [−1.24, −0.18]*, 93%	H4, H170
Paraesthesia	1 (118)	−0.02 [−0.11, 0.07], NA	H4
Insomnia	1 (118)	0.10 [−0.05, 0.25], NA	H4
Nervousness	1 (118)	0.04 [−0.05, 0.13], NA	H4
Melancholia	2 (178)	−0.14 [−0.36, 0.09], 88%	H4, H170
Vertigo	2 (178)	−0.09 [−0.20, 0.01], 64%	H4, H170
Weakness	1 (118)	−0.05 [−0.16, 0.06], NA	H4
Arthralgia	1 (118)	−0.11 [−0.18, −0.04]*, NA	H4
Headache	1 (118)	−0.05 [−0.12, 0.02], NA	H4
Palpitations	2 (178)	0.05 [−0.08, 0.17], 92%	H4, H170
Formication	1 (118)	−0.24 [−0.60, 0.12], NA	H4
Dyspareunia	1 (118)	−0.70 [−0.82, −0.58]*, NA	H4

*Statistically significant, see Chapter 4.
Abbreviations: CI, confidence interval; MD, mean difference; NA, not applicable.

Greene Climacteric Scale

Five studies (H27, H174–H177) measured menopause symptoms using the Green Climacteric Scale (GCS)[31]. The GCS includes 21 items scored zero to three, where lower scores indicate less bother. The sum of individual scores provides the total score and can be reported for the domains of psychological, physical and vasomotor. One item, relating to loss of interest in sex, is typically used only for the total score; however, four of the five included studies reported the mean score for this item.

Oral Chinese herbal medicine versus placebo

Three studies (H27, H174, H175) that compared oral CHM with placebo reported the total score and domain scores for GCS. Two hundred and eleven postmenopausal women were included in analysis for the total score and psychological domain, and data were available for 212 women for the physical, vasomotor and sexual domains. Oral CHM was no different to placebo in reducing bother from menopause symptoms overall (MD −4.41 points [−11.50, 2.67], I^2 = 98%; Table 5.20). No differences were seen between groups on the psychological domain (MD −1.94 points [−5.91, 2.03], I^2 = 97%), physical domain (MD −1.42 points [−2.95, 0.11], I^2 = 92%), vasomotor domain (MD −0.62 points [−1.35, 0.11], I^2 = 96%) and sexual domain (MD −0.09 points [−0.24, 0.06], I^2 = 18%). Statistical heterogeneity was detected for the total score, and for the psychological, physical and vasomotor domain scores. Subgroup analyses including studies judged as 'low' risk of bias for sequence

Table 5.20 Oral Chinese Herbal Medicine versus Placebo: Greene Climacteric Scale

Assessment	No. of Studies (Participants)	Effect Size (MD [95% CI], I^2)	Included Studies
Total score	3 (211)	−4.41 [−11.50, 2.67], 98%	H27, H174, H175
Subgroup: 'low' risk of bias SG	2 (161)	−4.84 [−16.51, 6.83], 99%	H27, H175
Psychological domain	3 (211)	−1.94 [−5.91, 2.03], 97%	H27, H174, H175
Psychological domain subgroup: 'low' risk of bais SG	2 (161)	−1.87 [−8.06, 4.33], 98%	H27, H175
Physical domain	3 (212)	−1.42 [−2.95, 0.11], 92%	H27, H174, H175
Physical domain subgroup: 'low' risk of bias SG	2 (161)	−1.68 [−4.28, 0.91], 96%	H27, H175
Vasomotor domain	3 (212)	−0.62 [−1.35, 0.11], 96%	H27, H174, H175
Vasomotor domain subgroup: 'low' risk of bias SG	2 (161)	−0.96 [−3.09, 1.17], 98%	H27, H175
Sexual domain	3 (212)	−0.09 [−0.24, 0.06], 18%	H27, H174, H175

Abbreviations: CI, confidence interval; MD, mean difference; SG, sequence generation.

did not reduce statistical heterogeneity. Other planned subgroup analyses were not able to be conducted due to the small number of studies included in the analyses; confidence in the results is limited as a result.

Oral Chinese herbal medicine versus pharmacotherapy

The GCS was used to assess menopause symptoms in two studies (H176, H177) that compared oral CHM with pharmacotherapy. One study (H176) involved 58 perimenopausal women, while the other study (H177) included 38 postmenopausal women. Meta-analysis showed no difference at the end of treatment between women who received oral CHM and women who received pharmacotherapy (MD −3.38 points [−18.57, 11.81], I^2 = 98%; Table 5.21). Results for perimenopausal women showed an improvement in symptoms with *Bu shen an shen fang* 补肾安神方 (MD −11.15 points [−13.46, −8.84]), while postmenopausal women who received treatment with conjugated oestrogen and medroxyprogesterone acetate reported lower GCS score at the end of treatment, indicating improvement in symptoms (MD 4.35 points [2.76, 5.94]).

Scores for GCS domains were reported by Chen *et al.* (H177). Women who received modified *Xiao yao san* 逍遥散 reported higher scores, indicating greater bother from symptoms, than women who

Table 5.21 Oral Chinese Herbal Medicine versus Pharmacotherapy: Greene Climacteric Scale

Assessment	No. of Studies (Participants)	Effect Size (MD [95% CI], I^2)	Included Studies
Total score	2 (96)	−3.38 [−18.57, 11.81], 98%	H176, H177
Psychological domain	1 (38)	2.51 [1.55, 3.47]*, NA	H177
Physical domain	1 (38)	1.07 [0.31, 1.83]*, NA	H177
Vasomotor domain	1 (38)	1.11 [0.63, 1.59]*, NA	H177
Sexual domain	1 (38)	−0.35 [−1.02, 0.32], NA	H177

*Statistically significant, see Chapter 4.

Abbreviations: CI, confidence interval; MD, mean difference; NA, not applicable.

received conjugated oestrogen and medroxyprogesterone acetate for the psychological, physical and vasomotor domains (Table 5.21), while no difference was seen between the two groups for the sexual domain.

Menopause Rating Scale

Seven studies used the Menopause Rating Scale (MRS)[32] to examine the impact of menopause symptoms on HRQoL. The MRS includes 11 items scored zero to four and the results can be summed to provide a total score, or can be reported for three dimensions: psychological, somatic and urogenital. Higher scores mean worse symptoms. Six RCTs (H18, H19, H24, H29, H125, H178) compared oral CHM with placebo and one (H44) compared oral CHM with pharmacotherapy.

Oral Chinese herbal medicine versus placebo

Six studies (H18, H19, H24, H29, H125, H178) reported the MRS total score, one study (H24) reported scores for the psychological, physical and vasomotor domains and two studies (H19, H125) reported scores for individual items. Meta-analysis was conducted where possible.

The MRS total at the end of treatment was 6.78 points lower in women who received oral CHM ([−11.08, −2.47], $I^2 = 92\%$; Table 5.22). Perimenopausal women received benefit with oral CHM (three studies, 278 women, MD −9.34 points [−16.35, −2.34], $I^2 = 94\%$; H18, H19, H29), while postmenopausal women did not obtain such benefit (three studies, 170 women, MD −4.14 points [−10.44, 2.15], $I^2 = 89\%$; H125, H24, H178). Studies assessed as 'low' risk of bias for sequence generation also showed benefit of oral CHM, and treatment duration of up to eight weeks or more than eight weeks did not appear to affect the outcome. All meta-analyses showed statistical heterogeneity and this lowers confidence in estimates of the treatment effect.

Table 5.22 Oral Chinese Herbal Medicine versus Placebo: Menopause Rating Scale

Assessment	No. of Studies (Participants)	Effect Size (MD [95% CI], I^2)	Included Studies
Total score at end of treatment	6 (448)	−6.78 [−11.08, −2.47]*, 92%	H18, H19, H24, H29, H125, H178
Subgroup: 'low' risk of bias SG	5 (336)	−5.66 [−10.24, −1.07]*, 88%	H18, H24, H29, H125, H178
Subgroup: treatment duration ≤8 w	1 (79)	−9.23 [−11.61, −6.85]*, NA	H178
Subgroup: treatment duration >8 w	5 (369)	−6.23 [−11.85, −0.61]*, 93%	H18, H19, H24, H29, H125
Total score at follow-up	3 (206)	−6.47 [−7.73, −5.20]*, 0%	H24, H29, H178

*Statistically significant, see Chapter 4.
Abbreviations: CI, confidence interval; MD, mean difference; NA, not applicable; SG, sequence generation; w, weeks.

The benefit seen with oral CHM continued after treatment ceased (MD −6.47 points [−7.73, −5.20], I^2 = 0%; Table 5.22). Interestingly, while oral CHM was not statistically different to placebo at the end of treatment in postmenopausal women, these women achieved a superior result to placebo at follow-up assessment (MD −5.94 points [−8.22, −3.66], I^2 = 0%). One study that included 108 perimenopausal women also showed ongoing benefit beyond the end of treatment (MD −6.70 points [−8.22, −5.18]; H29).

Scores for MRS dimensions were reported in a small study of 19 postmenopausal women (H24). Oral CHM formula *Zhi mu* 枳壳 14 was not statistically different to placebo on the psychological dimension (MD 0.40 points [−2.75, 3.55]), somatic dimension (MD −1.89 points [−4.96, 1.18]) and urogenital dimension (MD 0.00 points [−1.48, 1.48]) at the end of treatment. Follow-up assessment was conducted 12 weeks after the end of treatment and similar results were seen. Oral CHM was not superior to placebo on the psychological dimension (MD 0.50 points [−2.63, 3.63]) and urogenital dimension (MD −0.90 points [−2.80, 1.00]), but was superior to placebo on the somatic dimension (MD −3.92 points [−7.00, −0.84]).

Results for individual items of the MRS were reported in two studies (H19, H125). Meta-analysis showed oral CHM to be superior for improving hot flushes/sweating (184 women, MD −1.02 points [−1.97, −0.07], $I^2 = 93\%$), with benefits shown in both perimenopausal women (112 women, MD −1.50 points [−1.84, −1.16]; H19) and in postmenopausal women (72 women, MD −0.53 points [−0.91, −0.15]; H125). Kaszkin-Bettag *et al.* (H19) reported results for the remaining ten individual items. *Rheum rhaponticum* extract (ERr 731, from herb *shi yong da huang* 食用大黄) was superior to placebo in improving symptoms of sleep problems (MD −1.10 points [−1.40, −0.80]), heart complaints (MD −1.00 points [−1.33, −0.67]), depressive mood (MD −1.30 points [−1.62, −0.98]), irritability (MD −1.10 points [−1.36, −0.84]), anxiety (MD −1.20 points [−1.50, −0.90]), physical and mental exhaustion (MD −1.10 points [−1.38, −0.82]), sexual problems (MD −0.80 points [−1.14, −0.46]), bladder problems (MD −0.80 points [−1.14, −0.46]), vaginal dryness (MD −0.50 points [−0.78, −0.22]) and joint/muscular discomfort (MD −1.10 points [−1.42, −0.78]).

Oral Chinese herbal medicine versus pharmacotherapy

One study (H44) compared *Zi shui qing gan yin* 滋水清肝饮 with estazolam plus oryzanol (a rice bran oil) in 199 perimenopausal women. Women who received *Zi shui qing gan yin* 滋水清肝饮 scored 6.66 points lower than women who received estazolam plus oryzanol on the MRS total score ([−8.01, −5.31]). Scores on the psychological (MD −3.83 points [−4.62, −3.04]) and physical domains (MD −3.50 points [−4.23, −2.77]) were also lower with oral CHM.

Hot Flash Related Daily Interference

Two studies (H27, H80) with 92 postmenopausal women measured the impact of two oral CHM formulas used in combination on HRQoL using the Hot Flash Related Daily Interference Scale

(HFRDI).[33] The HFRDI focuses on the impact of hot flushes on quality of life in the previous week. Nine items are scored from zero to ten, higher scores indicate greater interference, and the sum of scores for all items provides a total score. Meta-analysis showed no difference between oral CHM and placebo in change from baseline (MD 9.84 points [−7.79, 27.48], $I^2 = 89\%$). Subgroup analyses to explore possible causes of statistical heterogeneity were not possible due to the small number of included studies.

Menopause-specific Quality of Life

The MENQOL[19] was used to assess the impact of menopause symptoms on HRQoL in ten studies (H5, H8, H16, H17, H26, H28, H29, H127, H138, H179). The MENQOL includes 29 items that are grouped into four domains: vasomotor, physical, psychosocial and sexual. Presence of symptoms is allocated a score of two; absence is allocated a score of one. Symptoms are then scored from zero to six, with higher scores indicating greater bother. The score for each item is the symptom score plus the score for presence/absence; the score range for each item is from one to eight. The mean score for each domain is calculated by dividing the sum of domain scores by the number of items in each domain. Variations in scoring have been noted in a review of the use of MENQOL by Sydora *et al.*,[34] including reporting of a total score in addition to, or in place of, domain scores; such variations were seen in studies included in this review. Standardised mean difference was used for meta-analysis where appropriate to account for such variation.

Oral Chinese herbal medicine versus placebo

Seven studies (H16, H17, H26, H28, H29, H127, H179) evaluated the effect of oral CHM on HRQoL using MENQOL. Two studies (H16, H127) reported change from baseline for each of the four domains and were analysed separately. One study (H179) included three treatment arms which were merged for analysis. Three studies (H26, H29, H179), all of which were assessed as 'low' risk of bias for

Table 5.23 Oral Chinese Herbal Medicine versus Placebo: Menopause-specific Quality of Life Questionnaire — Total Score

Assessment	No. of Studies (Participants)	Effect Size (MD/ SMD [95% CI], I^2)	Included Studies
Total score at end of treatment	3 (593)	SMD −0.52 [−1.10, 0.06], 89%	H26, H29, H179
Subgroup: treatment duration ≤8 w	2 (485)	SMD −0.49 [−1.41, 0.43], 94%	H29, H179
Subgroup: treatment duration >8 w	1 (108)	MD −11.70 [−18.98, −4.42]*, NA	H29
Total score at follow-up	2 (489)	SMD −1.05 [−1.88, −0.21]*, 91%	H29, H179

*Statistically significant, see Chapter 4.
Abbreviations: CI, confidence interval; MD, mean difference; NA, not applicable; SMD, standardised mean difference; w, weeks.

sequence generation, reported the total MENQOL score at the end of treatment. Oral CHM was not superior to placebo in reducing bother from menopause symptoms (593 women, SMD −0.52 [−1.10, 0.06], I^2 = 89%; Table 5.23). Perimenopausal women appeared to obtain some benefit from *Er xian tang* 二仙汤 in one study of 108 women (MD −11.70 points [−18.98, −4.42]; H29), while another that included both perimenopausal and postmenopausal women also reported benefit (one study, 104 women, MD −4.70 points [−6.56, −2.84]; H26). One study of 381 postmenopausal women showed no benefit of oral CHM over placebo (MD −1.09 points [−7.67, 5.49]; H179). Considerable statistical heterogeneity was detected in the main meta-analysis and subgroup meta-analysis according to duration of treatment. This lowered confidence in the results.

While no benefit of oral CHM was seen over placebo at the end of treatment, oral CHM appeared to be superior to placebo at follow-up assessment (489 women, SMD −1.05 [−1.88, −0.21], I^2 = 91%; Table 5.23). Benefits were seen in single studies of perimenopausal women (one study, 108 women, MD −26.40 points [−33.04, −19.76]; H29) and postmenopausal women (one study, 381 women, MD −16.55 points [−22.77, −10.33]; H179).

Table 5.24 Oral Chinese Herbal Medicine versus Placebo: Menopause-specific Quality of Life Questionnaire — Physical Domain

Assessment	No. of Studies (Participants)	Effect Size (SMD [95% CI], I^2)	Included Studies
Total score at end of treatment	5 (741)	−0.20 [−0.52, 0.13], 73%	H17, H26, H28, H29, H179
Subgroup: treatment duration ≤8 w	2 (445)	−0.14 [−0.35, 0.07], 0%	H28, H179
Subgroup: treatment duration >8 w	3 (296)	−0.18 [−0.79, 0.43], 85%	H17, H26, H29
Change score from baseline to end of treatment	2 (270)	−0.06 [−0.51, 0.38], 57%	H16, H127
Total score at follow-up	2 (445)	−0.14 [−0.35, 0.07], 0%	H28, H179

Abbreviations: CI, confidence interval; SMD, standardised mean difference; w, weeks.

Results were also reported for each of the four domains of MENQOL. All five studies that reported domain scores were assessed as 'low' risk of bias. There was no difference between groups in physical domain scores at the end of treatment (741 women, SMD −0.20 [−0.52, 0.13], I^2 = 73%; Table 5.24). Subgroup analysis showed results favouring oral CHM in two studies involving 172 perimenopausal women (SMD −0.39 [−0.69, −0.09], I^2 = 0%; H28, H29) and one study including 104 perimenopausal and postmenopausal women (MD −0.80 points [−1.32, −0.28]; H26). One study, which did not specify the menopausal status of participants, reported better results with placebo than with oral CHM (MD 0.59 points [0.07, 1.11], H17), while one study of 381 postmenopausal women found no statistical difference between oral CHM and placebo (MD −1.48 points [−5.18, 2.22]; H179).

Change from baseline was measured in two studies (H16, H127). Oral CHM was as effective as placebo in reducing bother from physical symptoms (270 women, SMD −0.06 [−0.51, 0.38], I^2 = 57%). The meta-analysis results were reflected in individual trial results according to menopausal status. One study of 55 postmenopausal women found no difference between groups (MD −0.40 points [−0.99, 0.19]; H16), while a second study that did not specify menopausal status reached the same conclusion (215 women, MD 1.60 points [−2.30, 5.50]; H127).

Follow-up assessment four weeks after the end of treatment found no difference between oral CHM and placebo in terms of bother from physical symptoms (445 women, SMD −0.14 [−0.35, 0.07], $I^2 = 0\%$). This finding held for perimenopausal women (one study, 64 women MD −0.13 points, [−0.59, 0.33]; H28) and postmenopausal women (one study, 381 women, MD −2.20 points [−5.73, 1.33]; H179).

Results for the psychosocial domain largely reflected those seen for the physical domain. Main analysis showed no benefit of oral CHM compared to placebo in scores at the end of treatment (741 women, SMD −0.16 [−0.51, 0.18], $I^2 = 77\%$) and at follow-up (445 women, SMD −0.13 [−0.34, 0.08], $I^2 = 0\%$), or in score change from baseline to end of treatment (215 women, MD −0.10 points [−2.33, 2.13]) (Table 5.25).

Table 5.25 Oral Chinese Herbal Medicine versus Placebo: Menopause-specific Quality of Life Questionnaire — Psychosocial Domain

Assessment	No. of Studies (Participants)	Effect Size (MD/ SMD [95% CI], I^2)	Included Studies
Total score at end of treatment	5 (741)	SMD −0.16 [−0.51, 0.18], 77%	H17, H26, H28, H29, H179
Subgroup: treatment duration ≤8 w	2 (445)	SMD −0.02 [−0.23, 0.19], 0%	H28, H179
Subgroup: treatment duration >8 w	3 (296)	SMD −0.25 [−0.88, 0.37], 86%	H17, H26, H29
Change score from baseline to end of treatment	1 (215)	MD −0.10 [−2.33, 2.13], NA	H127
Total score at follow-up	2 (445)	SMD −0.13 [−0.34, 0.08], 0%	H28, H179

Abbreviations: CI, confidence interval; MD, mean difference; NA, not applicable; SMD, standardised mean difference; w, weeks.

Analysis according to menopausal status showed no benefit at the end of treatment in two studies of 172 perimenopausal women (SMD −0.26 [−0.62, 0.10], I^2 = 27%; H28, H29), no benefit in one study of 381 postmenopausal women (MD −0.11 points [−2.17, 1.95]; H179) and no benefit in one study that did not specify menopausal status of 84 women (MD 0.54 points [−0.05, 1.13]; H17). One study of 104 perimenopausal and postmenopausal women showed oral CHM to be superior to placebo at the end of treatment (MD −1.20 points [−1.85, −0.55]; H26).

Findings for the vasomotor domain scores at the end of treatment were like those for the physical and psychosocial domains. Oral CHM was not statistically different to placebo in reducing bother from vasomotor symptoms at the end of treatment (741 women, SMD −0.25 [−0.66, 0.16], I^2 = 84%; Table 5.26), nor did oral CHM produce a greater change from baseline than placebo (215 women, MD 0.60 points [−0.69, 1.89]). The vasomotor domain score at follow-up four weeks after the end of treatment was lower among women who

Table 5.26 Oral Chinese Herbal Medicine versus Placebo: Menopause-specific Quality of Life Questionnaire — Vasomotor Domain

Assessment	No. of Studies (Participants)	Effect Size (MD/SMD [95% CI], I^2)	Included Studies
Total score at end of treatment	5 (741)	SMD −0.25 [−0.66, 0.16], 84%	H17, H26, H28, H29, H179
Subgroup: treatment duration ≤8 w	2 (445)	SMD −0.08 [−0.29, 0.13], 0%	H28, H179
Subgroup: treatment duration >8 w	3 (296)	SMD −0.37 [−1.12, 0.38], 90%	H17, H26, H29
Change score from baseline to end of treatment	1 (215)	MD 0.60 [−0.69, 1.89], NA	H127
Total score at follow-up	2 (445)	SMD −0.22 [−0.43, −0.01]*, 0%	H28, H179

*Statistically significant, see Chapter 4.

Abbreviations: CI, confidence interval; MD, mean difference; NA, not applicable; SMD, standardised mean difference; w, weeks.

received oral CHM than in women who received placebo (445 women, SMD −0.22 [−0.43, −0.01], I^2 = 0%).

No benefit of oral CHM at the end of treatment, compared to placebo, was found in studies that included perimenopausal women (two studies, 172 women, SMD −0.33 [−0.74, 0.08], I^2 = 43%; H28, H29), postmenopausal women (one study, 381 women, MD −0.26 points [−1.09, 0.57]; H179) or women with unspecified menopausal status (one study, 84 women, MD 0.56 points [−0.05, 1.17]; H17). Benefit was seen in the study that included both perimenopausal and postmenopausal women (one study, 104 women, MD −1.70 points [−2.37, −1.03]; H26).

Fewer studies reported results for the sexual domain of the MENQOL. In four studies, there was no difference in sexual domain scores between oral CHM and placebo at the end of treatment (360 women, SMD −0.19 [−0.44, 0.07], I^2 = 33%; Table 5.27). Results from individual studies showed no difference in change from baseline to end of treatment (215 women, MD 0.10 points [−1.21, 1.41]) or in score at four-week follow-up (64 women, MD −0.29 points [−1.02, 0.44]).

Analysis according to menopausal status produced similar outcomes to the physical, psychosocial and vasomotor domains: A benefit in one study of 104 perimenopausal and postmenopausal

Table 5.27 Oral Chinese Herbal Medicine versus Placebo: Menopause-specific Quality of Life Questionnaire — Sexual Domain

Assessment	No. of Studies (Participants)	Effect Size (MD/SMD [95% CI], I^2)	Included Studies
Total score at end of treatment	4 (360)	SMD −0.19 [−0.44, 0.07], 33%	H17, H26, H28, H29
Change score from baseline to end of treatment	1 (215)	MD 0.10 [−1.21, 1.41], NA	H127
Total score at follow-up	1 (64)	MD −0.29 [−1.02, 0.44], NA	H28

Abbreviations: CI, confidence interval; MD, mean difference; NA, not applicable; SMD, standardised mean difference.

women (MD −1.10 points [−1.91, −0.29]; H26) and no benefit in studies of perimenopausal women (two studies, 172 women, SMD −0.13 [−0.42, 0.17], $I^2 = 0\%$; H28, H29) and women with unspecified menopausal status (one study, 84 women, MD 0.13 points [−0.69, 0.95]; H17).

Oral Chinese herbal medicine versus pharmacotherapy

Three studies (H5, H8, H138) that compared oral CHM with pharmacotherapy reported MENQOL total or domain scores. Two studies (H5, H8) described scoring items from zero to six, with domain scores calculated as the sum of scores for items in that domain. The third study did not specify the method used for calculating scores. Results for 234 perimenopausal women were analysed. The total MENQOL score was not statistically different between *Kun tai jiao nang* 坤泰胶囊 and Premarin® at the end of treatment (MD 2.02 points [−5.74, 9.78]; Table 5.28). Similar results were seen for domain scores. Oral CHM was not superior to pharmacotherapy on the physical, psychosical, vasomotor and sexual domains (Table 5.28). One study that was assessed as 'low' risk of bias for sequence generation found that women who received oral CHM scored worse for the vasomotor domain than women who received Premarin®, but no difference was seen for the three other domains.

36-Item Short-Form Health Survey

The Medical Outcome Study 36-Item Short-Form Health Survey (SF-36)[35] was used to assess HRQoL in three studies (H45, H128, H180). The SF-36 includes eight domains: physical function, role functioning due to physical health problems, role functioning due to emotional problems, bodily pain, general health perceptions, vitality, social function and mental health. The score range for each doman is from zero to 100, with higher scores indicating better quality of life. All three studies that used the SF-36 to assess HRQoL compared oral CHM with pharmacotherapy.

Table 5.28 Oral Chinese Herbal Medicine versus Pharmacotherapy: Menopause-specific Quality of Life Questionnaire

Assessment	No. of Studies (Participants)	Effect Size (MD/ SMD [95% CI], I^2)	Included Studies
Total score	1 (57)	MD 2.02 [−5.74, 9.78], NA	H8
Physical domain	3 (234)	SMD −1.17 [−3.23, 0.88], 98%	H5, H8, H138
Physical domain subgroup: 'low' risk of bias SG	1 (57)	MD 0.46 [−3.15, 4.07], NA	H8
Psychosocial domain	3 (234)	SMD −1.01 [−2.94, 0.91], 98%	H5, H8, H138
Psychosocial domain subgroup: 'low' risk of bias SG	1 (57)	MD 0.65 [−2.11, 3.41], NA	H8
Vasomotor domain	3 (234)	SMD −0.27 [−1.48, 0.94], 95%	H5, H8, H138
Vasomotor domain subgroup: 'low' risk of bias SG	1 (57)	MD 1.05 [0.21, 1.89]*, NA	H8
Sexual domain	3 (234)	SMD −0.44 [−1.33, 0.46], 91%	H5, H8, H138
Sexual domain subgroup: 'low' risk of bias SG	1 (57)	MD −0.14 [−2.17, 1.89], NA	H8

*Statistically significant, see Chapter 4.

Abbreviations: CI, confidence interval; MD, mean difference; NA, not applicable; SG, sequence generation; SMD, standardised mean difference; w, weeks.

Two of the three studies included perimenopausal women (H45, H180), while the third did not specify menopausal status (H128). Only one of the studies reported scores for all domains (H180). Women who received oral CHM reported better scores than women who received pharmacotherapy on the physical function domain (214 women, MD 7.68 points [0.94, 14.42], I^2 = 82%), the role function due to emotional problems domain (147 women, MD 8.50 points [3.97, 13.02], I^2 = 18%) and social function domains (147 women, MD 4.82 points [1.27, 8.36], I^2 = 9%). Oral CHM was not statistically different to pharmacotherapy on the role functioning due

Table 5.29 Oral Chinese Herbal Medicine versus Pharmacotherapy: SF-36

Assessment	No. of Studies (Participants)	Effect Size (MD [95% CI], I^2)	Included Studies
Physical function	3 (214)	7.68 [0.94, 14.42]*, 82%	H45, H128, H180
Role function — physical	2 (147)	7.15 [−0.31, 14.61], 74%	H45, H180
Role function — emotional	2 (147)	8.50 [3.97, 13.02]*, 18%	H45, H180
Bodily pain	1 (74)	2.59 [−2.86, 8.04], NA	H180
General health	1 (74)	1.25 [−2.83, 5.33], NA	H180
Vitality	2 (147)	4.58 [−1.40, 10.56], 76%	H45, H180
Social function	2 (147)	4.82 [1.27, 8.36]*, 9%	H45, H180
Mental health	2 (147)	4.45 [−1.85, 10.75], 81%	H45, H180

*Statistically significant, see Chapter 4.
Abbreviations: CI, confidence interval; MD, mean difference; NA, not applicable.

to physical health problems, bodily pain, general health perceptions, vitality and mental health domains (Table 5.29).

Subgroup analysis according to menopausal status was possible for the physical function component of the SF-36. Two studies, which included 147 perimenopausal women, found oral CHM to be as effective as pharmacotherapy (MD 5.35 points [−1.36, 12.05], 84%; H45, H180). One study of 40 women with unspecified menopausal status found higher scores, indicating better outcomes, in women who received oral CHM (MD 14.60 points [5.77, 23.43]; H128).

Social Function Rating Scale

One study of 54 women (H96) assessed the impact of menopause symptoms on social function using the Social Function Rating Scale. The study authors described that the scale includes 24 items scored from zero to seven, where a lower score indicates better outcomes. The combination of oral CHM with pharmacotherapy produced a score 8.20 points lower than pharmacotherapy ([−10.53, −5.87]).

Modified Barthel Index

A modified version of the Barthel Index[36] was used to assess the impact of menopause symptoms on activities of daily living (H105). The Barthel Index is typically scored from zero to 100 and higher scores indicate greater independence and ability for self-care. Modifications used in this study were not described, aside from using a scoring system where a lower score means greater ability for self-care. In 92 perimenopausal women, oral CHM plus pharmacotherapy resulted in a lower score, meaning greater self-care, than pharmacotherapy alone (MD −7.28 points [−9.71, −5.85]).

Assessment Using Grading of Recommendations Assessment, Development and Evaluation

The Grading of Recommendations Assessment, Development and Evaluation (GRADE) approach was used to summarise results for clinically important questions. A consensus on items for inclusion in summary-of-findings tables was reached after following the process described in Chapter 4. The comparisons of oral CHM versus placebo and oral CHM versus HT were considered critically important. Three oral CHM formulas/products were also considered important for clinical practice: *Er xian tang* 二仙汤, *Tian wang bu xin dan* 天王补心丹 and *Kun tai jiao nang* 坤泰胶囊. We planned to prepare summary-of-findings tables for each of these formulas compared to HT and to placebo. None of the included studies tested the comparison of *Tian wang bu xin dan* 天王补心丹 versus HT, *Tian wang bu xin dan* 天王补心丹 versus placebo or *Kun tai jiao nang* 坤泰胶囊 versus placebo, so it was not possible to prepare summary-of-findings tables for these comparisons. The strength and quality ('certainty') of evidence for these important comparisons remain unclear.

Hot flush frequency, hot flush severity, GCS, PSQI, HAM-D and MENQOL domains and AEs were considered the most important outcomes to assess the effects of CHM on menopausal symptoms. While two studies (H70, H135) compared *Er xian tang* 二仙汤 with

HT, both reported outcomes other than those selected for summary-of-findings tables. The certainty of evidence for the comparison *Er xian tang* 二仙汤 with HT for important menopause outcomes is unclear.

Four summary-of-findings tables were prepared for oral CHM:

- Oral CHM versus placebo;
- Oral CHM versus HT;
- *Er xian tang* 二仙汤 versus placebo;
- *Kun tai jiao nang* 坤泰胶囊 versus HT.

Oral Chinese herbal medicine versus placebo

Oral CHM was compared with placebo in 32 RCTs (H16–H20, H22–H37, H80, H126, H127, H174, H175, H178, H179, H181–H184) that reported on pre-specified important outcomes. The certainty of the evidence was 'moderate' to 'low' (Table 5.30). Oral CHM resulted in fewer and less severe hot flushes than placebo ('moderate' certainty evidence) but was no different to placebo in scores for the psychological ('low' certainty evidence), physical ('low' certainty evidence), vasomotor ('low' certainty evidence) and sexual domains ('moderate' certainty evidence) of the GCS. Sleep quality on the PSQI was better in people who received oral CHM ('low' certainty evidence), while people who received oral CHM scored worse on the HAM-D ('moderate' certainty evidence).

Results for the four domains of MENQOL were reported as end-of-treatment scores (Table 5.30) or as change from baseline scores. 'Low' certainty evidence showed oral CHM was not statistically different to placebo at the end-of-treatment for the physical, psychosocial, vasomotor and sexual domains. The same result was seen in studies that reported change scores. 'Very low' certainty evidence showed no difference between oral CHM and placebo on the physical domain (two RCTs, 270 women, MD −0.06 points [−0.51, 0.38]; H16, H127), while 'low' certainty evidence from one study of 215 women (H127) showed no difference between oral CHM and placebo for the psychosocial (MD −0.01 points [−0.28, 0.26]),

Table 5.30 GRADE: Oral Chinese Herbal Medicine versus Placebo

Outcome; Treatment Duration	No. of Studies (Participants)	Relative Effect (MD/SMD [95% CI])	Certainty of the Evidence (GRADE)
Daily HF frequency; 4 w to 16 w	5 (474)	MD −2.33 [−4.02, −0.65]*	⊕⊕⊕◯ MODERATE[a]
Daily HF severity; 4 w to 16 w	5 (426)	MD −8.22 [−13.77, −2.67]*	⊕⊕⊕◯ MODERATE[c]
GCS-Psychol; 90 d to 12 m	3 (212)	MD −1.94 [−5.91, 2.03]	⊕⊕◯◯ LOW[a,b]
GCS-Ph; 90 d to 12 m	3 (212)	MD −1.42 [−2.95, 0.11]	⊕⊕◯◯ LOW[a,b]
GCS-V; 90 d to 12 m	3 (212)	MD −0.62 [−1.35, 0.11]	⊕⊕◯◯ LOW[a,b]
GCS-S; 90 d to 12 m	3 (212)	MD −0.09 [−0.24, 0.06]	⊕⊕⊕◯ MODERATE[b]
PSQI; 4 w to 8 w	3 (290)	MD −3.2 [−6.26, −0.14]*	⊕⊕◯◯ LOW[b,c]
HAM-D; 6 w	1 (56)	MD 2.71 [0.82, 4.6]*	⊕⊕⊕◯ MODERATE[b]
MENQOL-Ph; 8 w to 6 m	5 (741)	SMD −0.20 [−0.27, 0.37]	⊕⊕◯◯ LOW[c,d]
MENQOL-Psychosoc; 8 w to 6 m	5 (741)	SMD −0.16 [−0.51, 0.18]	⊕⊕◯◯ LOW[c,d]
MENQOL-V; 8 w to 6 m	5 (741)	SMD −0.25 [−0.25, 0.9]	⊕⊕◯◯ LOW[c,d]
MENQOL-S; 8 w to 6 m	4 (360)	SMD −0.19 [−0.44, 0.07]	⊕⊕◯◯ LOW[c,d]

*Statistically significant result.

Abbreviations: d, days; CI, confidence interval; GRADE, Grading of Recommendations Assessment, Development and Evaluation; GCS, Greene Climacteric Scale; HAM-D, Hamilton Rating Scale for Depression; HF, hot flush; m, months; MD, mean difference; MENQOL, Menopause-specific Quality of Life questionnaire; Ph, physical domain; PSQI, Pittsburgh Sleep Quality Index; Psychol, psychological domain; Psychosoc, psychosocial domain; S, sexual domain; SMD, standardised mean difference; V, vasomotor domain; w, weeks.

Notes

[a]Unexplained statistical heterogeneity.

[b]Small sample size.

[c]Unexplained statistical heterogeneity and differences in estimates of treatment effect.

[d]Unclear whether treatment effect includes no effect and clinically important effect.

Study references

Daily HF frequency: H19, H22, H23, H27, H29.

Daily HF severity: H22, H23, H27–H29.

GCS: H27, H174, H175.

PSQI: H35–H37.

HAM-D: H80.

MENQOL-Ph: H17, H26, H28, H29, H179.

MENQOL-Ps: H17, H26, H28, H29, H179.

MENQOL-V: H17, H26, H28, H29, H179.

MENQOL-S: H17, H26, H28, H29.

vasomotor (MD 0.12 points [−0.14, 0.39]) and sexual domains (MD 0.02 points, [−0.25, 0.29]).

Safety was reported in 31 RCTs (H16–H20, H23–H37, H80, H126, H127, H174, H175, H178, H179, H181–H184). One serious adverse event, dysplasia of the squamous epithelium, was reported among women who received oral CHM. This was not considered to be related to the trial. One participant withdrew due to headaches, nausea, excessive perspiration and intermittent aching in arms and legs which were considered to be related to the trial medication. One case of elevated alanine aminotransferase (ALT) was considered related to CHM.

Other AEs included 30 cases of diarrhoea, 17 cases of dry mouth/dental ulcers/swollen gums, 14 cases of rash/urticaria, 11 cases of nausea, 11 cases of dizziness, nine cases of constipation, eight cases of headache, eight cases of gastrointestinal symptoms, seven cases of palpitations, seven cases of breast tenderness, six cases of headache, joint pain or dizziness, five cases of nausea/stomach discomfort, five cases of unspecified menopause symptoms, four cases of flatulence, four cases of hypersomnia, four cases of joint pain, four cases of nervousness, three cases of dry mouth, three cases of insomnia, three cases of abdominal bloating and discomfort, and two cases each of vertigo, back pain, respiratory tract infection, lower abdominal pain and loose stools, abdominal pain, bloating and stomach pain, day-time drowsiness, sweating, worsening of depression and unspecified AEs. Single cases were reported of hypercholesterolaemia, bleeding per rectum, duodenal ulcer, cardiomyopathy, intercostal neuralgia, aggravation of dizziness, cervical dysplasia, weight gain, asthenia, depression, sleep disorder, pneumonia, hypoaesthesia, aggravation of asthma requiring steroids, bloating, allergic reaction, sensation of severe heat, hydrosalpinx, sore throat, distending pain in the chest and stomach-ache.

In the placebo groups, one serious AE of increased hepatic enzymes was reported. Two participants withdrew due to AEs of headache, abdominal bloating, constipation and dehydration. Other adverse events included 15 cases of nausea/stomach discomfort, ten cases of dry mouth/dental ulcers/swollen gums, nine cases of headache, joint pain or dizziness, seven cases of constipation, seven cases of dizziness, six cases of unspecified menopause symptoms, six cases of breast tenderness, five cases of headache, four cases of abdominal pain, bloating and stomach pain, four cases of nervousness, four cases of facial flushing, three cases of insomnia, three cases of abdominal bloating, and two cases each of palpitations, uterofibroma, gastrointestinal symptoms, daytime drowsiness, endometrial dysplasia, worsening of insomnia, dry mouth, hot flushes and epigastric pain. Single cases of stomach upset, skin tags, influenza, pituitary adenoma, viral infection of the upper respiratory tract, acute phlegmonous appendicitis, back pain, dysuria, weight gain, sweating, endometrial polyp, facial swelling, elevated blood pressure, diarrhoea, digestive problems, constipation, hypersomnia, herpes zoster, vaginal bleeding, elevated aspartate aminotransferase, sore throat, abdominal distension, deterioration of memory and nocturia were also reported.

Oral Chinese herbal medicine versus hormone therapy

Twenty-eight studies (H5–H8, H10, H21, H38, H46, H92, H93, H95, H139–H141, H143, H147, H149, H150, H153, H154, H156, H157, H160, H161, H163, H177, H182, H185) that compared oral CHM with HT reported on the selected outcomes. For many of these studies, the only pre-specified outcomes were AEs and not all studies reported clinical outcome data in a way that could be re-analysed. The certainty of evidence ranged from 'very low' to 'moderate' (Table 5.31). Oral CHM was not statistically different to HT in the change in daily hot flush frequency but produced a greater change (reduction) in hot flush severity ('moderate' certainty evidence). 'Low' certainty evidence showed HT was superior to oral CHM on the psychological, physical and vasomotor domains of the GCS, but oral CHM was not different to HT on the sexual domain. Oral CHM was not statistically different to HT in reducing depressive symptoms on the HAM-D ('very low' certainty evidence) and on all MENQOL domains ('low' certainty evidence).

Table 5.31 GRADE: Oral Chinese Herbal Medicine versus Hormone Therapy

Outcome; Treatment Duration	No. of Studies (Participants)	Relative Effect (MD [95% CI])	Certainty of the Evidence (GRADE)
Daily HF frequency (change score); 90 d	1 (52)	0.58 [−0.92, 2.08]	⊕⊕⊕◯ MODERATE[b]
Daily HF severity (change score); 90 d	1 (52)	1.12 [0.05, 2.19]*	⊕⊕⊕◯ MODERATE[b]
GCS-Psychol; 16 w	1 (38)	2.51 [1.55, 3.47]*	⊕⊕◯◯ LOW[a,b]
GCS-Ph; 16 w	1 (38)	1.07 [0.31, 1.83]*	⊕⊕◯◯ LOW[a,b]
GCS-V; 16 w	1 (38)	1.11 [0.63, 1.59]*	⊕⊕◯◯ LOW[a,b]
GCS-S; 16 w	1 (38)	0.35 [−1.02, 0.32]	⊕⊕◯◯ LOW[a,b]
HAM-D; mean 2.6 m	3 (167)	−6.35 [−13.81, 1.1]	⊕◯◯◯ VERY LOW[a,b,c]
MENQOL-Ph; mean 3 m	2 (147)	0.05 [−0.27, 0.37]	⊕⊕◯◯ LOW[a,b]
MENQOL-Psychosoc; mean 3 m	2 (147)	0.09 [−0.23, 0.42]	⊕⊕◯◯ LOW[a,b]
MENQOL-V; mean 3 m	2 (147)	0.33 [−0.25, 0.9]	⊕⊕◯◯ LOW[a,b]
MENQOL-S; mean 3 m	2 (147)	0.03 [−0.3, 0.35]	⊕⊕◯◯ LOW[a,b]

*Statistically significant result.

Abbreviations: d, days; CI, confidence interval; GRADE, Grading of Recommendations Assessment, Development and Evaluation; GCS, Greene Climacteric Scale; HAM-D, Hamilton Rating Scale for Depression; HF, hot flush; m, months; MD, mean difference; MENQOL, Menopause-specific Quality of Life questionnaire; Ph, physical domain; Psychol, psychological domain; Psychosoc, psychosocial domain; S, sexual domain; V, vasomotor domain; w, weeks.

Notes

[a]High risk of bias from lack of blinding.

[b]Small sample size.

[c]Unexplained statistical heterogeneity.

Study references

Daily HF frequency: H21.

Daily HF severity: H21.

GCS: H177.

HAM-D: H92, H93, H95.

MENQOL: H5, H161.

Safety was reported in 22 RCTs (H6–H8, H10, H21, H95, H139–H141, H143, H147, H149, H150, H153, H154, H156, H157, H160, H161, H163, H177, H182). Fewer AEs were reported with oral CHM. Adverse events in the intervention group included 23 cases of breast pain, 17 cases of vaginal bleeding, four cases of nausea, four cases of nausea and vomiting, three cases of unspecified digestive symptoms, three cases of abdominal discomfort, two cases of anorexia, two cases of bloating, and one case each of headache, increased vaginal discharge, cough and aggravation of asthma that required treatment with steroids. Adverse events with HT included 54 cases of vaginal bleeding, 45 cases of breast pain/tenderness, 19 cases of nausea, 13 cases of headache, abdominal pain, nausea and vomiting, nine cases of headache, seven cases of breast hyperplasia, six cases of abdominal pain/discomfort, six cases of gastrointestinal symptoms, five cases of endometrial thickening more than 5 mm, five cases of oedema, four cases of nausea and vomiting, two cases of abnormal liver function, two cases of weight gain, and one case each of mild abnormalities of liver and kidney function, and atypical endometrial hyperplasia.

Er xian tang 二仙汤 *versus placebo*

One study (H29) that compared *Er xian tang* 二仙汤 with placebo reported on the selected outcomes for summary-of-findings tables. This study provided 'moderate' certainty evidence for hot flushes and MENQOL (Table 5.32). *Er xian tang* 二仙汤 reduced frequency of hot flushes, but not severity, compared to placebo. Benefits were seen with *Er xian tang* 二仙汤 on the physical, psychosocial and vasomotor domains of MENQOL, while *Er xian tang* 二仙汤 was not statistically different to placebo in scores for the sexual domain at the end of treatment. Adverse events in the treatment group included two cases of headache, two cases of worsening of depression, one case of mild diarrhoea and one case of stomach-ache. Adverse events in the placebo group included three cases of worse hot flushes, two cases of worsening of insomnia and one case of mild headache.

Table 5.32 GRADE: *Er Xian Tang* 二仙汤 versus Placebo

Outcome; Treatment Duration	No. of Studies (Participants)	Relative Effect (MD [95% CI])	Certainty of the Evidence (GRADE)
Daily HF frequency; 12 w	1 (108)	−0.2 [−1.24, −0.84]*	⊕⊕⊕◯ MODERATE[a]
Daily HF severity; 12 w	1 (108)	−2.1 [−4.79, 0.59]	⊕⊕⊕◯ MODERATE[a]
MENQOL-Ph; 12 w	1 (108)	−6.4 [−12.36, −0.44]*	⊕⊕⊕◯ MODERATE[a]
MENQOL-Psychosoc; 12 w	1 (108)	−3.7 [−7.06, −0.34]*	⊕⊕⊕◯ MODERATE[a]
MENQOL-V; 12 w	1 (108)	−2.6 [−4.51, −0.69]*	⊕⊕⊕◯ MODERATE[a]
MENQOL-S; 12 w	1 (108)	−0.6 [−2.06, 0.86]	⊕⊕⊕◯ MODERATE[a]

*Statistically significant result.

Abbreviations: d, days; CI, confidence interval; GRADE, Grading of Recommendations Assessment, Development and Evaluation; HF, hot flush; MD, mean difference; MENQOL, Menopause-specific Quality of Life questionnaire; Ph, physical domain; Psychosoc, psychosocial domain; S, sexual domain; V, vasomotor domain; w, weeks.

Note

[a]Small sample size.

Study references

Daily HF frequency: H29.

Daily HF severity: H29.

MENQOL: H29.

Kun tai jiao nang 坤泰胶囊 versus hormone therapy

Five RCTs (H5–H8, H10) tested the product *Kun tai jiao nang* 坤泰胶囊, compared to HT, and reported on either MENQOL and/or AEs. 'Low' certainty evidence showed no difference between *Kun tai jiao nang* 坤泰胶囊 and HT in MENQOL scores for the physical, psychosocial, vasomotor and sexual domains at the end of treatment (Table 5.33). Four studies (H6–H8, H10) reported on safety. Adverse events with *Kun tai jiao nang* 坤泰胶囊 included 23 cases of breast pain, 15 cases of vaginal bleeding, four cases of nausea and vomiting,

Table 5.33 GRADE: *Kun Tai Jiao Nang* 坤泰胶囊 versus Hormone Therapy

Outcome; Treatment Duration	No. of Studies (Participants)	Relative Effect (SMD [95% CI])	Certainty of the Evidence (GRADE)
MENQOL-Ph; 8 w	2 (147)	0.05 [−0.27, 0.37]	⊕⊕◯◯ LOW[a,b]
MENQOL-Psychosoc; 8 w	2 (147)	0.09 [−0.23, 0.42]	⊕⊕◯◯ LOW[a,b]
MENQOL-V; 8 w	2 (147)	0.33 [−0.25, 0.9]	⊕⊕◯◯ LOW[a,b]
MENQOL-S; 8 w	2 (147)	0.03 [−0.3, 0.35]	⊕⊕◯◯ LOW[a,b]

Abbreviations: d, days; CI, confidence interval; GRADE, Grading of Recommendations Assessment, Development and Evaluation; MENQOL, Menopause-specific Quality of Life questionnaire; Ph, physical domain; Psychosoc, psychosocial domain; S, sexual domain; SMD, standardised mean difference; V, vasomotor domain; w, weeks.

Notes

[a]High risk of bias from lack of blinding.

[b]Small sample size.

Study reference

MENQOL: H5, H8.

three cases of abdominal discomfort and three cases of digestive tract symptoms. In the HT groups, AEs included 33 cases of vaginal bleeding, 30 cases of breast pain, six cases of gastrointestinal symptoms, four cases of nausea and vomiting, three cases of abdominal discomfort, and one case each of nausea, headache and abnormal liver function.

Randomised Controlled Trial Evidence for Individual Oral Formulas

Several studies tested the same formula for the same outcomes. Meta-analyses were able to be conducted for several formulas/products: *Gan mai da zao tang* 甘麦大枣汤, *Shu gan jie yu jiao nang* 疏肝解郁胶囊, *Kun tai jiao nang* 坤泰胶囊, *Qing xin zi shen tang* 清心滋肾汤 and *Zi shen sheng gan fang/ke li ji* 滋肾生肝方/颗粒剂. *Gan mai da zao tang* 甘麦大枣汤 was not superior to pharmacotherapy for end-of-treatment scores on the HAM-D (two RCTs, 201 women, MD −0.40 points [−1.86, 1.05], I^2 = 0%; H42, H87).

One study tested *Shu gan jie yu jiao nang* 疏肝解郁胶囊 alone and as an adjunct to pharmacotherapy. When used alone, *Shu gan jie yu jiao nang* 疏肝解郁胶囊 was not statistically different to pharmacotherapy in reducing depressive symptoms on the HAM-D (two RCTs, 180 women, MD −1.00 points [−3.54, 1.54], I^2 = 94%; H14, H15). However, when used as integrative medicine, *Shu gan jie yu jiao nang* 疏肝解郁胶囊 resulted in greater improvements in depressive symptoms on the HAM-D at the end of treatment compared with pharmacotherapy alone (two RCTs, 190 women, MD −3.36 points [−4.12, −2.60], I^2 = 0%; H12, H13).

Meta-analyses were possible for three formulas that measured the effects using the original or modified version of the KI. *Qing xin zi shen tang* 清心滋肾汤 was not statistically different to pharmacotherapy in KI scores at the end of treatment (three RCTs, 280 women, SMD −0.80 [−2.37, 0.77], I^2 = 97%; H83, H155, H156), nor was *Kun tai jiao nang* 坤泰胶囊 (four RCTs, 329 women, SMD −0.02 [−0.24, 0.19], I^2 = 0%; H5–H7, H10). There was a trend for *Zi shen sheng gan fang/ke li ji* 滋肾生肝方/颗粒剂 to reduce KI score, although this did not reach statistical significance (two RCTs, 540 women, SMD −0.17 [−0.34, −0.00], I^2 = 0%, p = 0.05; H152, H161). One study that tested *Kun tai jiao nang* 坤泰胶囊 as integrative medicine found no statistical difference in KI score at the end of treatment between the treatment and comparator groups (three RCTs, 498 women, SMD −0.62 [−1.27, 0.03], I^2 = 90%; H2–H4).

Frequently Reported Orally Used Herbs in Meta-analyses Showing Favourable Effect

Several of the meta-analyses for oral CHM have shown positive effects compared to placebo or pharmacotherapy. The herb ingredients of studies that were included in these meta-analyses were reviewed to identify the frequently used herbs that may contribute to the treatment effect. Analysis was conducted according to categories of outcomes, which included vasomotor, genitourinary, sleep and psychological symptoms, as well as global symptom scales and HRQoL. No meta-analyses showed favourable effects for genitourinary symptoms, so herb frequency analysis was not conducted for this outcome category.

Six studies were included in two meta-analyses for vasomotor symptoms (daily hot flush frequency/severity; see Tables 5.4, 5.5). Three herbs were used in two of the six studies: *huang bai* 黄柏, *xian mao* 仙茅 and *zhi mu* 知母. It is difficult to say whether these herbs contributed to the positive effects seen due to the small number of studies included in the herb frequency analysis.

Sleep symptoms were assessed using the PSQI, AIS, SDRS, SRSS and Spiegel Sleep Questionnaire, with meta-analysis possible for the PSQI, AIS and SRSS. Favourable results for oral CHM were seen in five meta-analyses involving 42 RCTs. Herbs that were found with high frequency in these studies were *suan zao ren* 酸枣仁, *gan cao* 甘草, *fu ling* 茯苓, *dang gui* 当归 and *zhi mu* 知母 (Table 5.34).

Table 5.34 Frequently Reported Orally Used Herbs in Meta-analyses Showing Favourable Effect for Sleep Symptoms

Herbs	Scientific Name	Frequency of Use
Suan zao ren 酸枣仁	*Ziziphus jujuba* Mill. var. spinosa (Bunge) Hu ex H. F. Chou	24
Gan cao 甘草	*Glycyrrhiza* spp.	19
Fu ling 茯苓	*Poria cocos* (Schw.) Wolf	15
Dang gui 当归	*Angelica sinensis* (Oliv.) Diels	14
Zhi mu 知母	*Anemarrhena asphodeloides* Bge.	14
Chai hu 柴胡	*Bupleurum* spp.	13
Bai shao 白芍	*Paeonia lactiflora* Pall.	12
Chuan xiong 川芎	*Ligusticum chuangxiong* Hort.	12
Sheng di huang 生地黄	*Rehmannia glutinosa* Libosch.	12
Shu di huang 熟地黄	*Rehmannia glutinosa* Libosch.	12

Notes: (1) Sleep symptoms: refer to Tables 5.7, 5.8 and 5.9, and sections 'Athens Insomnia Scale' and 'Self-rating Scale of Sleep'.
(2) The use of some herbs may be restricted in some countries. Readers are advised to comply with relevant regulations.

All ten of the most frequently used herbs in meta-analyses for sleep symptoms were found in the top 20 herbs in the overall pool. These herbs may have contributed to the positive results seen in meta-analyses and practitioners may wish to consider these herbs when prescribing treatments for menopausal women with sleep disturbances.

Psychological symptoms were assessed using the SDS, SAS, BDI, HAM-D, HAM-A and SCL-90, with meta-analysis results favouring oral CHM on the SDS, SAS, HAM-D and HAM-A. Four meta-analyses involving 49 RCTs showed favourable results with oral CHM for psychological symptoms. The most frequently used herbs in studies that contributed to positive findings for psychological symptoms were *gan cao* 甘草, *chai hu* 柴胡, *fu ling* 茯苓 and *dang gui* 当归 (Table 5.35). In fact, many of the herbs frequently used for psychological symptoms were the same as those used in studies for sleep symptoms and were largely reflective of the total pool. One herb, *yu jin* 郁金,

Table 5.35 Frequently Reported Orally Used Herbs in Meta-analyses Showing Favourable Effect for Psychological Symptoms

Herbs	Scientific Name	Frequency of Use
Gan cao 甘草	*Glycyrrhiza* spp.	21
Chai hu 柴胡	*Bupleurum* spp.	20
Fu ling 茯苓	*Poria cocos* (Schw.) Wolf	20
Dang gui 当归	*Angelica sinensis* (Oliv.) Diels	18
Suan zao ren 酸枣仁	*Ziziphus jujuba* Mill. var. spinosa (Bunge) Hu ex H. F. Chou	16
Yu jin 郁金	*Curcuma* spp.	16
Shu di huang 熟地黄	*Rehmannia glutinosa* Libosch.	14
Bai shao 白芍	*Paeonia lactiflora* Pall.	13
Chuan xiong 川芎	*Ligusticum chuangxiong* Hort.	10
Yin yang huo 淫羊藿	*Epimedium* spp.	10

Notes: (1) Psychological symptoms: see section 'Zung's Self-rating Anxiety Scale' and Tables 5.10, 5.11 and 5.12.

(2) The use of some herbs may be restricted in some countries. Readers are advised to comply with relevant regulations.

appears to be specific to psychological symptoms. This herb was used 28 times in the total pool of 191 oral CHM RCTs and was found/used 16 times in the 49 RCTs included in positive meta-analyses for psychological symptoms. This herb has the actions of clearing the Heart and regulating Blood,[37] which explains its frequent use for psychological symptoms.

Global symptom severity was assessed using the KI and GCS, with three meta-analyses showing favourable results for oral CHM on the KI. Seventy-nine RCTs were included in the three meta-analyses. The herbs used frequently in studies included in these meta-analyses match those in the total pool of oral CHM studies. This was not suprising, given that these studies comprised over 40% of the total pool. The most frequently used herbs in positive meta-analyses for global symptom scales were *shu di huang* 熟地黄, *fu ling* 茯苓, *bai shao* 白芍 and *dang gui* 当归 (Table 5.36). These herbs may contribute to the positive effects seen.

The number of studies in meta-analyses that demonstrated benefit of oral CHM on HRQoL was much smaller than for other outcome

Table 5.36 Frequently Reported Orally Used Herbs in Meta-analyses Showing Favourable Effect for Global Symptom Scales

Herbs	Scientific Name	Frequency of Use
Shu di huang 熟地黄	*Rehmannia glutinosa* Libosch.	45
Fu ling 茯苓	*Poria cocos* (Schw.) Wolf	40
Bai shao 白芍	*Paeonia lactiflora* Pall.	40
Dang gui 当归	*Angelica sinensis* (Oliv.) Diels	33
Shan yao 山药	*Dioscorea opposita* Thunb.	27
Shan zhu yu 山茱萸	*Cornus officinalis* Sieb. et Zucc.	27
Gan cao 甘草	*Glycyrrhiza* spp.	25
Chai hu 柴胡	*Bupleurum* spp.	23
Yin yang huo 淫羊藿	*Epimedium* spp.	21
Huang lian 黄连	*Coptis* spp.	20

Notes: (1) Global symptom scales: see Tables 5.14, 5.16 and 5.18.
(2) The use of some herbs may be restricted in some countries. Readers are advised to comply with relevant regulations.

Table 5.37 Frequently Reported Orally Used Herbs in Meta-analyses Showing Favourable Effect for Health-related Quality of Life

Herbs	Scientific Name	Frequency of Use
Bai shao 白芍	*Paeonia lactiflora* Pall.	3
Chai hu 柴胡	*Bupleurum* spp.	3
Dang gui 当归	*Angelica sinensis* (Oliv.) Diels	3
Gan cao 甘草	*Glycyrrhiza* spp.	3
Sheng di huang 生地黄	*Rehmannia glutinosa* Libosch.	3
Huang bai 黄柏	*Phellodendron chinense* Schneid.	2
Shi yong da huang 食用大黄	*Rheum rhaponticum*	2
Suan zao ren 酸枣仁	*Ziziphus jujuba* Mill. var. spinosa (Bunge) Hu ex H. F. Chou	2
Zhi mu 知母	*Anemarrhena asphodeloides* Bge.	2

Notes: (1) Health-related quality of life: see Tables 5.22, 5.23, 5.29.
(2) The use of some herbs may be restricted in some countries. Readers are advised to comply with relevant regulations.

categories. Health-related quality of life was assessed using the MRS, HFRDI, MENQOL, SF-36 and other activities of daily living scales. Oral CHM was found to be beneficial in five meta-analyses with nine RCTs for the outcomes MRS, MENQOL and SF-36. Five herbs were used in three of the nine studies: *bai shao* 白芍, *chai hu* 柴胡, *dang gui* 当归, *gan cao* 甘草 and *sheng di huang* 生地黄 (Table 5.37). These herbs may possibly have contributed to the positive effects seen in meta-analyses. However, due to the small number of studies in this analysis, we are unable to be certain about how much these herbs influenced the results.

Safety of Oral Chinese Herbal Medicine in Randomised Controlled Trials

Safety of oral CHM was reported in 92 RCTs (H2, H6–H11, H15–H21, H23–H37, H52, H55, H56, H58, H64, H68, H71, H72, H74–H76, H80, H81, H86, H87, H89, H90, H91, H94, H95, H101, H105, H107–H112, H114, H116, H117, H119, H120, H123, H126,

H127, H139–H141, H143, H147, H149, H150, H152–H154, H156, H157, H160, H161, H163, H172–H175, H177–H184). Nineteen RCTs reported that no AEs occurred during the trial (H9, H11, H23, H26, H31, H33, H35, H37, H71, H95, H107, H120, H123, H149, H156, H161, H163, H173, H175) with AEs occurring in the remaining studies. The adverse events were analysed where the nature and number of events were reported.

In total, 303 AEs occurred in women who received oral CHM alone. One serious AE of dysplasia of the squamous epithelium was reported, although this was considered not to be related to the trial medication (H24). One participant withdrew from the study by Van der Sluijs *et al.* (H27) due to a variety of AEs that included headaches, nausea, excessive perspiration and intermittent aching of the limbs. One case of elevated ALT was considered to be related to CHM (H28), while one case of moderate asthenia, vertigo and headache was judged possibly to be related to the intervention (H19). Other adverse events included 36 cases of diarrhoea, 30 cases of breast pain/tenderness, 24 cases of nausea and/or vomiting, 24 cases of gastrointestinal discomfort, 18 cases of dizziness, 17 cases of vaginal bleeding, 14 cases of insomnia/sleep disorder, 14 cases of rash, nine cases of constipation, nine cases of headache, eight cases of dry mouth, eight cases of palpitations/chest pain, six cases of fatigue, three cases of loss of appetite and 79 miscellaneous or combinations of AEs.

Eighty AEs were reported in women who received oral CHM as integrative medicine. Adverse events included 16 cases of gastrointestinal discomfort, 15 cases of nausea and/or vomiting, nine cases of vaginal bleeding, six cases of breast pain, six cases of headache, four cases of constipation, four cases of insomnia, four cases of dry mouth, four cases of loss of appetite, three cases of dizziness and fatigue, two cases of fatigue, two cases of diarrhoea, one case of palpitations and four miscellaneous/combinations of AEs.

The number of AEs in the comparator groups was 688, higher than in the intervention groups. One serious AE of elevated liver enzymes occurred in the comparator group of one study (H17).

In another study (H27), two participants withdrew due to AEs of headaches, abdominal bloating, constipation and dehydration.

Adverse events in the comparator groups included 79 cases of breast pain/tenderness, 73 cases of nausea and/or vomiting, 72 gastrointestinal pain/discomfort/symptoms, 72 cases of vaginal bleeding, 69 cases of fatigue, 62 cases of dry mouth, 49 cases of dizziness, 30 cases of headache, 20 cases of constipation, 14 cases of insomnia, 11 cases of palpitations/chest tightness, nine cases of loss of appetite, eight cases of diarrhoea, six cases of endometrial thickening, five cases of abnormal liver and/or kidney function and 178 miscellaneous/combinations of different symptoms.

Controlled Clinical Trials of Oral Chinese Herbal Medicine

Twenty-one CCTs (H186–H206) that evaluated oral CHM for menopause symptoms included 2,192 participants. All but one study compared an intervention group with a control group; in one three-arm study oral CHM was compared with tibolone (control group 1) and flupentixol/melitracen (control group 2; H203). The majority of studies were conducted in mainland China, with one study conducted in Japan (H206) and one recruiting women in both mainland China and the United Kingdom (H205). Studies were conducted in hospital outpatient departments (H188, H190, H194, H197, H198, H201, H203, H204), inpatient departments (H189), both inpatient and outpatient departments (H191, H202) and in a combination of hospital and community clinics (H205). The setting was not reported in nine studies (H186, H187, H192, H193, H195, H196, H199, H200, H206).

Three studies (H204 H206) did not report the menopausal status of women. The remaining studies (H197, H202, H203) included perimenopausal women; some described criteria relating to FSH and/or oestradiol levels and duration of amenorrhoea. The mean age of women in one study was lower than usually expected for menopausal women (mean age 44 years; H187). Other studies reported mean age as between 47 and 53 years. While some studies evaluated oral

CHM for menopause symptoms generally, others focused on women with comorbid depression (H187, H191, H193–H195, H200, H203), depression and anxiety (H201), depression and sleep disorders (H188), insomnia (H186, H206), psychological conditions (H199, H202) and genitourinary infection (H192). Duration of symptoms ranged from two months (H188) to 6.5 years (H198).

Treatment duration varied among included studies. Lian (2017; H187) provided treatment for 15 days, while four studies (H190, H195, H197, H204) reported treatment duration of three months/90 days. The median duration of treatment was eight weeks. Two studies described follow-up assessment after treatment ceased, which was conducted at four weeks (H203) or three months (H202). Three studies (H197, H204, H205) reported loss to follow-up. Twenty-one of the 2,192 participants were lost to follow-up assessment, and numbers were generally balanced between treatment and control groups.

Few studies used CM syndrome differentiation as an inclusion criterion or to guide treatment. Syndromes included Kidney *yin* deficiency (H197, H202, H204), Kidney deficiency and Liver stagnation (H190), Kidney and Liver deficiency, *yin* deficiency with excess Liver *yang*, Kidney *yin* and *yang* deficiency, and Heart and Kidney not communicating (H204). Oral CHM was used alone in 15 of the 21 studies (H187, H189–H191, H193, H194, H196–H198, H201–H206) and as IM in six (H186, H188, H192, H195, H199, H200). Two CHM formulas were included in multiple studies: *Zhi bai di huang wan* 知柏地黄丸 and Gan *mai da zao tang* 甘麦大枣汤 (Table 5.38). *Gan mai da zao tang* 甘麦大枣汤 was used in combination with *Gui pi tang* 归脾汤 in one study (H187). There was no overlap in other oral CHM formulas.

Seventy-three different herb ingredients were reported in the 21 CCTs. The most frequently used herb was *fu ling* 茯苓, used in 12 studies (Table 5.39). Other frequently used herbs included *bai shao* 白芍, *chai hu* 柴胡, *dang gui* 当归, *gan cao* 甘草 and *mu li* 牡蛎. Herbs used in CCTs were similar to those used in RCTs.

Comparators in the included studies included HT (H190, H192, H197, H198, H202–H205), antidepressants such as selective serotonin reuptake inhibitors, tricyclic antidepressants (H187–H189,

Table 5.38 Frequently Reported Oral Formulas in Controlled Clinical Trials

Most Common Formulas	No. of Studies	Ingredients
Zhi bai di huang wan 知柏地黄丸	3	*Zhi mu* 知母, *shu di huang* 熟地黄, *huang bai* 黄柏, *shan yu rou* 山萸肉, *shan yao* 山药, *mu dan pi* 牡丹皮, *fu ling* 茯苓 and *ze xie* 泽泻.
Gan mai da zao tang 甘麦大枣汤	2	*Gan cao* 甘草, *huai xiao mai* 淮小麦 and *da zao mei* 大枣枚 (H187, H193).

Notes: (1) Ingredients are referenced to the original studies where possible. If herb ingredients varied across studies, the herb ingredients were sourced from *Zhong Yi Fang Ji Da Ci Dian* 中医方剂大辞典. (2) The use of some herbs may be restricted in some countries. Readers are advised to comply with relevant regulations.

Table 5.39 Frequently Reported Orally Used Herbs in Controlled Clinical Trials

Most Common Herbs	Scientific Name	Frequency of Use
Fu ling 茯苓	*Poria cocos* (Schw.) Wolf	12
Bai shao 白芍	*Paeonia lactiflora* Pall.	11
Chai hu 柴胡	*Bupleurum* spp.	9
Dang gui 当归	*Angelica sinensis* (Oliv.) Diels	8
Gan cao 甘草	*Glycyrrhiza* spp.	7
Mu li 牡蛎	*Ostrea* spp.	7
Long gu 龙骨	Fossilised bones	7
Suan zao ren 酸枣仁	*Ziziphus jujuba* Mill. var. spinosa (Bunge) Hu ex H. F. Chou	6
Da zao 大枣	*Ziziphus jujuba* Mill.	5
Huang bai 黄柏	*Phellodendron chinense* Schneid.	5
Mu dan pi 牡丹皮	*Paeonia suffruticosa* Andr.	5
Shu di huang 熟地黄	*Rehmannia glutinosa* Libosch.	5
Yin yang huo 淫羊藿	*Epimedium* spp.	5
Zhi mu 知母	*Anemarrhena asphodeloides* Bge.	5
Gou qi zi 枸杞子	*Lycium barbarum* L.	4
Huang qin 黄芩	*Scutellaria baicalensis* Georgi	4
Shan zhu yu 山茱萸	*Cornus officinalis* Sieb. et Zucc.	4

Note: The use of some herbs may be restricted in some countries. Readers are advised to comply with relevant regulations.

H191, H193–H195, H199–H201, H203, H206) and benzodiazepines (H186, H196).

Outcomes

Thirteen of the 21 CCTs reported psychological outcomes; the most common psychological outcome measure was the HAM-D.[17] Nine studies reported global measures of menopause symptoms using the original or modified KI[16] or GCS,[31] and three studies reported sleep quality using either PSQI[18] or AIS.[22] One study reported vaginal symptoms and one reported HRQoL using MENQOL.[19] Adverse events were reported in 11 CCTs. None of the included studies reported vasomotor symptoms of hot flushes or night sweats, urinary tract infections, sexual symptoms or musculoskeletal symptoms. Not all studies reported data in a way that could be re-analysed and these were excluded from the analyses described below.

Vaginal Symptoms

Oral Chinese herbal medicine plus pharmacotherapy versus pharmacotherapy alone

Vaginal health was assessed in one study that combined oral CHM with Premarin® in the intervention group (H192). Vaginal moisture, pH, mucosa, discharge and rugae vaginales were scored from one to four. Scores for each item were summed to provide a total score, with higher score indicating better vaginal health. *Zhi bai di huang wan* 知柏地黄丸 was not statistically different to Premarin® (MD −0.14 points [−0.87, 0.59]).

Pittsburgh Sleep Quality Index

Oral Chinese herbal medicine plus pharmacotherapy versus pharmacotherapy alone

Two studies (H186, H188), of 186 perimenopausal women with sleep problems, used the PSQI to evaluate change in sleep. At the end of treatment, women who received oral CHM plus pharmacotherapy scored 4.51 points lower than those who received pharmacotherapy alone ([−6.44, −2.57], I^2 = 84%). While this difference was statistically significant, we were unable to examine potential sources of statistical heterogeneity. Thus, our confidence in this finding is limited.

Athens Insomnia Scale

Oral Chinese herbal medicine versus pharmacotherapy

One study (H196) evaluated sleep quality using the AIS in 72 women. The AIS score was 2.30 points lower in women who received *Yi shen tang* 挹神汤 compared to women who received estazolam ([−2.98, −1.62]).

Hamilton Rating Scale for Depression

Ten studies (H187, H188, H191, H193, H195, H199, H200, H201, H203, H206) with useable data measured depressive symptoms with the HAM-D. Results for studies that used oral CHM as integrative medicine were analysed separately to those that used oral CHM alone as the intervention.

Oral Chinese herbal medicine versus pharmacotherapy

Six studies (H187, H191, H193, H201, H203, H206) with 530 women used the 21- or 24-item version of HAM-D. Due to the different HAM-D versions used, results of these studies were analysed using SMD. The two control groups (HT and flupentixol/melitracen) of one study (H203) were merged for analysis. Women who received oral CHM alone had lower HAM-D scores at the end of treatment than women who received pharmacotherapy (SMD −1.02 units [−1.91, −0.14], I^2 = 95%). Considerable statistical heterogeneity was detected. Subgroup analysis for comparator type produced similar results for antidepressants, while only one study used HT (Table 5.40).

Table 5.40 Oral Chinese Herbal Medicine versus Pharmacotherapy: Hamilton Rating Scale for Depression

Subgroup	No. of Studies (Participants)	Effect Size (MD/SMD [95% CI], I^2)	Included Studies
All studies	6 (530)	SMD 1.02 [−1.91, −0.14]*, 95%	H187, H191, H193, H201, H203, H206
Antidepressants[#]	6 (494)	SMD −1.01 [−1.92, −0.09]*, 95%	H187, H191, H193, H201, H203, H206
Tibolone	1 (72)	MD −0.55 [−1.02, −0.08]*	H203
Treatment duration: ≥6 weeks	5 (450)	SMD −0.32 [−0.62, −0.01]*, 61%	H191, H193, H201, H203, H206

*Statistically significant, Chapter 4.

[#]Excludesone hormone therapy arm from study H203.

Abbreviations: CI, confidence interval; MD, mean difference; SMD, standardised mean difference.

One study (H187) provided treatment for 15 days, much shorter than the treatment duration in the remaining studies (range 6 to 12 weeks). When this study was excluded from analysis, statistical heterogeneity was reduced but remained above acceptable levels. The reason for statistical heterogeneity was not able to be identified by any of the planned subgroup analyses.

Oral Chinese herbal medicine plus pharmacotherapy versus pharmacotherapy alone

Depressive symptoms were measured using HAM-D in four studies (H188, H195, H199, H200). The HAM-D scores were 4.88 points lower in women who received oral CHM plus antidepressants compared with antidepressants alone (614 participants, [−5.87, −3.89], $I^2 = 77\%$). Subgroup analysis, according to treatment duration, found lower statistical heterogeneity in studies with treatment duration less than eight weeks (Table 5.41), but substantial heterogeneity in studies providing treatment for eight weeks or more. Even within these

Table 5.41 Oral Chinese Herbal Medicine plus Pharmacotherapy versus Pharmacotherapy: Hamilton Rating Scale for Depression

Subgroup	No. of Studies (Participants)	Effect Size (MD [95% CI], I^2)	Included Studies
All studies	4 (614)	−4.88 [−5.87, −3.89]*, 77%	H188, H195, H199, H200
Treatment duration: <8 w	2 (318)	−4.50 [−5.12, −3.89]*, 0%	H188, H199
Treatment duration: ≥8 w	2 (296)	−5.05 [−7.11, −2.99]*, 91%	H195, H200

* Statistically significant, see Chapter 4.
Abbreviations: CI, confidence interval; MD, mean difference; w, weeks.

subgroups there was diversity in treatment duration, so it seems unlikely that this is the sole reason for statistical heterogeneity. The reason for statistical heterogeneity is unclear and results should be interpreted with caution.

Hamilton Rating Scale for Anxiety

Five CCTs (H191, H194, H199–H201) measured anxiety using HAM-A. Three studies used oral CHM alone as the intervention, while two tested the combination of oral CHM with pharmacotherapy.

Oral Chinese herbal medicine versus pharmacotherapy

Two hundred and thirty-four women participated in the three CCTs (H191, H194, H201) that evaluated the impact of oral CHM on HAM-A. There was no statistical difference between oral CHM and antidepressants in HAM-A score at the end of treatment (MD −1.02 [−3.14, 1.10], I^2 = 89%). Planned subgroup analyses to examine potential causes of statistical heterogeneity were unable to be conducted due to the small number of studies in the meta analysis.

Oral Chinese herbal medicine plus pharmacotherapy versus pharmacotherapy alone

Two studies (H199, H200) tested the effect of oral CHM plus antidepressants compared with antidepressants alone on anxiety using the HAM-A. Four hundred and ninety-four women participated in these studies. The HAM-A scores were 2.64 points lower at the end-of-treatment in women who received the combination of oral CHM plus antidepressants ([−4.12, −1.16], I^2 = 97%). Again, subgroup analyses were not able to be conducted and the results should be considered in light of the substantial statistical heterogeneity.

Self-rating Depression Scale

Oral Chinese herbal medicine versus pharmacotherapy

One study (H190) evaluated depressive symptoms in 60 women using the SDS. *Zi shen shu kun tang* 滋肾舒坤汤 was more effective in improving SDS scores than tibolone at the end of treatment (MD −0.67 points [−1.19, −0.15]).

Self-rating Anxiety Scale

Oral Chinese herbal medicine versus pharmacotherapy

The study that evaluated SDS also measured SAS (H190). *Zi shen shu kun tang* 滋肾舒坤汤 was also more effective than tibolone at improving anxiety measured with the SAS (MD −0.65 [−1.17, −0.13]).

Kupperman Index

Seven studies (H190, H195, H197, H198, H202, H204, H205) that reported data on KI scores were able to be analysed. One CCT (H195) used the original 11-item version of KI and six used mKI that included additional items for urinary and sexual symptoms.

Oral Chinese herbal medicine versus pharmacotherapy

Meta-analysis was possible with five studies (H190, H197, H198, H202, H205), involving 547 women, that compared oral CHM with HT. Standardised mean difference was used for analysis. Oral CHM was more effective than pharmacotherapy in reducing mKI score (SMD −0.35 units [−0.55, −0.14], $I^2 = 0\%$). One of the studies included in the meta-analysis (H205) also reported scores for individual items of the mKI. *Zhi bai di huang wan* 知柏地黄丸 was more effective than tibolone at improving vertigo (MD −0.36 points [−0.51, −0.21]), headache (MD −0.31 points [−0.46, −0.16]), palpitations (MD −0.17 points [−0.31, −0.03]), formication (MD −0.60 points [−0.89, −0.31]), sexual symptoms (MD −0.42 points [−0.70, −0.14]) and urinary tract infections (MD −0.36 points [−0.63, −0.09]). No statistical difference was seen between groups in scores for vasomotor symptoms (MD 0.06 points [−0.55, 0.67]), paraesthesia (MD 0.16 points [−0.07, 0.39]), insomnia (MD 0.29 points [−0.01, 0.59]), nervousness (MD 0.25 points [−0.05, 0.55]), melancholia (MD −0.03 points [−0.18, 0.12]), weakness (MD 0.11 points [−0.03, 0.25]) and arthralgia (MD −0.09 points [−0.23, 0.05]).

One study (H204) reported the percentage of improvement in mKI. In this study of 60 women, there was no difference in the percentage of improvement in mKI between women who received *Tiao geng tang* 调更汤 and those who received tibolone (MD 0.00 points [−3.30, 3.30]).

Oral Chinese herbal medicine plus pharmacotherapy versus pharmacotherapy alone

One study (H195) evaluated the effect of oral CHM combined with flupentixol/melitracen on menopause symptoms using the KI. *Xiao yao san* 逍遥散 as integrative medicine was more effective in improving symptoms than flupentixol/melitracen (60 participants, MD −5.68 points [−6.67, −4.69]).

Greene Climacteric Scale

Oral Chinese herbal medicine versus pharmacotherapy

One study (H206) with 100 participants assessed menopause symptom severity using GCS. *Chai hu gui zhi gan jiang tang* 柴胡桂枝干姜汤 was not statistically different to antidepressants in reducing bother from menopause symptoms on GCS (MD 1.70 points [−0.70, 4.10]).

Menopause Rating Scale

Oral Chinese herbal medicine versus pharmacotherapy

The MRS was used to assess the impact of *Tiao geng tang* 调更汤 on menopause-related quality of life in 60 participants (H204). While not statistically significant, there appeared to be a trend for *Tiao geng tang* 调更汤 to be more effective than tibolone (MD −2.00 points [−4.02, 0.02]).

Menopause-specific Quality of Life

Oral Chinese herbal medicine versus pharmacotherapy

The CCT (H204) that used MRS as an outcome also measured quality of life using MENQOL. A score was calculated for each of the four domains by summing the scores for each item within the domain. This approach differs from the standard method (see Chapter 4), where the domain score is calculated by summing scores for each item, then dividing the number of items. The results of analysis presented here should be interpreted with this modification in mind. *Tiao geng tang* 调更汤 was not statistically different to tibolone in improving impact of menopause on the physical (MD −2.00 points [−6.05, 2.05]), psychosocial (MD 1.00 points [−1.02, 3.02]), vasomotor (MD −1.00 [−2.52, 0.52]) or sexual (MD 2.00 [−0.40, 4.40]) domains of the MENQOL.

Controlled Clinical Trial Evidence for Individual Oral Formulas

Despite there being little overlap in formulas used among the 21 CCTs, meta-analysis was possible for one formula: *Zhi bai di huang wan* 知柏地黄丸. Analysis of two studies involving 281 women found *Zhi bai di huang wan* 知柏地黄丸 was more effective than tibolone in improving mKI score at the end of treatment (SMD −0.26 [−0.49, −0.02], $I^2 = 0\%$).

Safety of Oral Chinese Herbal Medicine in Controlled Clinical Trials

Eleven CCTs reported on safety of oral CHM. Ten studies (H191, H193, H194, H196, H198, H201–H205) used oral CHM alone and one study (H200) combined oral CHM with pharmacotherapy. There were 635 participants who received oral CHM (either alone or as integrative medicine) and 623 participants who received pharmacotherapy. Three studies (H196, H202, H205) reported no AEs occurring during the study. There were 25 AEs in the oral CHM alone groups. Adverse events included five cases of nausea, five cases of lethargy, dry mouth and tremor, four cases of dry mouth, four cases of bloating, three cases of diarrhoea, two cases of dizziness, and one case each of sweating and constipation. Five AEs occurred in women who received oral CHM as integrative medicine; these included two cases of nausea and vomiting, two cases of headache and one case of blurred vision.

Ninety-three AEs were reported in the pharmacotherapy groups. These included ten cases of dry mouth, six cases of irregular vaginal bleeding, six cases of weight gain, six cases of sweating, six cases of constipation, four cases of early pregnancy symptoms, four cases of breast hyperplasia, four cases of dizziness, three cases of nausea, three cases of drowsiness and three cases of mild thickening of the endometrium. Adverse events with two cases included loss of appetite, insomnia, abdominal discomfort and pressure in the breast. Single AEs included restlessness, fatigue, vomiting, nausea and vomiting, and emotional instability. One study reported 13 adverse events that included nausea, vomiting, dizziness, insomnia, agitation, palpitations and others. Finally, there were an unspecified number of AEs that included breast pain and vaginal bleeding, dry mouth, loss of appetite and mild weakness.

Non-controlled Studies of Oral Chinese Herbal Medicine

Sixty-five non-controlled case series studies (H207–H271) involving 4,352 women evaluated oral CM for menopause symptoms. Thirty-two studies (H209, H212, H213, H215, H217, H219, H220, H223, H226–H228, H230, H233–H236, H238, H239, H242–H244, H246–H249, H252, H254–H256, H258–H260) used syndrome differentiation to select participants, with several describing multiple syndromes. The most frequent syndrome was Liver and Kidney *yin* deficiency, which was reported in 11 studies. Other syndromes found in multiple studies were Heart and Kidney not communicating (five studies) and Kidney deficiency and Liver depression/stagnation (two studies). Ten studies used syndrome differentiation to guide treatment; again, the syndromes described in multiple studies were Kidney *yin* deficiency (three studies) and Liver and Kidney *yin* deficiency (two studies).

In one study (H270) oral CHM was administered as integrative medicine with HT, while all other studies tested oral CHM alone. Many studies used an investigator-developed formulation, and these were excluded from formula frequency calculations. Only two formulas were evaluated in multiple studies: *Tian meng jiao nang* 甜梦胶囊 (H237, H241) and *Zi shui qing gan yin* 滋水清肝饮 (H213, H228). *Tian meng jiao nang* 甜梦胶囊 is a manufactured capsule containing 17 herbs (see Table 5.42), while *Zi shui qing gan yin* 滋水清肝饮 is a traditional formula used to nourish *yin* and clear Liver stagnation.

The most frequently reported herbs for oral use in non-controlled studies are described in Table 5.43. *Bai shao* 白芍 was the most

Table 5.42 Frequently Reported Oral Formulas in Non-controlled Studies

Most Common Formulas	No. of Studies	Ingredients
Tian meng jiao nang 甜梦胶囊	2	*Ci wu jia* 刺五加, *huang jing* 黄精, *can e* 蚕蛾, *sang shen* 桑椹, *dang shen* 党参, *huang qi* 黄芪, *sha ren* 砂仁, *gou qi zi* 枸杞子, *shan zha* 山楂, *shu di huang* 熟地黄, *yin yang huo* 淫羊藿, *chen pi* 陈皮, *fu ling* 茯苓, *ma qian zi* 马钱子, *fa ban xia* 法半夏, *ze xie* 泽泻 and *shan yao* 山药 (H237, H241).
Zi shui qing gan yin 滋水清肝饮	2	*Shu di* 熟地, *dang gui* 当归, *bai shao* 白芍, *suan zao ren* 酸枣仁, *shan yu rou* 山萸肉, *fu ling* 茯苓, *shan yao* 山药, *chai hu* 柴胡, *shan zhi zi* 山栀子, *mu dan pi* 牡丹皮 and *ze xie* 泽泻 (H213, H228).

Notes: (1) Ingredients are referenced to the original studies where possible. If herb ingredients varied across studies, the herb ingredients were sourced from *Zhong Yi Fang Ji Da Ci Dian* 中医方剂大辞典
(2) The use of some herbs may be restricted in some countries. Readers are advised to comply with relevant regulations.

Table 5.43 Frequently Reported Orally Used Herbs in Non-controlled Studies

Most Common Herbs	Scientific Name	Frequency of Use
Bai shao 白芍	*Paeonia lactiflora* Pall.	32
Shan yao 山药	*Dioscorea opposita* Thunb.	26
Shu di huang 熟地黄	*Rehmannia glutinosa* Libosch.	25
Fu ling 茯苓	*Poria cocos* (Schw.) Wolf	23
Shan zhu yu 山茱萸	*Cornus officinalis* Sieb. et Zucc.	22
Dang gui 当归	*Angelica sinensis* (Oliv.) Diels	21
Sheng di huang 生地黄	*Rehmannia glutinosa* Libosch.	19
Gou qi zi 枸杞子	*Lycium barbarum* L.	18
Mu dan pi 牡丹皮	*Paeonia suffruticosa* Andr.	17
Suan zao ren 酸枣仁	*Ziziphus jujuba* Mill. var. spinosa (Bunge) Hu ex H. F. Chou	17

(*Continued*)

Table 5.43 (*Continued*)

Most Common Herbs	Scientific Name	Frequency of Use
Gan cao 甘草	*Glycyrrhiza* spp.	16
Yin yang huo 淫羊藿	*Epimedium* spp.	16
Mu li 牡蛎	*Ostrea* spp.	15
Chai hu 柴胡	*Bupleurum* spp.	14
Nü zhen zi 女贞子	*Ligustrum lucidum* Ait.	14
Long gu 龙骨	Fossilised bones	13
Han lian cao 旱莲草	*Eclipta prostrata* L.	11
Tu si zi 菟丝子	*Cuscuta* spp.	11
Zhi mu 知母	*Anemarrhena asphodeloides* Bge.	11

Note: The use of some herbs may be restricted in some countries. Readers are advised to comply with relevant regulations.

common herb, followed by *shan yao* 山药, *shu di huang* 熟地黄, *fu ling* 茯苓 and *shan zhu yu* 山茱萸. The herbs in non-controlled studies were generally consistent with those seen in RCTs.

Safety of Oral Chinese Herbal Medicine in Non-controlled Studies

Ten non-controlled studies (H221, H243, H250, H253, H264–H269), including 1,234 women, reported on the safety of oral CHM in women with menopause symptoms. Three studies (H264, H265, H269) reported that no AEs occurred. There were 136 AEs reported in the remaining studies, including 105 cases of dry and thin vaginal mucosa, 15 cases of bitter taste in the mouth, five cases of increased menstruation, three cases of stomach discomfort when CHM was taken on an empty stomach, two cases of diarrhoea, and one case each of severe gastrointestinal reaction, postmenopausal bleeding, nausea, abdominal pain, abdominal fullness and mild vascular collapse unrelated to the intervention. The cases of nausea, abdominal pain, abdominal fullness and diarrhoea were considered likely to be related to treatment, with one participant withdrawing due to abdominal fullness. A further study (H268) reported mild stomach upset in two per cent of participants.

Topical Chinese Herbal Medicine

Four studies that evaluated topical CHM for menopause symptoms were included for further analysis. Three studies were RCTs (H272–H274) and one was a CCT (H275).

Randomised Controlled Trials of Topical Chinese Herbal Medicine

The three RCTs that evaluated topical CHM focused on sleep (H272) or vaginal symptoms of menopause (H273, H274). Studies were conducted in a hospital outpatient department in China (H272), a university hospital in Thailand (H274) and an unspecified setting in Iran (H273). One study (H272) included perimenopausal women with comorbid depression, while the other two included postmenopausal women (defined as more than 12 months of amenorrhoea) with vaginal symptoms. Two hundred and six women participated in these studies. The mean age of perimenopausal women was 48.8 years, while the mean age of postmenopausal women ranged from 52.9 to 56.4 years.

All studies included two parallel arms. None of the studies used CM syndrome differentiation for participant selection or for treatment. Interventions varied, as did the duration of treatment. One study used an investigator-developed multi-herb preparation consisting of the herbs *dang gui* 当归, *shu di* 熟地, *huang lian* 黄连 and *ye jiao teng* 夜交藤, which was applied as a foot bath for 28 days. Single herb preparations were used for a longer duration: fennel 5% cream (*xiao hui xiang* 小茴香) was used for eight weeks (H273), while *Pueraria mirifica* (*guo ye ge* 裹叶葛) was used for 12 weeks (H274). Comparators included diazepam (H272), placebo cream (H273) and CEE cream (H274).

All studies were described as using random allocation. One study (H274) used computer randomisation in blocks of four and was judged 'low' risk. Two studies did not describe the method of sequence generation and were judged as posing 'unclear' risk. None of the studies described how the allocation sequence was concealed ('unclear' risk). When topical CHM was compared with placebo (H273), participants, personnel and outcome assessors were blind to group allocation ('low' risk). Participants in the remaining two studies were not blind to group allocation, posing 'high' risk of bias. One study (H274) did not describe blinding of personnel ('unclear' risk), while the remaining study was judged 'high' risk as personnel were not blind to group allocation. Blinding of outcome assessors was not reported by Du *et al.* (H272). Suwanvesh *et al.* (H274) did not blind outcome assessors to group allocation and was judged as 'high' risk of bias. All studies were judged as 'low' risk for incomplete outcome data as there was no missing data (H272, H273) or statistical methods were used to account for missing data (H274).

Outcomes

One study (H272) evaluated the effect of topical CHM on sleep using the PSQI and two studies (H273, H274) measured various aspects of vaginal health.

Sleep Quality

One study (H272) applied topical CHM as a foot bath. At the end of 28 days of treatment with CHM, PSQI scores were 3.6 points higher than with diazepam (64 participants, [−4.73, −2.47]).

Vaginal Symptoms

The two studies that evaluated topical CHM for vaginal symptoms used different comparators and were not able to be pooled for meta-analysis. Yaralizadeh *et al.* (H273) assessed patient-reported vaginal burning, itching, dryness and dyspareunia in the 60 participants, which was assessed on a four-point scale. The authors found that fennel 5% cream increased the number of women who were symptom-free at the end of treatment for vaginal burning (RR 3.63 [2.00, 6.59]), itching (RR 1.97 [1.38, 2.81]), dryness (RR 20.33 [4.27, 96.93]) and dyspareunia (RR 57.00 [3.64, 892.83]), compared with placebo. None of the women in either the intervention or control group were symptom-free for physician-assessed vaginal pallor (also assessed on a four-point scale). This study also measured vaginal pH, which was reported as the number of women with a vaginal pH < 5, 5–5.49, 5.5–6.49, and > 6.5. As the normal pH range is 3.8 to 4.2 in reproductive women,[38] analysis was performed using the number of women with a vaginal pH less than 5. Fennel 5% cream was more effective than placebo in improving vaginal pH (RR 57.00 [3.64, 892.83]).

Vaginal cytology showed a higher proportion of superficial cells (MD 64.30% [58.12, 70.48]) and a lower proportion of intermediate (MD −54.00% [−60.30, −47.70]) and parabasal cells (MD −10.40%, [−12.93, −7.87]). The reduction in parabasal and intermediate cells and increase in proportion of superficial cells, indicate better vaginal health. Finally, the authors calculated a maturation value (MV) from vaginal cytology. The percentage of each cell type was multiplied by a factor (0 for parabasal cells, 0.5 for intermediate cells and 1.0 for superficial cells) and the MV was the sum of these values. All women had MV scores between 0 and 49 at baseline, indicating vaginal atrophy. At the end of treatment, all women who received fennel 5% cream had MV scores in the range of 65–100, while none of the women in the control group had MV score of 65–100.

Vaginal symptom scores were also assessed in the study by Suwanvesh *et al.* (H274). Vaginal symptoms of dryness, soreness, irritation, discharge and dyspareunia were scored on a four-point scale and scores were summed to provide a total score. *Guo ye ge* 裹叶葛 was not statistically different to CEE for the overall vaginal symptom score (82 participants, MD 0.27 points [−0.49, 1.03]) and for individual symptom scores for dryness (MD 0.02 points [−0.22,

0.26]), soreness (MD 0.07 points [−0.09, 0.23]), irritation (MD −0.03 points [−0.22, 0.16]), discharge (MD −0.02 points [−0.14, 0.10]) and dyspareunia (MD 0.20 points [−0.09, 0.49]).

Vaginal cytology reported as Vaginal Maturation Index found greater benefits with CEE than with *guo ye ge* 裹叶葛 (MD −19.34 points [−30.56, −8.12]). Vaginal health was assessed by a clinician during pelvic examination. The Vaginal Health Index (VHI) evaluates vaginal elasticity, pH, epithelial integrity, fluid volume and moisture on a scale of one to five. Women who received *guo ye ge* 裹叶葛 had a score 1.12 points higher at the end of treatment than women who received CEE ([0.30, 1.94]).

Safety of Topical Chinese Herbal Medicine in Randomised Controlled Trials

Two of the three RCTs (H273, H274) that evaluated topical CHM reported on AEs. No AEs occurred in these studies.

Controlled Clinical Trials of Topical Chinese Herbal Medicine

One non-randomised CCT (H275) met the inclusion criteria for this review. One hundred and twenty perimenopausal women with vaginitis were recruited from a hospital outpatient department in China. The average age of women was 62 years. Chinese medicine syndrome differentiation was not described. Women received treatment with *Bao fu kang shuan* 保妇康栓 (including the herbs *e zhu yu* 莪术油 and *bing pian* 冰片) for six days, and topical oestradiol benzoate was used in the comparator group. All women completed the follow-up assessment one week after the end of treatment.

The study assessed vaginal health for five items: rugae vaginales, vaginal moisture, vaginal pH, vaginal mucosa and vaginal discharge. Each item was scored from one to four and scores for all five items were summed to provide a total score (higher scores mean better vaginal health). The vaginal health score was 1.98 points higher in women who received *Bao fu kang shuan* 保妇康栓 compared with topical oestradiol benzoate ([1.36, 2.60]). No AEs occurred in the intervention group, while six cases of vaginal pain were reported in the comparator group.

Oral Plus Topical Chinese Herbal Medicine

One RCT (H276) evaluated the combination of oral and topical CHM, while none of the included CCTs or non-controlled studies evaluated this combination. The study was conducted in a hospital outpatient department in mainland China and involved 70 perimenopausal women. The mean age of women was 49 years and they had experienced menopausal symptoms for 17 months. The CM syndrome of Kidney *yin* deficiency was used as an inclusion criterion for the study and this diagnosis also guided treatment. Women in the intervention group received oral *Zhi bai di huang fang* 知柏地黄方 three times daily and washed daily with a CHM solution of herbs *di fu zi* 地肤子, *she chuang zi* 蛇床子, *ku shen* 苦参, *bai xian pi* 白鲜皮, *bai bu* 百部, *he shou wu* 何首乌, *bu gu zhi* 补骨脂, *dang gui* 当归, *he shi* 鹤虱, *rou cong rong* 肉苁蓉, *ku fan* 枯矾 and *er cha* 儿茶. Treatment was for two months. Women in the control group received Premarin® for 28 days followed by medroxyprogesterone acetate for four days; this constituted one cycle of treatment, which was repeated in the second month. No follow-up assessment was conducted once treatment ceased.

The study was described as using random allocation, but no details were provided for how this was done. Similarly, no information was described for how group allocation was concealed. The study was judged as 'unclear' risk of bias for sequence generation and allocation concealment. The study was judged to be 'high' risk for blinding of participants and personnel due to the nature of the interventions and comparators. It was unclear whether outcome assessors were blind to group allocation. All participants completed the study and data were available, posing 'low' risk of bias for incomplete outcome data. The study did not report trial registration and no trial protocol was identified. Subsequently, it was judged to be 'unclear' risk for the domain selective outcome reporting.

The study evaluated global change in menopause symptoms using mKI. Women who received the combination of oral plus topical CHM had a mean score 8.15 points lower at the end of treatment than women who received the Premarin®/medroxyprogesterone acetate combination ([−10.46, −5.84]). The study did not report on whether AEs occurred.

Clinical Evidence for Commonly Used Chinese Herbal Medicine Treatments

The clinical textbooks and guidelines that provided content for Chapter 2 have recommended the traditional formulas: *Zuo gui wan* 左归丸 plus *Er zhi wan* 二至丸, *You gui wan* 右归丸, *Er xian tang* 二仙汤, *Yi guan jian* 一贯煎 and *Tian wang bu xin dan* 天王补心丹. Commercially available manufactured products may also be selected according to CM syndrome differentiation. Manufactured products include *Liu wei di huang wan* 六味地黄丸, *Kun bao wan* 坤宝丸, *Geng nian an* 更年安, *Long feng bao jiao nang* 龙凤宝胶囊, *Kun tai jiao nang* 坤泰胶囊 and *Nü zhen ke li* 女珍颗粒. Several of these products have been tested in clinical studies. No clinical studies that met the inclusion criteria for this review tested *Zuo gui wan* 左归丸 plus *Er zhi wan* 二至丸, *You gui wan* 右归丸, *Tian wang bu xin dan* 天王补心丹, *Long feng bao jiao nang* 龙凤宝胶囊 or *Nü zhen ke li* 女珍颗粒. Results for other formulas are summarised below.

Er Xian Tang 二仙汤

Er xian tang 二仙汤 was used in eight RCTs (H27, H29, H70, H81, H86, H96, H135, H165). Three studies (H27, H29, H81) combined *Er xian tang* 二仙汤 with other formulas; evidence from these three studies will not be described here. The formula was modified when used alone.

One study (H29) compared *Er xian tang* 二仙汤 with placebo in 108 perimenopausal women. Modified *Er xian tang* 二仙汤 was not statistically different to placebo in terms of daily hot flush frequency at the end of treatment (MD −0.20 flushes [−1.24, 0.84]), but was more effective than placebo at follow-up (MD −0.70 flushes [−0.97, −0.43]). A similar result was seen for daily hot flush severity: MD −2.10 points [−4.79, 0.59] at end-of-treatment and MD −1.50 points [−2.69, −0.31] at follow-up. This trend was also seen on the MRS. The MRS total score at the end of treatment was not statistically different between the two groups (MD −2.50 points [−5.16, 0.16]) but was lower at follow-up in women who received modified *Er xian tang* 二仙汤 (MD −6.70 points [−8.22, −5.18]).

Modified *Er xian tang* 二仙汤 resulted in a lower MENQOL total score at the end of treatment compared to placebo (MD −11.70 points [−18.98, −4.42]); a finding that was also seen at follow-up (MD −26.40 points [−33.04, −19.76]). End-of-treatment domain scores were also lower with modified *Er xian tang* 二仙汤 for the physical (MD −6.40 points [−12.36, −0.44]), psychosocial (MD −3.70 points [−7.06, −0.34]) and vasomotor domains (MD −2.60 points [−4.51, −0.69]). No difference between groups was found on the sexual domain (MD −0.60 points [−2.06, 0.86]).

Three studies (H70, H86, H135) compared modified *Er xian tang* 二仙汤 with pharmacotherapy. One study of 80 perimenopausal women showed a greater improvement in sleep symptoms on the AIS with modified *Er xian tang* 二仙汤 than with HT (MD −2.01 points [−2.34, −1.68]; H70). Depression scores on the HAM-D were lower among women who received modified *Er xian tang* 二仙汤 compared to women who received fluoxetine (60 women, MD −3.30 points [−5.41, −1.19]; H86). Modified *Er xian tang* 二仙汤 was not statistically different to HT on mKI (MD −0.97 points [−7.18, 5.24]; H135).

Two studies (H96, H165) tested the combination of *Er xian tang* 二仙汤 plus pharmacotherapy. When *Er xian tang* 二仙汤 was combined with fluoxetine, women in the treatment group reported lower scores, meaning better outcomes, on the Social Function Rating Scale (54 women, MD −8.20 points [−10.53, −5.87]; H96), while fluoxetine alone was superior to the combination of fluoxetine and *Er xian tang* 二仙汤 on HAM-D (54 women, MD 10.70 points [9.47, 11.93]; H96). Women who recived *Er xian tang* 二仙汤 as integrative medicine reported lower scores on the KI than women who received HT alone (236 women, MD −1.48 points [−2.38, −0.58]; H165).

Three studies (H27, H81, H86) reported on safety with *Er xian tang* 二仙汤 used alone. Women who received *Er xian tang* 二仙汤 reported three cases of nausea and three cases of mild diarrhoea. One participant in the treatment group withdrew due to headaches, nausea, excessive perspiration and intermittent aching in the limbs.

Yi Guan Jian 一贯煎

One non-controlled study (H217) tested *Yi guan jian* 一贯煎 in menopausal women. The study did not report whether AEs occurred during treatment.

Liu Wei Di Huang Wan 六味地黄丸

Six RCTs (H54, H113, H154, H173, H184, H277) tested the formula *Liu wei di huang wan* 六味地黄丸. Three studies (H54, H113, H173) combined *Liu wei di huang wan* 六味地黄丸 with other formulas; results from these studies will not be presented here. Clinical outcomes were able to be analysed for one study (H154). *Liu wei di huang wan* 六味地黄丸 was not statistically different to HT in mKI scores at the end of treatment (50 women, MD 0.44 points [−1.20, 2.08]).

Kun Bao Wan 坤宝丸

Kun bao wan 坤宝丸 was tested in two RCTs (H136, H163). Meta-analysis was possible for the mKI, which showed no difference between *Kun bao wan* 坤宝丸 and HT (two RCTs, 101 women, SMD 0.27 [−0.31, 0.85], $I^2 = 50\%$). One study (H163) reported on safety, with no AEs occurring.

Geng Nian An 更年安

One RCT (H31) of 69 women tested *Geng nian an* 更年安 against placebo. The treatment resulted in a decrease in the proportion of parabasal cells (MD −2.50% [−3.17, −1.83]) and intermediate cells (MD −9.00% [−11.12, −6.88]) on the Vaginal Maturation Index, with a corresponding increase in the proportion of superficial cells (MD −11.50% [6.83, 16.17]). This shift to the right was not seen in the control group and suggests improvement of vaginal atrophy with *Geng nian an* 更年安. The study also reported on global symptom severity using the mKI. Total mKI score at the end of treatment was lower with *Geng nian an* 更年安 than with placebo (MD −2.33 points [−2.95, −1.71]).

Results for individual items of the mKI showed no difference between *Geng nian an* 更年安 and placebo in scores for melancholia (MD −0.08 points [−0.56, 0.41]) and formication (MD −0.23 points [−0.71, 0.26]). Benefits were seen with *Geng nian an* 更年安 compared to placebo for vasomotor symptoms (MD −3.11 points [−3.84, −2.38]), insomnia (MD −2.64 points [−3.31, −1.97]), vertigo (MD −2.20 points [−2.81, −1.58]), weakness (MD −2.43 points [−3.08, −1.79]), arthralgia (MD −1.55 points [−2.11, −1.00]), palpitations (MD −2.40 points [−3.05, −1.76]), tinnitus (MD −1.61 points [−2.17, −1.05]) and irritability (MD −2.12 points [−2.73, −1.51]). No AEs occurred during the trial.

Kun Tai Jiao Nang 坤泰胶囊

Ten RCTs (H1–H10) tested *Kun tai jiao nang* 坤泰胶囊. One study (H1) combined *Kun tai jiao nang* 坤泰胶囊 with another formula; the results for this study will not be presented here. *Kun tai jiao nang* 坤泰胶囊 was not statistically different to HT in improving menopausal symptoms on the KI (four RCTs, 329 women, SMD −0.02 [−0.24, 0.19], I^2 = 0%; Table 5.44). Meta-analysis of two studies with 145 women showed women who received HT reported lower scores, indicating greater improvement, on the vasomotor domain of the MENQOL (MD 0.89 points [0.14, 1.65], I^2 = 0%). No such differences were seen on the physical, psychosocial or sexual domains of the MENQOL.

Three studies (H2–H4) tested the effect of *Kun tai jiao nang* 坤泰胶囊 as integrative medicine with HT on KI. *Kun tai jiao nang* 坤泰胶囊 as integrative medicine was not statistically different to HT in KI

Table 5.44 *Kun Tai Jiao Nang* 坤泰胶囊 versus Hormone Therapy

Assessment	No. of Studies (Participants)	Effect Size (MD/SMD [95% CI], I^2)	Included Studies
KI	4 (329)	SMD −0.02 [−0.24, 0.19], 0%	H5–H7, H10
MENQOL — physical	2 (145)	MD 0.51 [−2.67, 3.68], 0%	H5, H8
MENQOL — psychosocial	2 (145)	MD 0.66 [−1.52, 2.84], 0%	H5, H8
MENQOL — vasomotor	2 (145)	MD 0.89 [0.14, 1.65]*, 0%	H5, H8
MENQOL — sexual	2 (145)	MD 0.08 [−1.40, 1.56], 0%	H5, H8

*Statistically significant, see Chapter 4.
Abbreviations: CI, confidence interval; KI, Kupperman Index; MD, mean difference; MENQOL, Menopause-specific Quality of Life questionnaire; SMD, standardised mean difference.

score at the end of treatment (three studies, 498 participants, SMD −0.62 [−1.27, 0.03], I^2 = 90%; H2–H4). One study (H4) of 118 women also reported results for each item of the KI. *Kun tai jiao nang* 坤泰胶囊 as integrative medicine was more effective than HT in improving vasomotor symptoms (MD −0.99 points [−1.23, −0.75]), melancholia (MD −0.26 points [−0.40, −0.12]), arthralgia (MD −0.11 points [−0.18, −0.04]) and dyspareunia (MD −0.70 points [−0.82, −0.58]). Hormone therapy alone was more effective than the combination of *Kun tai jiao nang* 坤泰胶囊 and HT in reducing palpitations (MD 0.11 points [0.06, 0.16]). No difference was seen between the two groups for the items paraesthesia (MD −0.02 points [−0.11, 0.07]), insomnia (MD 0.10 points [−0.05, 0.25]), nervousness (MD 0.04 points [−0.05, 0.13]), vertigo (MD −0.03 points [−0.14, 0.08]), weakness (MD −0.05 points [−0.16, 0.06]), headache (MD −0.05 points [−0.12, 0.02]) and formication (MD −0.03 points [−0.08, 0.02]).

Six studies (H2, H6–H10) reported on safety of *Kun tai jiao nang* 坤泰胶囊. Adverse events in people who received *Kun tai jiao nang* 坤泰胶囊 alone included 23 cases of breast pain, 15 cases of vaginal bleeding, six cases of gastrointestinal symptoms and four cases of nausea and vomiting. When *Kun tai jiao nang* 坤泰胶囊 was used as integrative medicine in one study (H2), AEs included 16 cases of gastrointestinal discomfort, five cases of irregular vaginal bleeding and four cases of breast pain.

Summary of Chinese Herbal Medicine Clinical Evidence

The symptoms that manifest during the menopausal transition are bothersome for women and can affect their quality of life. Hormone therapy is effective; however, some women may wish to use complementary treatments for symptom relief. Chinese herbal medicines have been tested for menopausal symptoms in many clinical studies, of which a selection have been presented in this review.

There appeared to be two natural groupings according to where the study was conducted. Studies conducted in China tended to describe women as 'perimenopausal', studied women with comorbidities such as depression, anxiety or insomnia, compared CHM with pharmacotherapy (HT or pharmacotherapy for comorbidities) and focused on global assessment of menopausal symptoms or symptoms related to comorbidities. Few studies reported criteria used to determine perimenopausal status. Studies conducted outside of China tended to focus on either perimenopausal or postmenopausal women, compared CHM with placebo, included assessment of vasomotor or vaginal symptoms in addition to global assessment of symptom severity, and assessed the impact of symptoms on HRQoL.

The difference in comparators according to the study location is likely to relate to cultural differences in the acceptability of CM. In China, CM is an established medical system and testing effectiveness against conventional medical treatments is more appropriate than testing efficacy against placebo. Outside of China, complementary therapies are not typically part of the mainstream medical system and the focus is largely on assessing efficacy.

The reasons for other differences between studies are less clear. Avis *et al.* (2001)[39] suggest there is no universal experience of menopause, and ethnic variations in menopausal symptoms have been identified.[40,41] For example, more Caucasian women experience hot flushes and sweating than Asian women.[40] In this review, the majority of studies that assessed vasomotor symptoms were conducted outside of China. It is possible that studies conducted in China are addressing the symptoms most bothersome to Chinese women, although further research would need to examine this in more detail.

The median duration of treatment in oral CHM RCTs, which comprised the majority of included studies, was eight weeks. This is typical for studies of CHM and reflects clinical practice. This may be sufficient to provide relief from symptoms. When considering that menopausal symptoms may persist for more than ten years,[42] the question of whether a (comparatively) short course of treatment can alleviate symptoms in the long term remains unanswered by this review.

Chinese medicine uses syndrome differentiation to tailor treatments according to each individual's signs, symptoms and concerns. Syndrome differentiation was described in 86 of the 281 included studies (30.6%). Syndromes related to the CM concepts of *yin* and/or *yang* deficiency and *qi* stagnation, and were often connected to the Kidney, Liver and Heart. The syndromes reported in clinical studies aligned with those described in contemporary clinical textbooks and guidelines (see Chapter 2).

Oral CHM is clearly the preferred route of administration tested in clinical studies, which reflects clinical practice for CM management of menopausal symptoms. Treatments tested in these studies were analysed to identify the most common formulas and herbs used. Analysis of formulas was conducted based on the formula name, not herb ingredients, due to the complexity of assessing similarity based on constituents. Diversity was seen in the treatments used, with more than 120 different CHM named formulas described in included studies. The most frequently tested formulas were the manufactured product *Kun tai jiao nang* 坤泰胶囊 and the traditional formulas *Xiao yao wan/san* 逍遥丸/散, *Er xian tang* 二仙汤 and *Suan zao ren tang* 酸枣仁汤, although none of these were tested in more than ten studies.

Given the diversity of CHM formulas, analysis of herb ingredients may provide a clearer picture of the actions of formulas. Some of the most frequently used herbs have actions that nourish the Kidneys, *yin* and *jing* 精 (for example, *shu di huang* 熟地黄, *sheng di huang* 生地黄 and *zhi mu* 知母), tonify Blood (for example, *dang gui* 当归) and nourish the Liver and Spleen (for example, *shan zhu yu* 山茱萸 and *shan yao* 山药). These actions address the CM syndromes described in the included studies and match the syndromes described in Chapter 2. The herbs that appeared with high frequency appear to have been influenced by the comorbidities reported in included studies. For example, *suan zao ren* 酸枣仁 was used 60 times among the 191 oral CHM RCTs. This herb has actions of constraining the Heart *qi* and calming the nerves and is often included in formulas for sleep disturbances. Many included studies focused on menopausal women with insomnia; hence it was not surprising that this herb appeared with high frequency.

Clinical outcomes were analysed in meta-analyses where possible or presented for individual studies if not possible. Results from meta-analyses of RCTs provided the best estimate of the treatment effect with CHM. Meta-analyses showed benefits with oral CHM, compared to placebo, in reducing daily hot flush frequency and severity, improving sleep quality on the PSQI, and improving global symptom severity on the original or mKI and the MRS. Favourable results for oral CHM in reducing daily hot flush frequency appeared to be influenced by one double-blind RCT (H19), although the reasons for this are unclear. The benefits found come with caveats — many studies were considered to have several potential sources of bias, and the certainty of results is limited.

Meta-analyses showed oral CHM was more effective than pharmacotherapy in improving sleep quality on the PSQI, AIS and SRSS, improving depressive symptoms on the HAM-D, improving anxiety symptoms on the HAM-A, improving global symptom severity on the original or mKI, and improving HRQoL on some domains of the SF-36. Benefits were also seen in meta-analyses when oral CHM was used as integrative medicine in improving sleep quality on the PSQI, improving anxiety on the SAS, improving depressive symptoms on the HAM-D, and improving global symptom severity on the original or mKI. Meta-analysis was not possible in studies that tested topical CHMs, or the combination of oral plus topical CHM.

Considerable statistical heterogeneity was seen in many of these analyses, which limits our confidence in the results. While positive effects of CHM were seen for some outcomes, no benefit of CHM was seen for many others. For example, CHM was not superior to placebo or pharmacotherapy in improving women's HRQoL when assessed using menopause-specific outcome scales. Furthermore, many studies had methodological shortcomings and/or incomplete reporting that raised questions about the accuracy and reliability of the data. As a result, confidence in the results of meta-analyses is lowered.

Many studies reported on safety of CHMs. Generally, AEs with CHMs were lower than with pharmacotherapy, although a lack of blinding may have contributed to this finding. The nature of AEs among women who received CHM and those who received pharmacotherapy was similar. It is possible that these may not be due to the treatments received but may be related to the menopausal transition (e.g., irregular vaginal bleeding) or may be due to natural ageing. Clinicians should continue to monitor patients for potential side effects of CHM.

There are several limitations of this review. While all studies involved menopausal women, only a small proportion of studies described criteria for menopausal status relating to FSH level or amenorrhoea. Subgroup analysis was conducted, where possible, to distinguish benefits according to menopausal status, but categorisation was based on the study description rather than according to any criteria described by study authors for menopausal status. Thus, we cannot be certain that the results found are truly reflective of outcomes for each stage of menopause.

Deviations were noted in the scoring for some outcomes such as the KI, MENQOL, MRS and SF-36. In the case of the SF-36, there is a strong argument against calculating a total score, as this produces a biased result.[43] Results for included studies that reported a total score for the SF-36 were not included in analysis. For scoring of MENQOL, the standard approach is to calculate the mean score of items within each of the four domains (see section 'Menopause-specific Quality of Life' for more details). Some studies included in this review calculated the sum score (not mean score) for each domain, while others calculated a total score by adding together the four domain scores. Lewis *et al.* (2005)[44] suggest that a total score for the MENQOL may be calculated as the mean of the four domain scores. Results for studies that made modifications to the scoring of the MENQOL were analysed using SMD to account for differences.

A similar approach was used for the KI, such that results of studies using the original and modified versions of the KI were analysed using SMD. The use of SMD is considered a reasonable approach when conducting meta-analysis of different outcome scales that measure the same concept. One disadvantage of this approach is that the absolute difference between groups cannot be found, making it impossible to determine whether the result represents a clinically important change.

None of the studies were free from bias and many meta-analyses were limited by considerable statistical heterogeneity that was not able to be explained through various subgroup analyses. This substantially limits our confidence in the results. Finally, few studies reported the impact of CHM on women's quality of life. Given the bother associated with menopausal symptoms and the long duration of the menopausal transition, it is important to assess HRQoL in future CHM clinical studies.

References

1. Chen HY, Cho WC, Sze SC, *et al.* (2008) Treatment of menopausal symptoms with Er-xian decoction: A systematic review. *Am J Chin Med* **36**(2): 233–244.
2. Lee HW, Choi J, Lee Y, *et al.* (2016) Ginseng for managing menopausal woman's health: A systematic review of double-blind, randomized, placebo-controlled trials. *Medicine (Baltimore)* **95**(38): e4914.

3. Taylor-Swanson L, Thomas A, Ismail R, *et al.* (2015) Effects of traditional Chinese medicine on symptom clusters during the menopausal transition. *Climacteric* **18**(2): 142–156.
4. Xu LW, Jia M, Cui XJ, *et al.* (2012) Chinese herbal medicine for menopausal symptoms. *For Immunopathol Dis Therap* **3**(1): 71–89.
5. Xu LW, Jia M, Salchow R, *et al.* (2012) Efficacy and side effects of Chinese herbal medicine for menopausal symptoms: A critical review. *Evid Based Complement Alternat Med* **2012**: 568106.
6. Zhou Q, Tao J, Song H, *et al.* (2016) Chinese herbal medicine Kuntai capsule for treatment of menopausal syndrome: A systematic review of randomized clinical trials. *Complement Ther Med* **29**: 63–71.
7. Zhu X, Liew Y, Liu ZL. (2016) Chinese herbal medicine for menopausal symptoms. *Cochrane Database Syst Rev* **3**: Cd009023.
8. Zhang Y, Xu L, Zheng Y, *et al.* (2017) Traditional Chinese herbal medicine for perimenopausal depression of Chinese women: A meta-analysis. *World J Tradit Chin Med* **3**(3): 51–57.
9. 高毅东, 张松涛, 黄俊山, *et al.* (2017) 从肝肾论治围绝经期失眠的临床疗效Meta分析. 北京中医药大学学报 **40**(02): 172–176.
10. 何霞霞, 刘笑梅, 尚成英. (2016) 中医药治疗围绝经期失眠症的系统评价. 西部中医药 **29**(11): 61–65.
11. 胡安琪, 李勇. (2016) 疏肝法联合激素替代疗法治疗围绝经期综合征的Meta分析. 中国药物评价 **33**(06): 498–503.
12. 李存存, 王晶晶, 陈潮, *et al.* (2013) 坤泰胶囊与激素替代疗法治疗更年期综合征有效性和安全性比较的Meta分析. 中国中西医结合杂志 **33**(09): 1183–1190.
13. 聂鹤云, 黄少桐, 陈晓凡, *et al.* (2015) 加味酸枣仁汤与西药治疗更年期失眠疗效比较的系统评价. 实用中西医结合临床 **15**(12): 22–24, 34.
14. 曾令烽, 蒙昌荣, 李滋平, *et al.* (2015) 中医药辅助治疗围绝经期失眠研究的Meta分析. 中国实验方剂学杂志 **21**(18): 195–201.
15. 张庆云, 王继伟, 余金明. (2013) 坤泰胶囊与雌激素治疗绝经综合征有效性与安全性的荟萃分析. 中华医学杂志 **93**(43): 3445–3449.
16. Kupperman HS, Wetchler BB, Blatt MH. (1959) Contemporary therapy of the menopausal syndrome. *J Am Med Assoc* **171**: 1627–1637.
17. Hamilton M. (1960) A rating scale for depression. *J Neurol Neurosurg Psychiatry* **23**: 56–62.
18. Buysse DJ, Reynolds CF 3rd, Monk TH, *et al.* (1989) The Pittsburgh Sleep Quality Index: A new instrument for psychiatric practice and research. *Psychiatry Res* **28**(2): 193–213.

19. Hilditch JR, Lewis J, Peter A, *et al.* (2008) A menopause-specific quality of life questionnaire: Development and psychometric properties. *Maturitas* **61**(1–2): 107–121.
20. Bachmann G, Notelovitz M, Gonzalez S, *et al.* (1991) Vaginal dryness in menopausal women: Clinical characteristics and nonhormonal treatment. *Clin Pract Sex* **9**: 25–32.
21. Abdo C. (2006) Development and validation of female sexual quotient: A questionnaire to assess female sexual function. *Revista Brasileira de Medicina* **63**(9): 477–482.
22. Soldatos CR, Dikeos DG, Paparrigopoulos TJ. (2000) Athens Insomnia Scale: Validation of an instrument based on ICD-10 criteria. *J Psychosom Res* **48**(6): 555–560.
23. 肖卫东, 刘平, 马弘, *et al.* (2007) 睡眠障碍评定量表的信度和效度分析. 中国心理卫生杂志 **21**(1): 41–42, 51.
24. 李建明. (2012) 睡眠状况自评量表(SRSS) 简介. 中国健康心理学杂志 **20**(12): 1851.
25. Spiegel R. (1981) *Sleep and Sleepiness in Advanced Age*. M.T.P. Press, Lancaster, UK.
26. Zung WW. (1965) A self-rating depression scale. *Arch Gen Psychiatry* **12**: 63–70.
27. Zung WW. (1971) A rating instrument for anxiety disorders. *Psychosomatics* **12**(6): 371–379.
28. Beck AT, Ward CH, Mendelson M, *et al.* (1961) An inventory for measuring depression. *Arch Gen Psychiatry* **4**: 561–571.
29. Hamilton M. (1959) The assessment of anxiety states by rating. *Br J Med Psychol* **32**(1): 50–55.
30. Derogatis LR, Lipman RS, Covi L. (1973) SCL-90: An outpatient psychiatric rating scale — preliminary report. *Psychopharmacol Bull* **9**(1): 13–28.
31. Greene JG. (1976) A factor analytic study of climacteric symptoms. *J Psychosom Res* **20**(5): 425–430.
32. Heinemann LA, Potthoff P, Schneider HP. (2003) International versions of the Menopause Rating Scale (MRS). *Health Qual Life Outcomes* **1**: 28.
33. Carpenter JS. (2001) The Hot Flash Related Daily Interference Scale: A tool for assessing the impact of hot flashes on quality of life following breast cancer. *J Pain Symptom Manage* **22**(6): 979–989.
34. Sydora BC, Fast H, Campbell S, *et al.* (2016) Use of the Menopause-Specific Quality of Life (MENQOL) questionnaire in research and

clinical practice: A comprehensive scoping review. *Menopause* **23**(9): 1038–1051.

35. Ware JJ, Sherbourne C. (1992) The MOS 36-item short-form health survey (SF-36). I. Conceptual framework and item selection. *Med Care* **30**: 473–483.
36. Mahoney FI, Barthel DW. (1965) Functional evaluation: The Barthel Index. *Md State Med J* **14**: 61–65.
37. Deadman P, Al-Khafaji M, Baker K. (2000) *A Manual of Acupuncture*. Journal of Chinese Medicine Publications, East Sussex, UK.
38. Goldstein I. (2010) Recognizing and treating urogenital atrophy in postmenopausal women. *J Womens Health (Larchmt)* **19**(3): 425–432.
39. Avis NE, Stellato R, Crawford S, *et al.* (2001) Is there a menopausal syndrome? Menopausal status and symptoms across racial/ethnic groups. *Soc Sci Med* **52**(3): 345–356.
40. Im EO, Ko Y, Chee W. (2014) Ethnic differences in the clusters of menopausal symptoms. *Health Care Women Int* **35**(5): 549–565.
41. Obermeyer CM, Reher D, Saliba M. (2007) Symptoms, menopause status, and country differences: A comparative analysis from DAMES. *Menopause* **14**(4): 788–797.
42. Freeman EW. (2014) Hot flushes and the menopause: How long should they be expected to last? *Maturitas* **78**(3): 153–154.
43. Lins L, Carvalho FM. (2016) SF-36 total score as a single measure of health-related quality of life: Scoping review. *SAGE Open Med* **4**: 2050312116671725.
44. Lewis JE, Hilditch JR, Wong CJ. (2005) Further psychometric property development of the Menopause-Specific Quality of Life questionnaire and development of a modified version, MENQOL-Intervention questionnaire. *Maturitas* **50**(3): 209–221.

References for Included Chinese Herbal Medicine Clinical Studies

Study No.	References
H1	钱碧霞, 刘姣, 雷先兰, 等. (2017) 丹栀逍遥丸联合坤泰胶囊治疗围绝经期睡眠障碍肝郁化火证临床观察. 新中医 **49**(09): 91–93.

(*Continued*)

Study No.	References
H2	王国荣, 韩延霞. (2017) 激素替代疗法联合坤泰胶囊治疗围绝经期综合征患者的疗效及安全性. 中国妇幼保健 **32**(21): 5364–5366.
H3	闫莉, 程娟, 张静, 杜文芳, 鲁耀华, 张习军, 李博. (2017) 替勃龙联合坤泰胶囊治疗绝经综合征的疗效观察. 中国生化药物杂志 **37**(10): 48–50.
H4	宫春兰. (2016) 坤泰胶囊联合替勃龙治疗更年期综合征 **59** 例. 中国药业 **25**(04): 125–127.
H5	任红娟, 杨春. (2015) 坤泰胶囊对比雌孕激素序贯疗法治疗围绝经期综合征的临床疗效及对生存质量的影响. 中国生化药物杂志 **29**(02): 116–118.
H6	陈继明, 高红艳, 李沁. (2015) 坤泰胶囊治疗围绝经期综合征患者 30 例临床观察. 中医杂志 **56**(03): 231–234.
H7	陈春娟. (2014) 坤泰胶囊治疗绝经综合症的临床观察. 中医临床研究 **6**(07): 48–49.
H8	周玲玲, 许良智, 刘宏伟, 等. (2009) 性激素与中成药治疗对绝经早期妇女生存质量的影响及其成本效用分析. 南方医科大学学报 **29**(11): 2182–2186. 李文娟,许良智,刘宏伟, 等. (2010) 坤泰胶囊与激素替代疗法对绝经早期妇女认知功能及心理状态影响的随机对照临床研究. 中西医结合学报 **8**(04): 321–327.
H9	龚莉莉, 张绍芬, 纪律. (2008) 绝经早期激素与中药治疗对认知记忆和生存质量的影响. 生殖与避孕 **28**(01): 26–31.
H10	陈蓉, 林守清, 杨欣, 等. (2005) 坤泰胶囊治疗妇女更年期综合征的临床研究. 中国新药杂志 **14**(12): 1472–1476.
H11	肖娟, 王彩娟, 孔祥芳, 等. (2017) 疏肝解郁胶囊联合西医治疗围绝经期失眠疗效观察. 现代中西医结合杂志 **26**(23): 2584–2586.
H12	谢娜, 张建春, 王彩娟, 等. (2017) 疏肝解郁治则对围绝经期睡眠障碍(焦虑抑郁型)心理及 BDNF 影响. 辽宁中医药大学学报 **19**(10): 135–138.
H13	喻俊, 钟远惠, 朱海兵, 等. (2016) 疏肝解郁胶囊合并草酸艾司西酞普兰治疗更年期综合征的临床效果观察. 内蒙古中医药 **35**(09): 85.
H14	吴辉. (2015) 舒肝解郁胶囊与舍曲林治疗围绝经期焦虑抑郁障碍疗效对比. 现代养生 (10): 95.
H15	梁杰. (2012) 舒肝解郁胶囊治疗围绝经期女性的抑郁症的研究. 中国药物滥用防治杂志 **18**(06): 336–337.

(*Continued*)

(***Continued***)

Study No.	References
H16	Davis SR, Briganti EM, Chen RQ, *et al.* (2001) The effects of Chinese medicinal herbs on postmenopausal vasomotor symptoms of Australian women: A randomised controlled trial. *Med J Aust* **174**(2): 68–71.
H17	Haines CJ, Lam PM, Chung TKH, *et al.* (2008) A randomized, double-blind, placebo-controlled study of the effect of a Chinese herbal medicine preparation (Dang Gui Buxue Tang) on menopausal symptoms in Hong Kong Chinese women. *Climacteric* **11**(3): 244–251.
H18	Heger M, Ventskovskiy BM, Borzenko I, *et al.* (2006) Efficacy and safety of a special extract of Rheum rhaponticum (ERr 731) in perimenopausal women with climacteric complaints: A 12-week randomized, double-blind, placebo-controlled trial. *Menopause* **13**(5): 744–759.
H19	Kaszkin-Bettag M, Ventskovskiy BM, Solskyy S, *et al.* (2009) Confirmation of the efficacy of ERr 731 in perimenopausal women with menopausal symptoms. *Altern Ther Health Med* **15**(1): 24–34.
H20	Kupfersztain C, Rotem C, Fagot R, Kaplan B. (2003) The immediate effect of natural plant extract, *Angelica sinensis* and *Matricaria chamomilla* (Climex) for the treatment of hot flushes during menopause: A preliminary report. *Clin Exp Obstet Gynecol* **30**(4): 203–206.
H21	Menati L, Khaleghinezhad K, Tadayon M, Siahpoosh A. (2014) Evaluation of contextual and demographic factors on licorice effects on reducing hot flashes in postmenopause women. *Health Care Women Int* **35**(1): 87–99.
H22	Nahidi F, Kariman N, Simbar M, Mojab F. (2012) The study on the effects of *Pimpinella anisum* on relief and recurrence of menopausal hot flashes. *Iran J Pharm Res* **11**(4): 1079–1085.
H23	Nahidi F, Zare E, Mojab F, Alavi-majd H. (2012) Effects of licorice on relief and recurrence of menopausal hot flashes. *Iran J Pharm Res* **11**(2): 541–548.
H24	Nedeljkovic M, Tian L, KJi P, *et al.* (2014) Effects of acupuncture and Chinese herbal medicine (Zhi Mu 14) on hot flushes and quality of life in postmenopausal women: Results of a four-arm randomized controlled pilot trial. *Menopause* **21**(1): 15–24.
H25	Plotnikoff GA, Watanabe K, Torkelson C, *et al.* (2011) The TU-025 keishibukuryogan clinical trial for hot flash management in postmenopausal women: Results and lessons for future research. *Menopause* **18**(8): 886–892.

(***Continued***)

Study No.	References
H26	Steels E, Steele ML, Harold M, Coulson S. (2017) Efficacy of a proprietary *Trigonella foenum-graecum* L. de-husked seed extract in reducing menopausal symptoms in otherwise healthy women: A double-blind, randomized, placebo-controlled study. *Phytother Res* **31**(9): 1316–1322.
H27	van der Sluijs CP, Bensoussan A, Chang S, Baber R. (2009) A randomized placebo-controlled trial on the effectiveness of an herbal formula to alleviate menopausal vasomotor symptoms. *Menopause* **16**(2): 336–344.
H28	Xia Y, Zhao YQ, Ren M, *et al.* (2012) A randomized double-blind placebo-controlled trial of a Chinese herbal medicine preparation (Jiawei Qing'e Fang) for hot flashes and quality of life in perimenopausal women. *Menopause* **19**(2): 234–244.
H29	Zhong LLD, Yong Y, Tang GWK, *et al.* (2013) A randomized, double-blind, controlled trial of a Chinese herbal formula (Er-Xian decoction) for menopausal symptoms in Hong Kong perimenopausal women. *Menopause* **20**(7): 767–776.
H30	Manonai J, Chittacharoen A, Theppisai U, Theppisai H. (2007) Effect of *Pueraria mirifica* on vaginal health. *Menopause* **14**(5): 919–924.
H31	Zhou J, Qu F, Nan R, Tang DY. (2007) The effect of Chinese medicinal herbs in relieving menopausal symptoms in ovariectomized Chinese women. *Explore (NY)* **3**(5): 478–484.
H32	Larmo PS, Yang B, Hyssala J, *et al.* (2014) Effects of sea buckthorn oil intake on vaginal atrophy in postmenopausal women: A randomized, double-blind, placebo-controlled study. *Maturitas* **79**(3): 316–321.
H33	Chang A, Kwak BY, Yi K, Kim JS. (2012) The effect of herbal extract (EstroG-100) on pre-, peri- and post-menopausal women: A randomized double-blind, placebo-controlled study. *Phytother Res* **26**(4): 510–516.
H34	Postigo S, Lima SMRR, Yamada SS, *et al.* (2016) Assessment of the effects of *Tribulus terrestris* on sexual function of menopausal women. *Rev Bras Ginecol Obstet* **38**(3): 140–146.
H35	Jokar A, Kargosha A, Akarzadeh M, *et al.* (2016) Comparing the influence of relaxation training and consumption of valerian on insomnia of menopause women: A randomized clinical trial. *Afr J Tradit Complement Altern Med* **13**(1): 40–44.

(*Continued*)

(***Continued***)

Study No.	References
H36	Kamalifard M, Farshbaf-Khalili A, Namadian M, *et al.* (2018) Comparison of the effect of lavender and bitter orange on sleep quality in postmenopausal women: A triple-blind, randomized, controlled clinical trial. *Women Health* **58**(8): 851–865.
H37	Taavoni S, Ekbatani N, Kashaniyan M, Haghani H. (2011) Effect of valerian on sleep quality in postmenopausal women: A randomized placebo-controlled clinical trial. *Menopause* **18**(9): 951–955.
H38	王飞峰, 段金莲, 王冰, 等. (2018) 甘麦大枣汤加减治疗肾虚肝郁型围绝经期失眠的临床观察. 中国中医药科技 **25**(01): 106–107.
H39	姚奏英, 陈慧, 朱丽萍. (2018) 滋肾解郁宁心方加减治疗围绝经期失眠临床观察. 中成药 **40**(01): 240–242.
H40	高志生, 倪烨, 肖晓, 等. (2017) 补肾柔肝解郁汤治疗围绝经期抑郁症的临床观察. 中国中医基础医学杂志 **23**(03): 364–366.
H41	赖瑜梅, 徐守权, 孙玉霞, 等. (2017) 归脾汤加麦冬治疗围绝经期妇女失眠临床观察. 陕西中医 **38**(07): 831–832.
H42	徐德毅, 赵洁, 易军. (2017) 加味甘麦大枣汤治疗阳虚型更年期抑郁症疗效及对神经内分泌系统的影响. 现代中西医结合杂志 **26**(17): 1910–1912.
H43	赵国鹏, 张红丽, 薛晨, 等. (2017) 酸枣仁汤治疗更年期失眠患者的疗效分析. 山西中医 **33**(02): 20–21, 31.
H44	郭亚利, 周岳君, 苏艳. (2017) 滋水清肝饮加减治疗更年期失眠 101 例. 江西中医药大学学报 **29**(01): 32–34, 68.
H45	李健, 魏格玲. (2016) 滋肾调肝法对围绝经期失眠的近期和远期疗效观察. 四川中医 **34**(06): 175–177.
H46	张秋霞, 杨茜, 武传颖. (2015) 激素替代与自拟安神丸治疗更年期综合征的对照研究. 中国生化药物杂志 **35**(12): 97–99.
H47	叶婉纯, 叶人, 袁拯忠, 王海波, 倪小芬, 方媚媚. (2015) 甲乙归藏汤加味治疗围绝经期失眠症临床观察. 广西中医药 **38**(02): 19–20.
H48	袁月平. (2015) 舒肝清胃养阴安神法治疗围绝经期失眠临床研究. 实用中医药杂志 **31**(06): 511.
H49	吴斐. (2015) 酸枣仁汤合左归丸治疗妇女更年期失眠 45 例. 河南中医 **35**(06): 1216–1218.
H50	刘宏娜. (2015) 酸枣仁汤加味辅治更年期失眠的临床疗效观察. 家庭心理医生 **1:** 344–345.

(***Continued***)

Study No.	References
H51	白桦, 王静, 刘法. (2014) 补肾乐眠汤治疗围绝经期妇女顽固性失眠临床观察. 陕西中医 **35**(06): 666–668.
H52	王俊. (2014) 更年期不寐患者应用加味酸枣仁汤治疗的临床效果观察. 中国卫生产业 **11**(25): 180–181.
H53	陈萍, 王淼, 吴佳璇. (2014) 李氏引火汤治疗女性更年期不寐 58 例. 西部中医药 **27**(08): 57–58.
H54	李桦, 项颗, 马琳. (2014) 六味地黄汤合四逆散治疗女性更年期失眠症 22 例. 中国中医药现代远程教育 **12**(23): 30–31.
H55	韩丽娟, 王思明, 李胜前. (2014) 宁心安神汤治疗女性更年期失眠 67 例临床观察. 海峡药学 **26**(09): 84–86.
H56	张文静. (2014) 中药足部熏蒸治疗更年期失眠症的临床观察. 内蒙古中医药 **33**(18): 79–80.
H57	李清媛, 冀德才, 乔宇. (2013) 酸枣仁汤加减治疗更年期失眠症疗效观察. 中国实用医药 **8**(07): 154–155.
H58	杜巧琳, 王小云. (2009) 舒肝胶囊对更年期抑郁症妇女抑郁情绪及睡眠障碍的影响研究. 中国广东广州.
H59	曹腊梅, 郭旭琴, 朱普贤, 等. (2018) 清心镇肝方对围绝经期失眠患者血清性激素及 5-羟色胺水平影响. 临床军医杂志 **46**(02): 139–141.
H60	沈涌, 王志伟. (2018) 疏肝健脾汤治疗围绝经期睡眠障碍的疗效观察及对 Kupperman, SAS, SDS 评分影响. 中华中医药学刊 **36**(02): 496–498.
H61	芮绵, 王丽, 王彩娟, 等. (2017) 清肝泻心汤加减治疗围绝经期失眠临床疗效及对血清 5-HT 水平的影响研究. 现代中西医结合杂志 **26**(26): 2904–2906.
H62	邓建平, 沈咏慧, 孙丹, 等. (2017) 舒心滋肾方配合舒乐安定治疗围绝经期女性失眠伴焦虑疗效观察. 浙江临床医学 **19**(5): 885–886, 888.
H63	郑捷. (2017) 酸枣仁汤治疗女性更年期失眠 60 例效果观察. 中国校医 **31**(07): 522, 525.
H64	肖高红. (2017) 调冲安神汤对更年期综合征伴失眠患者睡眠质量的影响. 临床医学研究与实践 **2**(25): 111–112.
H65	张新成. (2017) 逍遥散加减联合抗焦虑药治疗更年期失眠症的疗效观察. 实用中西医结合临床 **17**(11): 84–85.
H66	刘曲慧, 孙小翠. (2016) 更年舒片联合替勃龙片对围绝经期综合征患者血脂代谢及激素水平的影响. 中医学报 **31**(06): 889–891, 895.

(*Continued*)

(*Continued*)

Study No.	References
H67	郑艳辉. (2016) 桂枝加龙骨牡蛎汤治疗围绝经期焦虑性失眠障碍患者的疗效观察. 中国初级卫生保健 **30**(11): 59–60.
H68	刘娜娜, 王赛, 康斐. (2016) 调冲安神汤治疗更年期综合征伴失眠临床研究. 河南中医 **36**(10): 1775–1777.
H69	柳芬. (2014) 酸枣仁汤加减与黛力新治疗更年期抑郁症的临床疗效观察. 中华中医药学刊 **32**(12): 3044–3046.
H70	石国令. (2017) 二仙汤加味方治疗更年期综合征临床观察. 四川中医 **35**(01): 125–127.
H71	张亚敏, 陈雷. (2009) 固元宁神汤治疗心肾不交型围绝经期失眠症临床观察. 上海中医药杂志 **43**(05): 39–40.
H72	张蓉, 宋李冬. (2012) 柴胡加龙骨牡蛎汤治疗围绝经期患者失眠的疗效. 中国临床医学 **19**(02): 175–176.
H73	程梦婕, 胡剑卓. (2017) 加味酸枣仁汤合温胆汤治疗女性更年期失眠疗效观察. 实用中医药杂志 **33**(10): 1131–1133.
H74	姚憬, 王忠建, 朱微微, 等. (2014) 膏方调治肝肾阴虚型围绝经期失眠症临床研究. 辽宁中医杂志 **41**(09): 1921–1922.
H75	居跃君. (2011) 从肝肾论治围绝经期失眠症临床观察. 光明中医 **26**(07): 1403–1404.
H76	叶玉妹, 杨慰, 张晓丹, 等. (2010) 宁神合剂治疗妇女更年期失眠症临床观察. 上海中医药杂志 **44**(02): 47–48, 80.
H77	王桂英, 冯绍明, 田力铭. (2015) 补肾疏肝汤治疗围绝经期综合征 56 例临床观察. 河北中医 **37**(05): 676–678.
H78	郝焕妮, 蒋海玲, 康志媛. (2017) 中西医结合治疗更年期抑郁症临床研究. 中医学报 **32**(06): 1018–1020.
H79	孙艳明. (2013) 滋水清肝饮加减治疗围绝经期综合征相关情绪障碍的临床观察. 天津中医药 **30**(11): 660–662.
H80	Kashani L, Esalatmanesh S, Eftekhari F, *et al.* (2018) Efficacy of *Crocus sativus* (saffron) in treatment of major depressive disorder associated with post-menopausal hot flashes: A double-blind, randomized, placebo-controlled trial. *Arch Gynecol Obstet* **297**(3): 717–724.

(Continued)

Study No.	References
H81	黄敏琪. (2017) 二仙汤合柴胡加龙骨牡蛎汤治疗围绝经期女性抑郁症的研究. 南京中医药大学.
H82	徐志男. (2017) 加味乌梅丸汤剂治疗围绝经期抑郁的临床观察. 中国中医科学院.
H83	施凤, 李素, 张婧. (2017) '清心滋肾汤'加味对围绝经期抑郁症的临床效果分析. 中国现代医药杂志 **19**(11): 10–13.
H84	周之人. (2016) 酸枣仁汤联合氟哌噻吨美利曲辛与谷维素治疗围绝经期抑郁随机平行对照研究. 实用中医内科杂志 **30**(09): 55–57.
H85	唐贺利, 田霖, 闫昕. (2016) 调更解郁方治疗更年期抑郁症 30 例临床研究. 江苏中医药 **48**(9): 41–43.
H86	李光义. (2014) 加味二仙汤治疗更年期抑郁症的临床研究. 山东中医药大学.
H87	马小娟, 冯振宇, 赵杰, 王虹娟, 董馨德. (2014) 加味甘麦大枣汤对更年期抑郁症患者血清单胺类神经递质的影响. 山西中医学院学报 **15**(05): 42–44. 冯振宇, 赵杰. (2014) 加味甘麦大枣汤治疗女性更年期抑郁症的临床疗效观察. 内蒙古中医药 **33**(18): 9–10.
H88	许凤全, 张莹, 张琳园. (2013) 补肾疏肝化瘀汤治疗围绝经期抑郁症 82 例临床研究. 河北中医 **35**(03): 333–334.
H89	邵晓林. (2011) 解郁丸与米安色林治疗更年期抑郁的临床观察. 中国民康医学 **23**(09): 1107–1109.
H90	陈力, 杨广野, 王荷琴. (2011) 乌灵胶囊联合逍遥丸治疗更年期抑郁症的疗效观察. 中国实用医药 **6**(19): 179–180.
H91	李英杰. (2010) 加减柴胡加龙骨牡蛎汤治疗围绝经期抑郁症 36 例疗效观察. 河北中医 **32**(11): 1654–1655.
H92	何军琴. (2008) 补肾调肝清心方对围绝经期抑郁症患者睡眠障碍的治疗机理探讨. 中国中医药信息杂志 **15**(06): 16–18.
H93	张瑞芬. (2007) 消更解郁汤治疗肾虚肝郁型围绝经期抑郁症的临床研究. 山东中医药大学.
H94	高楠. (2010) 乐心汤治疗围绝经期抑郁症的临床观察. 黑龙江中医药大学.
H95	Qu F, Cai XF, Gu Y, *et al.* (2009) Chinese medicinal herbs in relieving perimenopausal depression: A randomized, controlled trial. *J Altern Complement Med* **15**(1): 93–100.

(Continued)

(***Continued***)

Study No.	References
H96	杨军. (2018) 加味二仙汤联合盐酸氟西汀胶囊治疗更年期抑郁症 27 例. 中医研究 **31**(01): 36–37.
H97	李克建, 郭娟, 陈云. (2017) 补肾解郁清心汤治疗更年期抑郁症疗效及对 DA, NE, 5-HIAA 的影响. 现代中西医结合杂志 **26**(26): 2864–2866, 2954.
H98	夏松柏, 虞冬辉. (2017) 甜梦口服液联合帕罗西汀治疗围绝经期抑郁症的临床观察. 中国药房 **28**(03): 344–347.
H99	孙利东. (2016) 中西医结合治疗更年期抑郁症效果探讨. 中外医疗 **35**(08): 153–154.
H100	赵冰, 赵瑞君, 张桂敏. (2016) 中药联合帕罗西汀治疗围绝经期抑郁症 40 例效果. 药物与临床 **55**: 122.
H101	张学团. (2016) 自拟解郁方联合艾司西酞普兰治疗更年期综合征的效果观察. 社区医学杂志 **14**(04): 51–52.
H102	王勇, 康明秀, 马静, 毛稚霞, 程娟, 窦光茜. (2015) 度洛西汀联合百合地黄汤加减治疗围绝经期抑郁症对照研究. 临床心身疾病杂志 **21**(5): 44–46.
H103	虞红霞. (2015) 归脾汤联合黛力新治疗更年期抑郁症临床观察. 新中医 **47**(12): 140–141.
H104	王海岭, 王传升. (2015) 文拉法辛联合九味镇心颗粒治疗围绝经期焦虑抑郁症的临床研究. 中国医药导报 **12**(02): 86–88.
H105	王春钢, 梅静, 张燕, 张红. (2015) 中药联合帕罗西汀治疗围绝经期抑郁症 46 例. 河南中医 **35**(3): 578–579.
H106	张慧珍, 山书玲, 赵纯. (2014) 四二五合方合甘麦大枣汤治疗围绝经期抑郁症临床观察. 中国中医基础医学杂志 **20**(09): 1256–1257.
H107	李彬, 李桂荣, 董立娜. (2013) 解忧汤联合西药治疗更年期抑郁症的疗效研究. 中国当代医药 **20**(06): 136–137.
H108	张翠花, 姚武斌. (2011) 帕罗西汀联合乌灵胶囊治疗女性围绝经期抑郁症临床疗效评价. 求医问药 **9**(12): 545–546.
H109	陈慧, 姚奏英, 卢俊明, 赵丽芬, 朱丽萍. (2011) 中西医联合治疗围绝经期抑郁症的临床观察. 中国中医药科技 **18**(05): 429–430.
H110	任凯, 姜晓岩, 赵希武. (2009) 帕罗西汀联合大补阴丸治疗女性更年期抑郁症疗效观察. 中国医药 **4**(3): 223–224.
H111	张广强, 张广普, 艾长明, 谢永强, 赵文学, 岳春芝. (2009) 枣仁补血汤联合氟西汀治疗更年期抑郁症 38 例临床观察. 北京中医药 **28**(11): 873–874.

(*Continued*)

Study No.	References
H112	刘茹. (2007) 中西医结合治疗更年期抑郁症的对照研究. 北京中医 **26**(08): 512–513.
H113	熊辉, 张倩平, 陶玉玲, 汤翔群, 关红. (2008) 中西医结合与单纯性激素治疗围绝经期抑郁症. 中国生育健康杂志 **19**(02): 76–78.
H114	王全利, 姚石安. (2012) 静顺袋泡茶治疗女性围绝经期焦虑疗效观察. 现代中西医结合杂志 **21**(05): 515–516.
H115	吴海芬. (2012) 中医药治疗更年期焦虑症 44 例. 福建中医药 **43**(05): 44–45.
H116	杨洪波, 冯丽平. (2011) 甘麦巴芪汤治疗女性更年期焦虑症 78 例临床观察. 中国中医药科技 **18**(02): 142–143.
H117	霍军, 于海亭, 孔德荣, 等. (2008) 女性更年期焦虑的中西医对比治疗研究. 医药论坛杂志 **29**(12): 61–62.
H118	吕梦亮, 彭思菡, 何淑娴. (2017) 桂枝甘草龙骨牡蛎汤加减治疗围绝经失眠的临床分析. 光明中医 **32**(09): 1262–1263.
H119	张艳敏, 廖辉. (2013) 柴胡加龙骨牡蛎汤联合黛力新治疗围绝经期妇女广泛性焦虑状态 30 例临床观察. 四川中医 **31**(04): 88–89.
H120	Qian LQ, Wang B, Niu JY, *et al.* (2010) Assessment of the clinical effect of Chinese medicine therapy combined with psychological intervention for treatment of patients of peri-menopausal syndrome complicated with hyperlipidemia. *Chin J Integr Med* **16**(2): 124–130.
H121	杨琪. (2015) 更年安神胶囊治疗围绝经期综合征(肾阴阳两虚证)的随机对照临床观察. 湖北中医药大学.
H122	倪爽, 李佶, 张莉, 戴熠婷, 伍睿昕, 韩小丽. (2015) 更年宁心颗粒治疗围绝经期综合征随机, 双盲, 安慰剂对照临床观察. 上海中医药杂志 **49**(03): 35–37.
H123	唐逍. (2013) 知柏地黄丸治疗女性更年期综合征阴虚火旺证临床研究. 青岛大学.
H124	刘海红, 卢苏, 施亚平. (2011) 滋阴降火方治疗绝经综合征阴虚火旺证. 中国实验方剂学杂志 **17**(19): 268–270.
H125	Kim SY, Seo SK, Choi YM, *et al.* (2012) Effects of red ginseng supplementation on menopausal symptoms and cardiovascular risk factors in postmenopausal women: A double-blind randomized controlled trial. *Menopause* **19**(4): 461–466.

(*Continued*)

(*Continued*)

Study No.	References
H126	Park JY, Kim KH. (2016) A randomized, double-blind, placebo-controlled trial of *Schisandra chinensis* for menopausal symptoms. *Climacteric* **19**(6): 574–580.
H127	Yang HY, Yang J, Wen ZH, *et al.* (2012) Effect of combining therapy with traditional Chinese medicine-based psychotherapy and herbal medicines in women with menopausal syndrome: A randomized controlled clinical trial. *Evid Based Complement Alternat Med* **2012:** 354145.
H128	郭育兰, 张云. (2017) 黄芪赤风汤加减治疗围绝经期潮热多汗症临床研究. 河北中医药学报 **32**(05): 18–20.
H129	陈惠清, 伍朝霞, 杨林波. (2017) 焦宁汤治疗围绝经期焦虑症的临床观察. 河北中医 **39**(04): 529–532.
H130	刘姣, 卢益中, 江松平, 等. (2016) 滋肾平肝调冲法治疗围绝经期综合征临床观察. 新中医 **48**(06): 130–132.
H131	何洁. (2016) 滋肾养巢方治疗肾阴虚型绝经前后诸证的临床研究. 福建中医药大学.
H132	张玉蓉, 陈小平, 谢波, 曾科学. (2015) 补肾安冲方治疗肾阴虚型围绝经期综合征 30 例临床观察. 湖南中医杂志 **31**(05): 1–3.
H133	吴西志. (2015) 补肾安神汤治疗围绝经期妇女顽固性失眠症 45 例. 河南中医 **35**(09): 2142–2144.
H134	张弦, 叶璐, 鲁佩佩, 傅丹旦, 骆丽娜, 何若苹. (2015) 癫狂梦醒汤合逍遥散治疗气滞血瘀型围绝经期综合征 36 例观察. 浙江中医杂志 **50**(12): 896–897.
H135	李晓曼, 周英. (2015) 二仙汤治疗围绝经期综合征的疗效观察. 中国中医药现代远程教育 **13**(17): 24–26.
H136	郭睿, 刘砚韬. (2015) 坤宝丸治疗更年期综合征 32 例疗效及安全性分析. 中国药业 **24**(24): 223–224.
H137	沈敏. (2015) 秦伯未膏方治疗肝肾阴虚型绝经前后诸证的临床疗效观察. 南京中医药大学.
H138	赵伟. (2015) 中医辨证治疗围绝经期综合征的临床疗效. 医药 (7): 204–204.
H139	孙建华, 张晓丹, 翟沛. (2015) 自拟更年安汤治疗阴虚型绝经综合征 40 例临床观察. 中医临床研究 **7**(16): 20–22.

(*Continued*)

Study No.	References
H140	罗志娟, 吴剑兰, 吴媛媛, 等. (2014) 安脏汤与替勃龙治疗绝经综合征的临床疗效对比研究. 时珍国医国药 **25**(01): 128–129.
H141	孙迎春. (2014) 补肾活血法治疗肾虚血瘀型围绝经期综合征及对心脏变时功能影响的临床研究. 山东中医药大学.
H142	严春玲, 王辉皪, 刘普勇, 曹亚芳, 魏智慧, 李苹. (2014) 当归六黄汤治疗更年期综合征的临床研究. 四川中医 **32**(05): 95–97.
H143	杜冠华, 王颖, 尚敏捷. (2014) 更宁汤治疗绝经综合征 56 例疗效观察. 新中医 **46**(06): 135–137.
H144	张素, 徐莲薇, 张天嵩, 等. (2014) 和坤汤治疗围绝经期综合征临床观察. 上海中医药杂志 **48**(12): 59–60+62.
H145	莫达瑜. (2014) 宁更培元汤治疗肝肾阴亏型围绝经期综合征的临床观察. 中国中医药科技 **21**(06): 664–665.
H146	代杰. (2014) 调更补益汤治疗更年期综合征的作用评价. 内蒙古医学杂志 **46**(09): 1093–1094.
H147	吴翊群, 陈明, 叶丽华, 卜新华. (2014) 香芍颗粒治疗女性围绝经期综合征的疗效分析. 中国医药导刊 **16**(12): 1475–1476.
H148	王国彧, 陈小雪, 李滨. (2013) 安乐片治疗更年期综合症的临床研究. 中医药信息 **30**(04): 91–93.
H149	李淑娟. (2013) 熙坤汤治疗肾阴虚型绝经前后潮热的临床观察. 山东中医药大学.
H150	李丽, 杨岚, 彭灿. (2012) 补肾调冲法联合激素替代疗法治疗围绝经期综合征的临床研究. 中国医药科学 **2**(11): 83–84+91.
H151	杨立波. (2012) 黑逍遥散治疗肝肾阴虚型绝经前后诸症 50 例. 山东中医杂志 **31**(11): 797–798.
H152	马东玉, 刘明, 李实, 等. (2012) 滋肾生肝法治疗肝肾阴虚型更年期综合征临床研究. 中国医药导报 **9**(29): 123–125.
H153	张鸿宇, 罗晓. (2012) 左归丸合逍遥丸治疗围绝经期综合征. 中国实验方剂学杂志 **18**(12): 295–297.
H154	朱旭华, 程玲, 富冬梅. (2011) 补肾活血中药治疗围绝经期综合征肾虚血瘀型的临床研究. 成都中医药大学学报 **34**(01): 24–26.
H155	何惠玲, 李红, 邢瑞佳. (2011) 清心滋肾汤治疗围绝经期综合征 30 例. 陕西中医 **32**(11): 1450–1451.

(*Continued*)

(Continued)

Study No.	References
H156	冯艳. (2010) 清心滋肾汤治疗更年期综合征阴虚火旺证的临床研究. 南京中医药大学.
H157	王秋梅, 关秋云, 马丽爽. (2010) 益肾清心汤治疗肾阴虚型围绝经期综合征35 例疗效观察及对生殖激素的影响. 河北中医 **32**(11): 1618–1620.
H158	许新, 管凤刚, 周玉春, 金保方. (2009) 星状神经节阻滞术联合中医药治疗围绝经期综合征的临床观察. 南京中医药大学学报 **25**(04): 261–264.
H159	周玲玲, 许良智, 刘宏伟, 等. (2009) 性激素与中成药治疗对绝经早期妇女生存质量的影响及其成本效用分析. 南方医科大学学报 **29**(11): 2182–2186.
H160	高琦, 程慧莲. (2007) 舒更宁心汤治疗肾阴阳俱虚型围绝经期综合征疗效分析. 新疆医科大学学报 **30**(03): 290–292.
H161	王秋平. (2010) 滋肾生肝颗粒治疗肝肾阴虚型更年期综合征的临床研究. 南京中医药大学.
H162	于金凤, 高学娟, 贾桐, 张广美. (2005) 益坤宁治疗围绝经期综合征的临床观察. 中医药学报 **33**(02): 24–26.
H163	Azizi H, Liu YF, Du L, *et al.* (2011) Menopause-related symptoms: Traditional Chinese medicine versus hormone therapy. *Altern Ther Health Med* **17**(4): 48–53.
H164	陶朝慧. (2017) 补肾化瘀汤联合雌激素治疗肾虚血瘀型围绝经期综合征疗效观察. 时珍国医国药 **28**(04): 915–916.
H165	康建颖, 陆月红. (2017) 二仙汤治疗围绝经期综合症患者的临床疗效及对性激素的影响. 健康研究 **37**(03): 321–323.
H166	屈兴玲, 张艳, 李刚. (2017) 更年安神开郁方联合西药治疗肾虚肝郁型更年期综合征临床观察. 中医临床研究 **9**(09): 26–29.
H167	杨晓慧, 沈兰. (2017) 更年顺安汤为主治疗女性更年期综合征 92 例观察. 浙江中医杂志 **52**(01): 41.
H168	梁贵萍. (2017) 克龄蒙结合疏肝补肾中药对围绝经期综合征的临床研究. 中国现代药物应用 **11**(01): 27–29.
H169	陈永新, 李涛, 韩亚琼, 黄素培, 张瑞岭. (2017) 乌灵胶囊联合米氮平对更年期抑郁症患者神经内分泌的影响. 中药药理与临床 **33**(02): 200–203.
H170	张艺, 江南. (2016) 自拟凝神疏肝汤治疗围绝经期综合征(心肝火盛证)临床观察. 四川中医 **34**(01): 86–88.

(*Continued*)

Study No.	References
H171	袁野. (2015) 地贞颗粒治疗女性更年期综合征效果分析. 中外医学研究 **13**(31): 142–143.
H172	杨浩昭. (2015) 中西医结合治疗更年期综合征的临床疗效观察. 国际医药卫生导报 **21**(4): 533–535.
H173	刘洪, 郑桃晓, 郑小莉, 周贤刚. (2012) 中西医结合治疗更年期综合征 88 临床观察. 中医药导报 **18**(02): 47–49.
H174	Hsu CC, Kuo HC, Chang SY, *et al.* (2011) The assessment of efficacy of *Diascorea alata* for menopausal symptom treatment in Taiwanese women. *Climacteric* **14**(1): 132–139.
H175	Shamshad Begum S, Jayalakshmi HK, Vidyavathi HG, *et al.* (2016) A novel extract of fenugreek husk (FenuSMARTtm) alleviates postmenopausal symptoms and helps to establish the hormonal balance: A randomized, double-blind, placebo-controlled study. *Phytother Res* **30**(11): 1775–1784.
H176	古衍, 姚吉龙, 姜向坤. (2007) 补肾安神方治疗围绝经期失眠(阴虚火旺型) 32 例疗效观察. 新中医 **39**(09): 28–29.
H177	Chen LC, Tsao YT, Yen KY, *et al.* (2003) A pilot study comparing the clinical effects of Jia-Wey Shiau-Yau San, a traditional Chinese herbal prescription, and a continuous combined hormone replacement therapy in postmenopausal women with climacteric symptoms. *Maturitas* **44**(1): 55–62.
H178	Rahimikian F, Rahimi R, Golzareh P, *et al.* (2017) Effect of *Foeniculum vulgare* Mill. (fennel) on menopausal symptoms in postmenopausal women: A randomized, triple-blind, placebo-controlled trial. *Menopause* **24**(9): 1017–1021.
H179	Fu SF, Zhao YQ, Ren M, *et al.* (2016) A randomized, double-blind, placebo-controlled trial of Chinese herbal medicine granules for the treatment of menopausal symptoms by stages. *Menopause* **23**(3): 311–323.
H180	张其慧. (2006) 调肝理脾中药治疗围绝经期失眠 36 例临床观察. 中医杂志 **47**(09): 678–680.
H181	de Souza KZD, Vale FBC, Geber S. (2016) Efficacy of *Tribulus terrestris* for the treatment of hypoactive sexual desire disorder in postmenopausal women: A randomized, double-blinded, placebo-controlled trial. *Menopause* **23**(11): 1252–1256.

(*Continued*)

(*Continued*)

Study No.	References
H182	Kwee SH, Tan HH, Marsman A, Wauters C. (2007) The effect of Chinese herbal medicines (CHM) on menopausal symptoms compared to hormone replacement therapy (HRT) and placebo. *Maturitas* **58**(1): 83–90.
H183	Oh KJ, Chae MJ, Lee HS, *et al.* (2010) Effects of Korean red ginseng on sexual arousal in menopausal women: Placebo-controlled, double-blind crossover clinical study. *J Sex Med* **7**(4 Pt 1): 1469–1477.
H184	Qu F, Zhou J. (2009) Chinese medicinal herbs in relieving perimenopausal depression: A randomized, placebo-controlled trial. *Maturitas* **63:** S114.
H185	Tsuyoshi H, Iino K, Tarakida A, *et al.* (2011) Effects of Kamishoyosan (Japanese herbal medicine) for climacteric disorders compared with HT. *Climacteric* **14:** 139.
H186	李克建. (2017) 柏子养心汤加减治疗中老年围绝经期失眠症. 吉林中医药 **37**(12): 1219–1222.
H187	连利霞. (2017) 甘麦大枣汤合归脾汤加减治疗更年期抑郁症疗效观察. 临床医药文献电子杂志 **4**(39): 7701.
H188	刘艳, 王红艳, 宋威, 李蒙蒙. (2016) 帕罗西汀联合丹栀逍遥丸治疗合并睡眠障碍的女性围绝经期抑郁症患者的疗效. 神经疾病与精神卫生 **16**(4): 434–437.
H189	郭利红, 姚华强, 王芳. (2016) 清心解郁汤治疗围绝经期综合征抑郁症的临床观察. 陕西中医 **37**(09): 1203–1204.
H190	王芳. (2016) 滋肾舒坤汤治疗肾虚肝郁型绝经综合征情志异常的临床研究. 山东中医药大学.
H191	马荣, 葛桂敏. (2016) 自拟更年解七方对肝郁血虚型更年期抑郁症与艾司西太普兰的疗效对照观察. 中西医结合心血管病电子杂志 **4**(12): 109–110.
H192	石明晴, 韩克, 夏玉兰, 等. (2015) 倍美力软膏及知柏地黄丸治疗绝经妇女复发性泌尿生殖道感染临床观察. 光明中医 **30**(10): 2185–2187.
H193	贾丽红, 马建梅. (2015) 舍曲林合并甘麦大枣饮治疗更年期抑郁症对照研究. 山西职工医学院学报 **25**(06): 38–40.
H194	赵志成. (2015) 酸枣仁汤加减治疗更年期抑郁症的疗效研究. 中国医学工程 **23**(10): 80–83.

(*Continued*)

Study No.	References
H195	陈青微, 陈慧. (2015) 逍遥散联合黛力新中西医结合治疗围绝经期抑郁症的临床观察. 中国现代医生 **53**(02): 141–143.
H196	刘蕊, 曲丹, 刘欢. (2015) 抱神汤加减治疗女性围绝经期失眠症 36 例的临床研究. 中国医药导刊 **17**(01): 52–53.
H197	范萌. (2015) 知柏地黄方加减汤剂治疗肾阴虚型围绝经期综合征临床观察. 北京中医药 **34**(12): 974–976.
H198	雷金平. (2014) 滋肾静心汤治疗围绝经期综合征临床观察. 中国健康心理学杂志 **22**(02): 189–191.
H199	蒋培荣, 孙宗顺, 汪彬. (2013) 中西医结合治疗急性更年期神经症 128 例. 辽宁中医杂志 **40**(09): 1876–1877.
H200	张晓玲, 付善萍, 彭春林, 张慧玲. (2013) 中西医结合治疗围绝经期焦虑抑郁症临床研究. 中国妇幼保健 **28**(26): 4331–4333.
H201	叶庆红, 陈志斌, 唐锴, 黄碧艳. (2012) 舒肝解郁胶囊与舍曲林治疗围绝经期焦虑抑郁障碍疗效. 临床精神医学杂志 **22**(03): 216.
H202	李贺琦. (2011) 益坤饮对围绝经期综合征患者情志调节及血清 5-羟色胺影响的临床研究. 南京中医药大学.
H203	李英杰. (2011) 围绝经期及绝经后抑郁不同治疗方式疗效分析. 中国误诊学杂志 **11**(04): 834–835.
H204	Jia M, Kluwe L, Liu HC, *et al.* (2015) Efficacy and side-effects of a semi-individualized Chinese herb mixture 'Tiao Geng Tang' for menopausal syndrome in China. *In Vivo* **29**(1): 109–115.
H205	Jiang D, Zhou JH, Zhou J, *et al.* (2015) Zhi-bai-di-huang-wan, a classic Chinese medicinal formula in relieving menopausal symptoms: A multi-centre and controlled trial from UK and China. *Afr J Tradit Complement Altern Med* **12**(S1): 45–51.
H206	Ushiroyama T, Ikeda A, Sakuma K, Ueki M. (2005) Chai-hu-gui-zhi-gan-jiang-tang regulates plasma interleukin-6 and soluble interleukin-6 receptor concentrations and improves depressed mood in climacteric women with insomnia. *Am J Chin Med* **33**(5): 703–711.
H207	侯莉娟, 姚艳丽, 丁象宸. (2017) 回医方二胶复经汤治疗围绝经期综合征 60 例临床观察. 中国民族医药杂志 **23**(08): 12–13.

(*Continued*)

(*Continued*)

Study No.	References
H208	程佳丽, 雷福云. (2017) 舒神调更丸治疗围绝经期综合征疗效观察. 湖北中医杂志 **39**(05): 42–44.
H209	徐伟. (2017) 五加丹加减治疗肝肾阴虚型经断前后诸证的临床观察. 黑龙江省中医药科学院.
H210	李晓倩, 折娜, 米艳荣, 等. (2016) 中药更年乐汤治疗妇女围绝经期综合征的临床研究. 临床医学专集: 1860–1862.
H211	关素珍, 尹金鹏, 潘妍, 蒋赟. (2015) 归芍地黄汤合生脉散治疗围绝经期综合征临床研究. 中药材 **38**(01): 206–208.
H212	胡俊攀. (2015) 益肾填精法治疗肾阴虚型围绝经期综合征的临床观察. 河南中医学院.
H213	龙旭, 李淑芬, 杨卓, 等. (2015) 滋水清肝饮治疗肾虚肝郁型围绝经期综合征 94 例临床观察. 实用中医内科杂志 **29**(04): 36–38.
H214	唐昌丽. (2014) 丹栀逍遥散治疗更年期综合征的有效性和安全性研究. 成都医学院学报 **9**(01): 61–64.
H215	涂轶佳, 朱燕芬, 陈理, 张士芬. (2014) '更眠安汤'治疗肾阴虚型女性更年期失眠的临床疗效. 上海医药 **35**(22): 36–38.
H216	李莹鸿, 靳利利. (2014) 桂枝汤加减治疗更年期失眠的临床观察. 内蒙古中医药 **33**(35): 44.
H217	王苏醒. (2014) 一贯煎加味治疗绝经前后诸证的临床研究. 云南中医学院.
H218	严晓丽, 许红, 王惠茹, 等. (2014) 益肾平肝安神法治疗更年期失眠 60 例. 陕西中医 **35**(02): 159–161.
H219	皮璐. (2014) 中药治疗女性更年期焦虑 50 例观察. 成都中医药大学学报 **37**(03): 76–78.
H220	吴艳. (2014) 滋阴补肾更年方治疗围绝经期综合征 36 例临床观察. 药物与人 **27**(7): 120–121.
H221	宋志宇, 庞剑月, 隋净净, 等. (2013) 舒肝颗粒治疗更年期焦虑症的机制研究. 中药药理与临床 **29**(03): 183–185.
H222	从羽. (2013) 调肝安更汤治疗经断前后诸症 40 例. 光明中医 **28**(04): 726–727.
H223	李鹏. (2013) 养阴安神汤对肾阴虚型绝经前后诸证睡眠障碍患者血清性激素与 5-HT 影响的临床研究. 福建中医药大学.
H224	缪宏珠, 马红雨, 李莹, 董玲, 郝淑娟. (2012) 安坤汤治疗围绝经期综合征 43 例临床观察. 中国妇幼保健 **27**(04): 556–557.

(Continued)

Study No.	References
H225	岳小鹏. (2012) 补肾化瘀汤治疗肾虚血瘀型围绝经期综合征的临床研究. 山东中医药大学.
H226	陈琰, 王赛莉, 赵燕宁. (2012) 益肾清心汤治疗围绝经期睡眠障碍 46 例. 辽宁中医杂志 **39**(05): 859–861.
H227	杨文. (2012) 滋肾清心法治疗围绝经期综合征 40 例. 中国中医药咨讯 **4**(3): 131–131.
H228	张黎. (2012) 滋水清肝饮加减治疗肾阴虚肝郁型围绝经期综合征临床观察. 成都中医药大学.
H229	李俊箐. (2011) 保更汤治疗围绝经期综合征疗效观察. 上海中医药杂志 **45**(02): 41–43.
H230	徐玉慧. (2011) 青蒿鳖甲汤合知柏地黄汤加减治疗肾阴虚型围绝经期综合征的临床分析. 成都中医药大学.
H231	黄月芳. (2011) 调天葵法治疗更年期抑郁症 50 例. 浙江中西医结合杂志 **21**(5): 356–357.
H232	王艳东. (2011) 益经汤治疗绝经综合征 56 例. 陕西中医 **32**(03): 327–328.
H233	王俊, 陈霞. (2011) 益坤饮治疗绝经综合征 64 例临床疗效观察. 实用老年医学 **25**(05): 404–405, 408.
H234	温利娟. (2010) 安宁颗粒治疗更年期综合征的临床观察. 北京中医药大学.
H235	孙津津, 盛晓园, 傅萍. (2010) 欢乐宁方治疗心肾不交型围绝经期综合征 36 例临床观察. 中华中医药学刊 **28**(11): 2391–2392.
H236	李丽. (2010) 肾阴虚型围绝经期综合征妇女外周血 IL-6 TNFα 的变化及大补阴煎加味治疗的临床观察. 辽宁中医药大学学报 **12**(03): 136–137.
H237	曾永青. (2010) 甜梦胶囊治疗更年期综合征失眠的临床观察. 亚太传统医药 **6**(07): 29–31.
H238	李芳芳. (2010) 滋肾涵肝汤治疗肝肾阴虚型围绝经期综合征的临床研究. 山东中医药大学.
H239	李苇苇. (2011) 更安汤治疗肾虚肝郁型围绝经期综合征的临床研究. 临床合理用药杂志 **4**(32): 49–50.
H240	池雷. (2009) 宁心敛阴汤治疗更年期综合征 20 例. 河南中医 **29**(12): 1201.
H241	洪育萍, 谌剑飞. (2009) 甜梦胶囊治疗围绝经期综合征临床观察. 现代中西医结合杂志 **18**(11): 1248–1249.
H242	马云枝, 朱世瑞. (2009) 镇肝熄风汤治疗更年期综合征 50 例临床观察. 中国实用神经疾病杂志 **12**(01): 91, 94.

(*Continued*)

(Continued)

Study No.	References
H243	陈蔚. (2009) 滋肾养肝汤治疗围绝经期综合征 168 例疗效观察. 中国现代药物应用 **3**(02): 142–143.
H244	柳静, 卢苏. (2009) 滋阴降火方治疗阴虚火旺型绝经综合征 33 例临床分析. 四川中医 **27**(08): 95–96.
H245	甘柏柳, 苏惠萍, 周平 廖丹梅, 李惠珍, 何海宁. (2008) 安更方治疗围绝经期综合征 60 例疗效观察. 广西医学 **30**(02): 194–195.
H246	杜巧琳, 王小云. (2008) 舒肝胶囊治疗更年期妇女抑郁症 36 例临床观察. 新中医 **40**(10): 61–62, 68.
H247	杜巧琳. (2008) 疏肝补肾法治疗更年期妇女抑郁症 42 例. 辽宁中医杂志 **35**(11): 1698–1699.
H248	刘艳玲, 丁雨, 罗美玉, 董国娟, 宋卓敏. (2008) 一解合方治疗更年期抑郁症 42 例临床观察. 上海中医药杂志 **42**(07): 53–54.
H249	吕丽丽. (2008) 滋阴潜阳法治疗更年期综合征的临床疗效观察. 北京中医药大学.
H250	朱旭华, 程玲, 富冬梅. (2007) 补肾活血法治疗围绝经期综合征 62 例. 成都中医药大学学报 **30**(02): 16–18.
H251	邹蕴珏. (2007) 菖蒲郁金汤治疗围绝经期抑郁症 35 例. 中医研究 **20**(01): 36–37.
H252	王丽. (2006) 补肾安更汤治疗围绝经期综合症的临床研究. 山东中医药大学.
H253	郑真, 吕晔, 马红, 等. (2006) 宁心红杞胶囊对绝经妇女保健作用的临床研究. 空军总医院学报 **22**(03): 162–164.
H254	程巍. (2010) 一贯煎加减治疗肝肾阴虚型绝经综合征的临床观察. 长春中医药大学.
H255	王丹, 刘格, 韩延华. (2005) 延灵丹治疗围绝经期综合征 28 例临床观察. 中医药学报 **33**(03): 23–24.
H256	薛赛琴, 姜坤. (2004) 改良 Kupperman 评分法对更年舒治疗更年期综合征 85 例疗效分析. 中国中西医结合杂志 **24**(02): 152–154.
H257	张雯婷. (2004) 滋肾清心汤治疗更年期综合征 32 例. 福建中医药 **35**(03): 12–13.
H258	李相玉. (2004) 滋肾养肝, 交通心肾法治疗女性更年期综合征的临床研究. 北京中医药大学.

(*Continued*)

Study No.	References
H259	柴丽娜. (2003) 辨证治疗更年期综合征的临床总结. 北京中医 **22**(02): 32–33.
H260	马红, 吕晔, 孙浩, 等. (2002) 立春胶囊治疗女性围绝经期综合征 74 例临床观察. 天津中医 **19**(04): 55–56.
H261	武权生, 唐怡, 陈红. (2001) 复方精血归治疗绝经后阴道干涩症 32 例疗效观察. 新中医 **33**(05): 18–19.
H262	孙丽珍. (1997) 地黄汤加味治疗更年期综合征 32 例疗效观察. 浙江中医学院学报 **21**(02): 50.
H263	Chan CCW, Lau WNT, Chiu SP, *et al.* (2006) A pilot study on the effects of a Chinese herbal preparation on menopausal symptoms. *Gynecol Endocrinol* **22**(2): 70–73.
H264	Hasper I, Ventskovskiy BM, Rettenberge R, *et al.* (2009) Long-term efficacy and safety of the special extract ERr 731 of *Rheum rhaponticum* in perimenopausal women with menopausal symptoms. *Menopause* **16**(1): 117–131.
H265	Hidaka T, Yonezawa R, Saito S. (2013) Kami-shoyo-san, Kampo (Japanese traditional medicine), is effective for climacteric syndrome, especially in hormone-replacement-therapy-resistant patients who strongly complain of psychological symptoms. *J Obstet Gynaecol Res* **39**(1): 223–228.
H266	Kaszkin-Bettag M, Beck S, Richardson A, *et al.* (2008) Efficacy of the special extract ERr 731 from rhapontic rhubarb for menopausal complaints: A 6-month open observational study. *Altern Ther Health Med* **14**(6): 32–38.
H267	Lai JN, Hwang JS, Chen HJ, Wang JD. (2005) Finished herbal product as an alternative treatment for menopausal symptoms in climacteric women. *J Altern Complement Med* **11**(6): 1075–1084.
H268	Liu D, Lu Y, Ma H, *et al.* (2009) A pilot observational study to assess the safety and efficacy of Menoprogen for the management of menopausal symptoms in Chinese women. *J Altern Complement Med* **15**(1): 79–85.
H269	Namiki T, Sato H, Matsumoto Y, *et al.* (2014) Identification of a predictive biomarker for the beneficial effect of Keishibukuryogan, a Kampo (Japanese traditional) medicine, on patients with climacteric syndrome. *Evid Based Complement Alternat Med* **2014:** 962109.
H270	Terauchi M, Hiramitsu S, Akiyoshi M, *et al.* (2014) Effects of the Kampo formula Tokishakuyakusan on headaches and concomitant depression in middle-aged women. *Evid Based Complement Alternat Med* **2014:** 593560.

(*Continued*)

(Continued)

Study No.	References
H271	Ushiroyama T, Yoshida S, Tadaki K, *et al.* (2004) A pilot study of a Kampo formula, EH0202, with intriguing results for menopausal symptoms. *J Altern Complement Med* **10**(2): 397–399.
H272	杜言辉, 彭小星. (2014) 中药药浴治疗围绝经期失眠 32 例临床分析. 中国妇幼保健 **29**(16): 2588–2589.
H273	Yaralizadeh M, Abedi P, Najar S, *et al.* (2016) Effect of *Foeniculum vulgare* (fennel) vaginal cream on vaginal atrophy in postmenopausal women: A double-blind randomized placebo-controlled trial. *Maturitas* **84:** 75–80.
H274	Suwanvesh N, Manonai J, Sophonsritsuk A, Cherdshewasart W. (2017) Comparison of *Pueraria mirifica* gel and conjugated equine estrogen cream effects on vaginal health in postmenopausal women. *Menopause* **24**(2): 210–215.
H275	徐丽. (2011) 康妇特栓治疗老年性阴道炎 140 例疗效观察. 中国中医药咨讯 **3**(10): 176–176.
H276	冯华, 顾晓芳. (2017) 中药内服外洗法用于肾阴虚型围绝经期综合征患者治疗的临床效果. 现代医学 **45**(12): 1779–1780.
H277	董燕. (2014) 六味地黄汤对女性更年期综合征糖脂代谢及内分泌水平的影响. 四川中医 **32**(12): 68–70.
H278	王凯丽, 闫西鹏, 赵颖颖, 等. (2017) 安神解郁汤联合黛力新治疗女性更年期轻中度抑郁症 40 例. 山东中医杂志 **36**(03): 204–206.
H279	李长甫. (2017) 四逆四物汤治疗阴阳两虚型更年期综合征临床研究. 亚太传统医药 **13**(24): 154–156.
H280	Lima SMRR, Postigo S, Reis BF, *et al.* (2011) The effects of *Tribulus terrestris* on sexuality in post-menopausal women. *Menopause* **18**(12): 1363.
H281	Parhizkar S, Manzouri L. (2015) A randomised controlled trial on climacteric symptoms management and quality of life improvement of *Nigella sativa* seeds powder in menopausal women. *Maturitas* **81**(1): 179.
H282	Taavoni S, Ekbatani NN, Haghani H. (2017) Effect of *Tribulus terrestris,* ginger, saffron, and Cinnamomum on menopausal symptoms: A randomised, placebo-controlled clinical trial. *Przeglad Menopauzalny* **16**(1): 19–22.

6

Pharmacological Actions of Frequently Used Herbs

OVERVIEW

Many plant products contain phytoestrogens, which may alleviate symptoms of menopause. Experimental studies can provide insight into possible biological activities and mechanisms of herbal medicines. This chapter reviews a selection of *in vivo* and *in vitro* studies of the ten most frequently used Chinese herbs from randomised clinical trials in Chapter 5.

Introduction

A number of systematic reviews have reviewed the potential effects of Chinese herbal medicine (CHM) for menopausal symptoms with some promising results found.[1–3] The evidence from clinical studies included in Chapter 5 has also shown benefits of CHM in reducing the physical and psychological symptoms of menopause. If such treatments are to play a role in clinical management of menopause, it is important to examine how they exert their clinical effects. This chapter reviews experimental evidence from *in vitro* and *in vivo* experimental models for some of the most frequently used herbs in clinical trials.

The pathological processes and mechanisms of menopause have been described in Chapter 1. The change of ovarian structure and function is the key factor contributing to the progression of menopause, which results in a change in hormonal balance, such as a decrease in oestrogen and progesterone hormones and an increase in follicle-stimulating hormone (FSH) and luteinising hormone (LH). This change in hormones can contribute to health problems after menopause such as heart disease, metabolic disease, osteoporosis and urinary dysfunction.

Various animal models of menopause are well-established, such as the intact ageing rodent model, the ovariectomised (OVX) rodent model with undetectable oestrogen levels (most widely used for menopause-related laboratory studies) and the recently established chemical 4-vinylcyclohexene diepoxide (VCD)-induced menopausal rodent model. Compared to the VCD rodent model of menopause, which is a follicle-deplete, ovary-intact animal showing the natural progression from pre- to postmenopause, the intact ageing and OVX models lack two important aspects of human menopause: very low oestrogen levels and a menopause transition.[4–6] Despite this, they are both frequently used in experimental studies of menopause.

Methods

The most frequently cited herbs in randomised controlled trials (RCTs) were selected by the research team and expert gynaecologists. The key herbs reviewed were *shu di huang* 熟地黄, *fu ling* 茯苓, *gan cao* 甘草, *shan yao* 山药, *bai shao* 白芍, *chai hu* 柴胡, *dang gui* 当归, *shan zhu yu* 山茱萸, *suan zao ren* 酸枣仁 and *zhi mu* 知母. Experimental studies on their pharmacological actions relevant to menopause were identified and the activities of each herb and/or main compounds were examined to identify their therapeutic effects on hormone regulation (such as oestrogen, progesterone, FSH and LH), adrenergic/serotonergic/dopaminergic activity and thermoregulation.

The constituent compounds were identified by searching herbal monographs, high-quality reviews of CHM, *materia medica* and PubMed. To identify pre-clinical studies, a literature search in PubMed, Google Scholar and PubMed Central was undertaken. Search terms included the scientific names of the plant as well as the Chinese *pinyin* and the names of the main compounds found in the herb. These were combined with terms for menopause, climacteric, phytoestrogens, oestrogen, progesterone, FSH, LH, anti-androgen, thermoregulation, anti-osteoporosis, sedative, hypnotic effects and ovarian failure rodent models.

Experimental Studies on *Shu Di Huang* 熟地黄

Shu di huang 熟地黄, the processed/steamed rhizome of *Rehmannia glutinosa* Libosch, has been used for treatment of a variety of disorders. Currently, approximately 140 compounds have been identified, including monoterpenoids, polysaccharides, triterpenes, flavonoid glycosides, phenethyl alcohol glycosides, phenolic acid glycosides and lignans. Iridoid glycosides, such as catalpol, aucubin and acetoside, are considered to be the most abundant monoterpenoids,[7] and polysaccharides are one of the main active constituents of *R. glutinosa*.[7,8] *R. glutinosa* exhibits beneficial activities on the blood, immune, endocrine, cardiovascular and nervous systems.[7,8]

Hormone Regulation

Oestrogenic effects are essential to alleviate menopausal symptoms, especially hot flushes and night sweats. Studies have suggested that oestrogen receptor alpha (ERα) has a more prominent role on the mammary gland and uterus, and ERα-dependent oestrogenic activity may enhance tissue proliferation and hormonal carcinogenesis. In contrast, oestrogen receptor beta (ERβ)-dependent oestrogenic effects may counteract the ERα-promoted cell hyperproliferation in tissues such as breast and uterus.[9]

The beneficial effect of *R. glutinosa* on regulation of reproductive hormones was attributed to its active compounds. Catalpol has showed an ovarian failure-resistant effect on senile female rats *in vivo*, supported by significantly rejuvenating the granulocytic ultrastructure of follicles that are responsible for the generation of hormones and nourishing ovarian tissues by modulating the apoptosis-related molecules. These improvements, in both the quality and quantity of follicles, resulted in a rebalance of hormones in the aged rats with an increase of serum 17β-estradiol (E_2) and progesterone (P_4) and decreased levels of FSH and LH.[10]

Menoprogen (MPG), a commercially prepared oral Chinese medicine (CM) formula that includes *R. glutinosa*, is used in China for the management of menopause-related symptoms. Menoprogen could significantly increase endogenous levels of E_2 and P_4, and reduce levels of FSH and LH *in vitro* and *in vivo* in an aged rat model of menopause.[11,12] Similar findings were observed in OVX rats. Menoprogen administered daily for two weeks could recover uterine and adrenal gland atrophy and restore serum E_2 and P_4 levels.[13] The proposed mechanism of MPG was through reducing ovarian granulosa cell (GC) apoptosis via involvement of insulin-like growth factor-1 (IGF-1) and insulin-like growth factor binding protein-1 (IGFBP-1), thereby increasing E_2 and P_4 production.[11,14]

Antidepressant-like Activity

In addition to the various physiological changes, menopause also results in a wide range of psychological and neurobiological disorders. Low or depressed mood is one of the more common psychological and neurobiological symptoms of menopause. Current understanding of the pathogenesis of depression relates to dysfunction of the hypothalamic–pituitary–adrenal [HPA] axis (an interactive neuroendocrine unit consisting of the hypothalamus, the pituitary gland and the adrenal glands), abnormal expression of neurotransmitters (such as serotonin [5-hydroxytryptamine, 5-HT], norepinephrine [NE] and dopamine [DA]) or their receptors, and abnormal expression of synaptic regulators, such as brain-derived neurotrophic factor (BDNF)/tropomyosin receptor kinase B (TrkB) and *N*-methyl-D-aspartate (NMDA).[15,16]

R. glutinosa and its active component, catalpol, have been extensively investigated in terms of their functions in modulating the HPA axis, activating specific neurotransmitters, and modulating the expression of synaptic regulators to improve symptoms of depression and anxiety. Ethanol extracts of *R. glutinosa* have been shown to possess an antidepressant-like effect on a mouse behavioural despair depression model, as indicated by the shorter immobility time during the forced swim test (FST) and tail suspension test (TST).[17] This finding was further explored in a rat model of depression evoked by chronic unpredictable mild stress (CUMS, a well-validated animal model of depression), suggesting that the antidepressant-like action of *R. glutinosa* partially involved restoring HPA axis dysfunction, enhancing monoaminergic nervous systems and upregulating BDNF and TrkB expression.[18] More recently, the antidepressant and anxiolytic effects of *R. glutinosa* confirmed in OVX mice exposed to CUMS are believed to be largely associated with modulation of brain neurotransmitters, regulation of neurotrophins and activation of ERβ.[19]

In addition to the crude extracts of *R. glutinosa,* the antidepressant-like effects of catalpol have also been examined. The administration of catalpol could reduce the duration of immobility in the TST and FST, increase levels of central monoamine neurotransmitters (such as 5-HT and its metabolite 5-hydroxyindoleacetic acid [5-HIAA]) without affecting NE or DA in mice, and antagonise the reserpine-induced ptosis, akinesia and hypothermia in a dose-dependent manner comparable to the clinical antidepressant fluoxetine hydrochloride (FH).[20] This suggested actions involving upregulation of the central serotonergic system, but not noradrenergic or dopaminergic systems.

Experimental Studies on *Fu Ling* 茯苓

Fu ling 茯苓 (*Poria cocos*) is a well-known medicinal fungus that has been used in CM for its diuretic, sedative and tonic effects. The major phytochemical compounds present in *P. cocos* are triterpenoids and polysaccharides.[21,22] Pharmacological activities include anti-inflammatory, antioxidant, antiviral and antibacterial activities.[21,22] Several studies have examined the actions of multi-herb CHM formulas, of which *fu ling* is one ingredient. Such studies that describe actions relevant to the pathogenesis of menopause have been summarised below.

Hormone Regulation

Gui zhi fu ling wan 桂枝茯苓丸 (GZFLW, also known as Keishi-bukuryo-gan) is a classic CHM formula comprising five herbal ingredients: *fu ling* (*Poria cocos*), *gui zhi* (*Cinnamomum cassia* Presl.), *shao yao* (*Paeonia lactiflora* Pall. or *Paeonia veitchii* Lynch), *mu dan pi* (*Paeonia suffruticosa* Andr.) and *tao ren* (*Prunus persica* (L.) Batsch or *Prunus davidiana* (Carr.) Franch.). *Gui zhi fu ling wan* has been reported to relieve menopausal hot flushes (MHF) which are strongly associated with calcitonin gene-related peptide (CGRP).

Calcitonin gene-related peptide is a widely expressed sensory neuropeptide and is believed to be a potent vasodilator neuropeptide responsible for MHFs.[23] The lower concentration of plasma CGRP due to ovarian hormone deficiency in OVX rats could induce an elevation of skin temperature and arterial vasorelaxation through upregulating the number of CGRP receptors.[24] These OVX-induced CGRP-related responses could be prevented by oestrogen supplement and administration of GZFLW.[25,26]

Further studies on the effects of GZFLW in female rats treated with the gonadotrophin releasing hormone (GnRH) analogue leuprorelin confirmed that both GZFLW and 17b-estradiol significantly inhibited the CGRP-induced elevation of the skin temperature, but GZFLW did not affect E_2, LH and FSH levels. This was validated *in vitro* in oestrogen receptor-positive human breast cancer (MCF-7) cells that are specifically stimulated by oestrogen or oestrogen-like substances.[27]

Antidepressant-like Activity

Xiao yao san 逍遥散 (XYS) is a well-known CHM formula used for a wide variety of depression-like symptoms. It is composed of *fu ling* (*Poria cocos* [Schw.] Wolf), *chai hu* (*Bupleurum chinense* DC.), *dang gui* (*Angelica sinensis* [Oliv.] Diel), *bai shao* (*Paeonia lactiflora* Pall.), *bai zhu* (*Atractylodes macrocephala* Koidz), *bo he* (*Mentha haplocalyx* Briq.), *sheng jiang* (*Zingiber officinale* Rosc.) and *gan cao* (*Glycyrrhiza uralensis* Fisch.). In the CUMS model of depression, antidepressant effects of high dose XYS were observed to be greater than amitriptyline and were time-dependent.[28] Furthermore, the active petroleum ether fraction of XYS responsible for the most effective antidepressant effect was identified, suggesting that lipophilic components are largely associated with the antidepressant effect of XYS.[29]

Experimental Studies on *Gan Cao* 甘草

The three plant sources of *gan cao* 甘草 (licorice) are *Glycyrrhiza uralensis* Fisch., *Glycyrrhiza inflata* Bat. and *Glycyrrhiza glabra* L. More than 400 compounds have been isolated from *gan cao*, and the main bioactive constituents of licorice include triterpene saponins (more than 20 identified) and flavonoids (more than 300 identified).[30–32] Pharmacological activities include anti-inflammatory, antiallergic, antioxidant, antiviral, anticarcinogenic, antithrombotic, antiulcer, immunoregulatory, hepatoprotective and cardioprotective effects.[30–33] Other pharmacological effects in relation to menopause are discussed.

Hormone Regulation

There are a large number of *in vitro* and/or *in vivo* studies that have demonstrated that various crude extracts and/or compounds of licorice possess strong oestrogen-like effects and antiprogestogenic-like effects. The crude extracts of *G. uralensis* could effectively induce oestrogenic activity in a concentration-dependent manner.[34] The oestrogenic activity of crude methanol (MeOH) extracts of the three licorice species have been examined *in vitro*. The results demonstrated that *Glycyrrhiza* species had varying levels of oestrogenic activities, with *G. uralensis* showing the highest oestrogenic properties, followed by *G. inflata*.[35] When comparative ER subtype selectivity was examined, researchers found that *G. uralensis* and *G. inflata* could be more oestrogenic and had nanomolar potency for ERβ.[36] This suggests they might be better choices for the menopausal formulations, with an enhanced safety profile, as ERβ-dependent oestrogenic effects can oppose ER α-dependent proliferation and hormonal carcinogenesis.

Glabridin, a major isoflavan from licorice, could bind to human ER with comparable affinity to genistein (the best-known phytoestrogen), and could activate creatine kinase (CK) activity (a known marker for oestrogen responsive genes), in oestrogen-responsive tissues *in vivo. Glabridin* also inhibited growth of breast cancer cells independently of ERs, indicating that glabridin is a phytoestrogen.[37] Further, glabrene and isoliquiritigenin (ILC) had a higher affinity to bind to human ER as an agonist for ER-mediated transcription than glabridin and stimulated CK with similar stimulatory effects as oestradiol in oestrogen-responsive tissues *in vivo.*[38] In addition, the glycosylated form of the dihydroflavanone, liquiritigenin (LigF) and its precursor chalcone, isoliquiritigenin (LigC) and 8-prenylapigenin from *G. inflata,* also demonstrated oestrogenic properties with LigF for ERβ selective ligand, LigC for dual oestrogenic/chemopreventive activities and 8-prenylapigenin for ERβ effect along with ERα activities.[35] Liquiritigen was also reported to regulate ERα, ERβ and aryl hydrocarbon receptor (AhR) target genes in human breast cancer (MCF-7) and hepatoma cells.[39,40] In addition to the oestrogen-like effects, *G. uralensis* has also demonstrated dose-dependent inhibition of progesterone activity.[41]

Antidepressant-like Activity

Antidepressant-like effects of *G. glabra* were seen in a mouse model of depression. The aqueous extracts significantly decreased the immobility times in both the FST and TST without affecting locomotor activity of mice. The efficacy was comparable to that of imipramine and fluoxetine and was attenuated by sulpiride (a selective dopamine D2 receptor antagonist) and prazosin (an alpha1-adrenoceptor antagonist), but not by p-chlorophenylalanine (an inhibitor of 5-HT synthesis). This indicates that the main antidepressant mechanism might involve the adrenergic and dopaminergic systems.[42]

Liquiritin and isoliquiritin from *G. uralensis* exerted significant antidepressant-like activity in agreement with the above findings in both the FST and TST in mice, but showed increases in 5-HT and NE that were similar to that of fluoxetine, and a decrease in the ratio of 5-HIAA/5-HT in the mouse hippocampus, hypothalamus and cortex. This indicates that the mechanisms of action might be associated with the increase in 5-HT and NE in the mouse CNS.[43]

Sedative Actions

Sleep disturbance is common during menopause. The γ-aminobutyric acid type A-benzodiazepine ($GABA_A$-BZD) receptor is considered the most important target for the development of sedative-hypnotic drugs.[44] Ethanol extracts of *G. glabra* showed hypnotic effects on pentobarbital-induced sleep in mice. The dose-dependent decrease in sleep latency and increase in sleep duration were similar to diazepam. Furthermore, ethanol extract of *G. glabra* showed an increase in the amount of non-rapid eye movement (NREM) sleep, without a decrease of delta activity, in a manner similar to that of physiological sleep. This effect could be completely suppressed by flumazenil, a specific $GABA_A$-BZD receptor antagonist.[45] These findings were further extended to the flavonoid glabrol, as a large number of flavonoids have been reported to exert hypnotic activity, indicating *G. glabra*- and glabrol-induced sleep changes occur through a positive allosteric modulation of $GABA_A$-BZD receptors.[45]

The effects of glabridin, another major flavonoid component from licorice, on γ-aminobutyric acid (GABA) responses have been examined in acutely isolated dorsal raphe neurons of the rat using the patch-clamp technique. Glabridin showed GABA-induced responses with a biphasic concentration-potentiation relationship similar to those of zolpidem, a hypnotic drug. The glabridin-induced potentiation could not be suppressed by flumazenil, a benzodiazepine receptor antagonist, implying that the sedative and hypnotic effects of glabridin are largely due to potentiation of GABAergic suppression in dorsal raphe neurons by $GABA_A$ receptor actions.[46] In addition, isoliquiritigenin was also reported to suppress cocaine-induced extracellular DA release in the rat brain through modulating $GABA_B$ receptors, which might benefit sleep in menopausal women.[47]

Experimental Studies on *Shan Yao* 山药

Shan yao 山药, the rhizome of *Dioscorea opposita* Thunb., also called Chinese yam, is one of the well-known edible and pharmaceutical foods in China. It contains various chemical components and nutrients, including polysaccharides, flavonoids, allantoin, adenosine, arbutin DA, batatasin and other active ingredients. Pharmacological activities include anti-inflammatory, antioxidant, antitumour, anticoagulant and immunostimulatory effects.[48,49] Other pharmacological effects in relation to menopause are discussed.

Hormone Regulation

The physiological and pathological effects of oestrogen are mediated by two types of ER: the genomic nuclear ERα and ERβ and the non-genomic oestrogen receptor (GPR30). Aqueous extracts of *D. opposita* could promote proliferation of MCF-7 cells similar to 17β-E_2. This *D. opposita*-induced proliferation could be completely abolished by the blockade of ER and GPR30.[50] Aqueous extracts of *D. opposita* could significantly increase the uterus coefficient and serum levels of E_2 and FSH in immature female Swiss mice comparable to oestradiol valerate and enhance the expression of oestrogen receptors ERα, ERβ and GPR30 in the uterus. These *in vitro* and *in vivo* findings suggested that ERα, ERβ and GPR30 play important roles in mediating the *D. opposita*-stimulated proliferation in MCF-7 cells and an oestrogen-like effect *in vivo*. Furthermore, adenosine and arbutin, two compounds isolated from *D. opposita*, were identified to be responsible for these proliferation and oestrogen-like effects.[50]

Additionally, a bioactive protein isolated from *D. opposita*, designated DOI, demonstrated potent oestrogen-stimulating activity shown by increasing oestradiol biosynthesis and aromatase expression levels in a rat ovarian granulosa cell model. Confirmation of the oestradiol-stimulating effect of DOI *in vivo* revealed that DOI upregulated expression of ovarian aromatase — but not breast aromatase — thereby increasing secretion of oestradiol and progesterone in aged female Sprague Dawley rats.[51] More importantly, as it is believed that the level of ERβ is higher than ERα in the normal ovary,[52] bioactive DOI-like proteins could increase the translational expression of ERβ protein levels without a change in the expression of ERα, implying a potential reduction of the risk of oestrogen-induced ovarian cancer.[53] In addition to the oestrogen-like effects, *D. opposita* also demonstrated inhibition of progesterone activity in a dose-response manner.[41]

Experimental Studies on *Bai Shao* 白芍

Bai shao 白芍 (white peony) is sourced from the dried root without bark of *P. lactiflora* Pall. The main characteristic constituents of *P. lactiflora* include monoterpenoids, triterpenoids, flavonoids, phenols and tannins. It consists of more than 15 components, with the main bioavailable compounds being paeoniflorin, pentagalloylglucose, gallic acid, albiflorin and benzoic acid. Among them, paeoniflorin is the most abundant, accounting for the pharmacological activities.[54,55] Pharmacological activities include anti-inflammatory, antioxidant, antiviral, antibacterial, antifungal, antitumour, anti-arthritis, anticoagulant, antiplatelet and immunomodulatory activities.[54,55] Other pharmacological effects in relation to menopause are discussed.

Hormone Regulation

Radix Paeoniae alba (RPA), the dried root of *P. lactiflora* Pall, has been reported to have potent oestrogenic activity in *in vivo* models of immature and OVX mice, and in *in vitro* studies. In 21-day-old immature female mice, water extracts of RPA could stimulate development of the uterus and vagina, while in OVX mice, RPA could restore the oestrus cycle and reverse atrophy of the uterus and vagina. Furthermore, RPA resulted in an increase in serum oestradiol and a decrease in serum LH and FSH, by upregulating the expression of ERα and ERβ in the reproductive target tissues. Moreover, RPA significantly reduced the OVX-induced high rectal temperature and relieved hot flushes due to oestrogen decline in OVX mice. *In vitro*, RPA could induce proliferation of ER-positive MCF-7 cells, but not ER-negative MDA-MB-231 cells (human epithelial breast tissue cells) and significantly induced ERα/β-oestrogen response element (ERE) luciferase expression. The oestrogenic activities of RPA could be significantly suppressed by ICI-182,780, a specific ER antagonist, *in vivo* and *in vitro*, implying that its potent oestrogenic activity occurs by enhancing biosynthesis of oestrogen and ER expression through ER-ERE-dependent pathways.[56]

Antidepressant-like Activity

The antidepressant effect of *P. lactiflora* was studied in mouse models of depression and was attributed to its total glycosides, including paeoniflorin and albiflorin. Treatment with total glycosides could antagonise reserpine-induced ptosis and suppress the activities of monoamine oxidases in mouse cerebrum, indicating that the antidepressant effects of total glycosides might be partly associated with the inhibition of monoamine oxidases.[57]

More recently, the paeoniflorin isomer albiflorin was reported to have antidepressant-like activity in the CUMS-induced rat model of depression. Oral administration of albiflorin increased levels of 5-HT and 5-HIAA in serum and the hypothalamus, while decreasing expressions of 5-HT_{1A} and 5-HT_{2A} receptors in the hypothalamus. This indicates the albiflorin-mediated antidepressant-like effects in the CUMS-induced rat model of depression might be associated with the normalisation of the serotonergic system. In addition to involvement of the serotonergic system, treatment with albiflorin could remarkably improve CUMS-induced decreases in DA and noradrenalin concentration in serum and the hypothalamus and restore the altered levels of tyrosine hydroxylase (TH), DA D2 receptors and DA transporter (DAT) back to normal levels in the hypothalamus. This indicates albiflorin-mediated antidepressant-like effects might also be associated with normalisation of the dopaminergic system.[58]

Experimental Studies on *Chai Hu* 柴胡

The botanical source of *chai hu* 柴胡 *(Radix Bupleuri)* is the dried roots of *Bupleurum chinense* DC., *Bupleurum scorzonerifolium* Willd and *Bupleurum falcatum*.[59,60] The chemical constituents include triterpenoid saponins, lignins, essential oils, flavones, phenylpropanols, coumarins, polyynes, polyacetylenes and polysaccharides. Among them, the major bioactive compounds include over 100 different triterpenoid saponins; indeed, two saikosaponins — saikosaponins a and d — are used to evaluate the quality of *Radix Bupleuri*.[59,60] Pharmacological activities include anti-inflammatory, antioxidant, antiviral, antibacterial, antitumour, anti-arthritis, anticoagulant, antiplatelet and immunomodulatory activity.[59,60] Other pharmacological effects in relation to menopause are discussed.

Hormone Regulation

Saikosaponin-d (SSd), with a similar structure to oestradiol, demonstrated its oestrogen-like activity by stimulating the proliferation of MCF-7 cells and inducing ERE luciferase activity which could be significantly abolished by the specific ER antagonist ICI-182,780 in MCF-7 cells. Further evaluation of involvement of ERα and/or ERβ in mediating the actions of SSD in ER-negative human cervical carcinoma (HeLa) cells suggested that SSd could dose-dependently activate ERE luciferase activity via the ERα-mediated pathway.[61]

Antidepressant-like Activity

Dopamine, 5-HT and GABA are very important CNS neurotransmitters. The water extract of *Radix Bupleuri* was found to interact with DA D1 and D2, 5-HT_{1A} receptors and GABA site with moderate affinity in male Institute of Cancer Research (ICR) mice.[62] Oral administration of *B. falcatum* could significantly decrease the total duration of immobility in the TST. This antidepressant-like activity of *B. falcatum* was inhibited by pre-treatment with p-chlorophenylalanine (PCPA, a 5-HT synthesis inhibitor) and alpha-methyl-p-tyrosine (AMPT, a catecholamine synthesis inhibitor) in the TST. This inhibition could be reversed by fluoxetine for PCPA and bupropion for AMPT in the TST. This indicates that antidepressant activity may occur through the serotonergic and noradrenergic systems.[63]

Furthermore, the antidepressant-like effect of *B. falcatum* was assessed in a repeated restraint stress rat model. Repeated restraint stress can produce increases in depression and anxiety behaviours and change the expression of corticotrophin releasing factor in the hypothalamus. Pre-treatment with *B. falcatum* significantly decreased immobility in the FST and increased open-arm exploration in the elevated plus maze test, accompanied with inhibition of the restraint stress-induced increase in TH expression in the locus coeruleus. This implies that the reduced depression and anxiety-like behaviours with *B. falcatum* is possibly through central adrenergic mechanisms.[64]

Experimental Studies on *Dang Gui* 当归

Dang gui 当归, mainly derived from the dried root of *Angelica sinensis*, consists of over 70 compounds. Ferulic acid, *Z*-Ligustilide, butylidenephthalide, butyl-phthalide and polysaccharide are thought to be the main biologically active components.[65,66] Pharmacological activities include anti-inflammatory, antioxidant, anti-atherosclerosis, antithrombotic, antiplatelet, antihepatotoxic, anticardiovascular and immunomodulatory activities.[65,66] Pharmacological effects relevant to menopause are described.

Hormone Regulation

The oestrogenic activity of ethanol extracts of *A. sinensis* was assessed *in vivo*. Ethanol extract could increase uterine weight, stimulate the uterine histo-architecture, promote cornification of the vaginal epithelium, selectively suppress LH secretion and further reduce serum LH concentration in OVX rats. It also produced a great modification of the vaginal smear, leading to a change of the oestrous cycle with a prolonged oestrus stage and a temporary reduction of the regular cyclicity in intact female rats.[67] In addition to the oestrogen-like effects, *A. sinensis* also demonstrated dose-dependent inhibition of progesterone activity.[41]

Antidepressant-like Activity

The water extracts of *A. sinensis* were reported to have high affinity to GABA sites and moderate affinity on 5-HT_{1A} receptors.[62] By using a 5-HT receptor (5-HT_7) binding assay, five fractionations from ethanol extracts of *A. sinensis* (*p*-hydroxyphenethyl *trans*-ferulate, 11(*S*),16(*R*)-dihydroxy-octadeca-9*Z*,17-dien-12,14-diyn-1-yl acetate, (3*R*,8*S*)-falcarindiol, imperatorin and 8-hydroxy-1-methoxy-, *Z*-9-heptadecene-4,6-diyn-3-one) demonstrated competitive binding activity with inhibitory effects on [3H] lysergic acid diethylamide (LSD) binding to the 5-HT_7 receptors. This indicates that these compounds might partially contribute to the serotonergic activity of *A. sinensis*.[68]

Experimental Studies on *Shan Zhu Yu* 山茱萸

Shan zhu yu 山茱萸, the fruit of *Cornus officinalis* Sieb. et Zucc. (CO), is also known as *Corni Fructus,* Asiatic Dogwood and Japanese Cornel Dogwood. *Shan zhu yu* contains 305 compounds including alkaloids, iridoids, flavones, polysaccharides, phenylpropanoids, organic acid, tannins, morroniside, loganin terpenoids, carboxylic acids and essential oils. Among them, iridoids are believed to be the major bioactive compounds.[69,70] Pharmacological activities include anti-inflammatory, antioxidant, antibacterial, anti-ageing, antidiabetic, cardioprotective and neuroprotective effects.[69,70]

Sedative Actions

Loganin, a major iridoid glycoside of *shan zhu yu,* has been reported to possess sedative and hypnotic activity. It significantly decreased locomotor activity in normal mice and reduced the hypnotic effect of sodium pentobarbital but did not improve the caffeine-induced short sleep time. Loganin recovered PCPA-induced insomnia, exerted a synergistic hypnotic effect with 5-hydroxytryptophan, improved sleep onset with a sub-hypnotic dose of pentobarbital, decreased sleep latency and prolonged sleep time induced by a hypnotic dose of pentobarbital in mice. In line with these findings, loganin decreased the concentration of 5-HT and DA, and their metabolites 3,4-dihydroxyphenylacetic acid, and increased the 5-HIAA/5-HT ratio in the prefrontal cortex. This indicates that loganin may exert its hypnotic effects through serotonergic and dopaminergic pathways. Moreover, loganin also remarkably promoted NREM sleep and total sleep, and significantly shortened wakefulness without reducing the electroencephalograph (EEG) power of delta which was compatible with physiological sleep. Additionally, loganin increased the ratio of c-Fos (+) in glutamic acid decarboxylase (GAD) (+) neurons in the ventrolateral preoptic nucleus (VLPO), a necessary component of sleep circuitry, at a hypnotic dose.[71] This suggests loganin may also have hypnotic actions by activating GABAergic neurons in the VLPO.

Experimental Studies on *Suan Zao Ren* 酸枣仁

Suan zao ren 酸枣仁 (the dried seed of *Ziziphus jujuba* Mill. var. spinosa) contains triterpenic acids, flavonoids, cerebrosides, amino acids, phenolic acids, mineral constituents and polysaccharides. Pharmacological activities include anti-inflammatory, antioxidant, anticancer, anti-obesity, immunostimulatory, hepatoprotective and gastrointestinal protective activities.[72,73] *Z. jujuba* seed has attracted much attention for the treatment of patients with sleep disorders, anxiety, nervous exhaustion and night sweats due to its significant effects against disturbances of the central nervous system.

Antidepressant-like Activity

The water extracts of *Z. jujuba* were reported to interact with DA D1 and D2 receptors, 5-HT_{1A} and 5-HT_2 receptors, and GABAergic sites with moderate affinity in male ICR mice.[62] The formula *Suan zao ren he huan* 酸棗仁合歡 (SHF), consisting of *Z. jujuba* and other herbs, such as *he huan pi* (*Albizia julibrissin* Durazz.), *bai shao* (*P. lactiflora* Pall) and *bai zi ren* (*Platycladus orientalis* (L.) Franco), displayed antidepressant-like effects in the CUMS depressive mouse model.

The ethanolic extracts of SHF could produce a significant decrease in the immobility period in TST and FST, accompanied with an increase in 5-HT levels in mice hippocampus, NE levels in mice hippocampus and frontal cortex, and the inhibition of monoamine oxidase-A and monoamine oxidase-B. The mechanism of action may involve the serotonergic, noradrenergic and monoamine oxidase enzyme systems.[74] The saponins part of the SHF extracts was believed to contribute to the antidepressant effect, which achieved the same antidepressant effect as SHF through the same mechanisms of action.[75]

Furthermore, the combination of *Z. jujuba* and the lily bulb (a traditional formula used for depressive disorder patients in CM), has been found to alleviate depressive behaviours in the rat model of chronic depression. The combination was found to change three indexes in the FST, such as immobility time, swimming time and climbing time, improve the CUMS-induced decrease in sucrose consumption and rearing movement in the open field test (OFT), and attenuate the CUMS-induced increase in faecal granules. Meanwhile, elevated serum 5-HT and brain 5-HIAA were observed, indicating the antidepressant-like effect of the combination of these two herbs might be associated with the increase of serum 5-HT in peripheral blood and 5-HIAA in the brain.[76]

Sedative Actions

Fifty percent ethanol extracts of *Z. jujuba* inhibit locomotor activity, prolong pentobarbital-induced sleeping time and inhibit amphetamine-induced locomotor stimulatory responses in mice.[77] Sanjoinine A was identified as the bioactive compound responsible for the hypnotic effects through the GABAergic systems.[78] The anxiolytic-like effects of sanjoinine A were also demonstrated in male mice. In cultured cerebellar granule cells, sanjoinine A increased chloride influx and expression of α- and γ-subunits of $GABA_A$ receptors and glutamic acid decarboxylase (GAD65/67), suggesting these effects might be mediated by GABAergic transmission.[79]

In addition to sanjoinine A, cyclopeptide alkaloid fraction from *Z. jujuba* (CAFZ) played an important role in the enhancement of hypnotic effects through GABA receptor Cl–channel activation examined in pentobarbital-treated mice and in cultured cerebellar granule cells.[80]

Spinosin, a C-glycoside flavonoid from *Z. jujuba*, showed significant potentiation of the hypnotic effect of pentobarbital on sleep in mice, as measured by increased sleep duration and increased rate of sleep onset. Additionally, spinosin reversed PCPA-induced suppression of the hypnotic effect of pentobarbital, suggesting that the potentiating mechanism of spinosyn might be associated with the serotonergic system.[81] Furthermore, postsynaptic 5-HT1A receptors were reported to be the responsible receptor.[82]

Experimental Studies on *Zhi Mu* 知母

Zhi mu 知母, the dried rhizomes of *Anemarrhena asphodeloides* Bunge., contains more than 108 compounds including steroidal saponins, flavonoids, phenylpropanoids, alkaloids, steroids, organic acids, anthraquinones and benzophenones. Among them, the most remarkable of the bioactive ingredients are the steroidal saponins (such as timosaponins AI, AII, AIII and AIV, and timosaponins BI and BII).[83] Pharmacological activities include anti-inflammatory, antioxidant, antimicrobial, antiviral, anti-osteoporosis, antitumour, antidiabetic, anticoagulant, antihypertensive and antidepressant effects; neuroprotective properties; and actions against skin ageing and damage.[83] Activities relevant to menopause have been identified.

Hormone Regulation

The steroidal saponins are major compounds from *A. asphodeloides* and their structures are similar to that of mammalian oestrogens. Indeed, it was reported that the ethanolic extracts of *A. asphodeloides* showed mild oestrogenic activity by increasing the uterine weight and E_2 level in serum in OVX rats.[84]

Antidepressant-like Activity

There are a great number of *in vitro* and/or *in vivo* studies that have demonstrated that various crude extracts and/or compounds of *A. asphodeloides* possess strong antidepressant-like effects. Treatment with sarsasapogenin in rodents could significantly reduce the duration of immobility in the FST without affecting locomotor activity. It also showed monoamine oxidase inhibitory activity in the mouse brain with a sharp increase of noradrenaline and 5-HT levels in the hypothalamus and hippocampus, indicating the antidepressant activity of sarsasapogenin might involve the central monoaminergic neurotransmitter systems.[85,86]

In addition to sarsasapogenin, timosaponin B-II (TB-II) and B-III (TB-III) have been considered important for the main antidepressive activity of timosaponins. TB-II demonstrated significant antidepressant bioactivity shown by effectively shortening the immobility time in TST and FST through 5-HT and DA pathways in the brain.[87] Additionally, TB-III and its two derivatives displayed modest antidepressive activity by reducing the duration in the OFT, TST and FST.[88] Furthermore, YY-23, a modified metabolite of TB-III, could affect NMDA receptors in acutely dissociated rat hippocampal CA1 neurons *in vitro*. In the CUMS and chronic social defeat stress (CSDS) mouse models, treatment of the stressed mice with YY-23 could rapidly and significantly reverse CUMS and CSDS-induced depressive behaviours, such as the CUMS-induced immobility deficit of TST and the deficiency of sucrose consumption in the sucrose preference test, and CSDS-induced reduction of social interaction, without affecting locomotor activity. These data indicated that YY-23 could act as a novel non-competitive NMDA receptor antagonist with rapid antidepressant-like effects in mouse models of CUMS and CSDS depression.[89]

Summary of Pharmacological Actions of the Common Herbs

Each of these ten herbs has attracted research attention in experimental models relevant to menopause. Most herbs, with the exception of *shan zhu yu* 山茱萸 and *suan zao ren* 酸枣仁, exhibited hormone regulatory actions through modulating the genomic nuclear ERα and ERβ, and the non-genomic oestrogen receptor (GPR30). In particular, *shu di huang* 熟地黄, *gan cao* 甘草 and *shan yao* 山药 exerted very strong oestrogen-like effects due to the fact that they contain phytoestrogens.

Phytoestrogens, known as selective oestrogen receptor modulators (SERMs), are both structurally and functionally similar to mammalian oestrogens, can act as weak agonists by stimulating oestrogen receptors to exert oestrogenic effects in the low-oestrogen environment of postmenopause and anti-oestrogenic effects in the high-oestrogen environment of premenopause.[90,91] Many plants have been identified as containing phytoestrogens; the most common types of phytoestrogens are coumestans, lignans and isoflavones. Phytoestrogens have been explored as a natural alternative to hormone therapy to improve menopausal symptoms by inhibiting or stimulating oestrogen-like actions in a cell-type, tissue-specific and dose-dependent manner, but with fewer side effects.[90,91]

Antidepressant-like actions were observed with most herbs, with the exception of *shan yao* 山药 and *shan zhu yu* 山茱萸. Powerful antidepressant properties were shown by restoring HPA axis dysfunction, modulating abnormal expression of neurotransmitters or receptors, and recovering abnormal expression of synaptic regulators. Sedative and hypnotic actions were observed with *gan cao* 甘草, *shan zhu yu* 山茱萸 and *suan zao ren* 酸枣仁. *Suan zao ren* 酸枣仁, in particular, showed excellent sedative and hypnotic properties due to its significant effects against disturbances of the central nervous system via modulation of the GABAergic system.

The crude extracts and/or pure compounds of *shu di huang* 熟地黄, *shan yao* 山药, *bai shao* 白芍, *chai hu* 柴胡, *dang gui* 当归 and *zhi mu* 知母 have been assessed in OVX rodent models. As highlighted above, the OVX rodent model does not model the menopause transition and rodents continue to have very low oestrogen levels. Further studies using the VCD rodent model could provide more guidance on the potential mechanisms of action for CHMs used in clinical practice.

These *in vitro* and *in vivo* studies examined herb actions specific to menopause and provide potential explanations for the clinical benefits of some of the common herbs. The findings highlight that CHMs have multiple components that can act on multiple pathways relevant to menopause. This fully reflects the multiple targets synergy characteristic of *CM generally.*

References

1. Xu LW, Jia M, Salchow R, *et al.* (2012) Efficacy and side effects of Chinese herbal medicine for menopausal symptoms: A critical review. *Evid Based Complement Alternat Med* **2012**: 568106.
2. Zhang Y, Xu L, Zheng Y, *et al.* (2017) Traditional Chinese herbal medicine for perimenopausal depression of Chinese women: A meta-analysis. *World J Tradit Chin Med* **3**(3): 51–57.
3. Zhu X, Liew Y, Liu ZL. (2016) Chinese herbal medicine for menopausal symptoms. *Cochrane Database Syst Rev* **3**: Cd009023.
4. Brooks HL, Pollow DP, Hoyer PB. (2016) The VCD mouse model of menopause and perimenopause for the study of sex differences in cardiovascular disease and the metabolic syndrome. *Physiology (Bethesda)* **31**(4): 250–257.
5. Diaz Brinton R. (2012) Minireview: Translational animal models of human menopause: Challenges and emerging opportunities. *Endocrinology* **153**(8): 3571–3578.
6. Van Kempen TA, Milner TA, Waters EM. (2011) Accelerated ovarian failure: A novel, chemically induced animal model of menopause. *Brain Res* **1379**: 176–187.
7. Zhang RX, Li MX, Jia ZP. (2008) Rehmannia glutinosa: Review of botany, chemistry and pharmacology. *J Ethnopharmacol* **117**(2): 199–214.
8. Liu C, Ma R, Wang L, *et al.* (2017) *Rehmanniae radix* in osteoporosis: A review of traditional Chinese medicinal uses, phytochemistry, pharmacokinetics and pharmacology. *J Ethnopharmacol* **198**: 351–362.
9. Paterni I, Granchi C, Katzenellenbogen JA, *et al.* (2014) Estrogen receptors alpha (ERalpha) and beta (ERbeta): Subtype-selective ligands and clinical potential. *Steroids* **90**: 13–29.
10. Wei M, Lu Y, Liu D, *et al.* (2014) Ovarian failure-resistant effects of catalpol in aged female rats. *Biol Pharm Bull* **37**(9): 1444–1449.

11. Li Y, Ma H, Lu Y, *et al.* (2016) Menoprogen, a TCM herbal formula for menopause, increases endogenous E2 in an aged rat model of menopause by reducing ovarian granulosa cell apoptosis. *Biomed Res Int* **2016**: 2574637.
12. Lu Y, Ma H, Liu D. (2008) Pharmacological investigations of the unique herbal formula Menoprogen in rats: Estrogenic activity and mechanism. *Gynecol Endocrinol* **24**(3): 161–170.
13. Ma H, Chung MH, Lu Y, *et al.* (2010) Estrogenic effects of the herbal formula, menoprogen, in ovariectomized rats. *Biol Pharm Bull* **33**(3): 455–460.
14. Wei M, Zheng SZ, Lu Y, *et al.* (2015) Herbal formula menoprogen alters insulin-like growth factor-1 and insulin-like growth factor binding protein-1 levels in the serum and ovaries of an aged female rat model of menopause. *Menopause* **22**(10): 1125–1133.
15. Juruena MF, Bocharova M, Agustini B, *et al.* (2018) Atypical depression and non-atypical depression: Is HPA axis function a biomarker? A systematic review. *J Affect Disord* **233**: 45–67.
16. Zhang Z, Deng T, Wu M, *et al.* (2019) Botanicals as modulators of depression and mechanisms involved. *Chin Med* **14**: 24.
17. Wang JM, Cui Y, Zhang YY, *et al.* (2014) Antidepressant-like effect of extracts from dried root of *Rehmannia glutinosa* (Dihuang). *J Chin Pharm Sci* **49**(23): 2073–2076.
18. Wang JM, Pei LX, Zhang YY, *et al.* (2018) Ethanol extract of Rehmannia glutinosa exerts antidepressant-like effects on a rat chronic unpredictable mild stress model by involving monoamines and BDNF. *Metab Brain Dis* **33**(3): 885–892.
19. Zhou XD, Shi DD, Zhang ZJ. (2019) Ameliorative effects of *Radix rehmanniae* extract on the anxiety- and depression-like symptoms in ovariectomized mice: A behavioral and molecular study. *Phytomedicine* **63**: 153012.
20. Wang J, Cui Y, Feng W, *et al.* (2014) Involvement of the central monoaminergic system in the antidepressant-like effect of catalpol in mice. *Biosci Trends* **8**(5): 248–252.
21. Rios JL. (2011) Chemical constituents and pharmacological properties of *Poria cocos*. *Planta Med* **77**(7): 681–691.
22. Sun Y. (2014) Biological activities and potential health benefits of polysaccharides from *Poria cocos* and their derivatives. *Int J Biol Macromol* **68**: 131–134.

23. Chen JT, Shiraki M. (2003) Menopausal hot flash and calciotonin gene-related peptide; effect of Keishi-bukuryo-gan, a kampo medicine, related to plasma calciotonin gene-related peptide level. *Maturitas* **45**(3): 199–204.
24. Noguchi M, Yuzurihara M, Ikarashi Y. (2002) Effects of the vasoactive neuropeptides calcitonin gene-related peptide, substance P and vasoactive intestinal polypeptide on skin temperature in ovariectomized rats. *Neuropeptides* **36**(5): 327–332.
25. Noguchi M, Ikarashi Y, Yuzurihara M, *et al.* (2003) Effects of the Japanese herbal medicine Keishi-bukuryo-gan and 17beta-estradiol on calcitonin gene-related peptide-induced elevation of skin temperature in ovariectomized rats. *J Endocrinol* **176**(3): 359–366.
26. Noguchi M, Ikarashi Y, Yuzurihara M, *et al.* (2003) Effects of 17 beta-estradiol and the Japanese herbal medicine Keishi-bukuryo-gan on the release and synthesis of calcitonin gene-related peptide in ovariectomized rats. *J Pharmacol Sci* **93**(1): 80–86.
27. Noguchi M, Ikarashi Y, Yuzurihara M, *et al.* (2005) Skin temperature rise induced by calcitonin gene-related peptide in gonadotropin-releasing hormone analogue-treated female rats and alleviation by Keishi-bukuryo-gan, a Japanese herbal medicine. *Life Sci* **76**(18): 2079–2090.
28. Dai Y, Li Z, Xue L, *et al.* (2010) Metabolomics study on the anti-depression effect of xiaoyaosan on rat model of chronic unpredictable mild stress. *J Ethnopharmacol* **128**(2): 482–489.
29. Zhou Y, Lu L, Li Z, *et al.* (2011) Antidepressant-like effects of the fractions of Xiaoyaosan on rat model of chronic unpredictable mild stress. *J Ethnopharmacol* **137**(1): 236–244.
30. Asl MN, Hosseinzadeh H. (2008) Review of pharmacological effects of *Glycyrrhiza* sp. and its bioactive compounds. *Phytother Res* **22**(6): 709–724.
31. Ji S, Li Z, Song W, *et al.* (2016) Bioactive constituents of *Glycyrrhiza uralensis* (Licorice): Discovery of the effective components of a traditional herbal medicine. *J Nat Prod* **79**(2): 281–292.
32. Zhang Q, Ye M. (2009) Chemical analysis of the Chinese herbal medicine Gan-Cao (licorice). *J Chromatogr A* **1216**(11): 1954–1969.
33. Peng F, Du Q, Peng C, *et al.* (2015) A review: The pharmacology of isoliquiritigenin. *Phytother Res* **29**(7): 969–977.
34. Kang SC, Lee CM, Choi H, *et al.* (2006) Evaluation of oriental medicinal herbs for estrogenic and antiproliferative activities. *Phytother Res* **20**(11): 1017–1019.

35. Hajirahimkhan A, Simmler C, Yuan Y, *et al.* (2013) Evaluation of estrogenic activity of licorice species in comparison with hops used in botanicals for menopausal symptoms. *PLoS One* **8**(7): e67947.
36. Hajirahimkhan A, Mbachu O, Simmler C, *et al.* (2018) Estrogen receptor (ER) subtype selectivity identifies 8-prenylapigenin as an ERbeta agonist from *Glycyrrhiza inflata* and highlights the importance of chemical and biological authentication. *J Nat Prod* **81**(4): 966–975.
37. Tamir S, Eizenberg M, Somjen D, *et al.* (2000) Estrogenic and antiproliferative properties of glabridin from licorice in human breast cancer cells. *Cancer Res* **60**(20): 5704–5709.
38. Tamir S, Eizenberg M, Somjen D, *et al.* (2001) Estrogen-like activity of glabrene and other constituents isolated from licorice root. *J Steroid Biochem Mol Biol* **78**(3): 291–298.
39. Gong P, Madak-Erdogan Z, Flaws JA, *et al.* (2016) Estrogen receptor-alpha and aryl hydrocarbon receptor involvement in the actions of botanical estrogens in target cells. *Mol Cell Endocrinol* **437**: 190–200.
40. Gong P, Madak-Erdogan Z, Li J, *et al.* (2014) Transcriptomic analysis identifies gene networks regulated by estrogen receptor alpha (ERalpha) and ERbeta that control distinct effects of different botanical estrogens. *Nucl Recept Signal* **12**: e001.
41. Ahmed HM, Yeh JY, Tang YC, *et al.* (2014) Molecular screening of Chinese medicinal plants for progestogenic and anti-progestogenic activity. *J Biosci* **39**(3): 453–461.
42. Dhingra D, Sharma A. (2006) Antidepressant-like activity of *Glycyrrhiza glabra* L. in mouse models of immobility tests. *Prog Neuropsychopharmacol Biol Psychiatry* **30**(3): 449–454.
43. Wang W, Hu X, Zhao Z, *et al.* (2008) Antidepressant-like effects of liquiritin and isoliquiritin from *Glycyrrhiza uralensis* in the forced swimming test and tail suspension test in mice. *Prog Neuropsychopharmacol Biol Psychiatry* **32**(5): 1179–1184.
44. Erman MK. (2005) Therapeutic options in the treatment of insomnia. *J Clin Psychiatry* **66**(Suppl 9): 18–23; quiz 42–43.
45. Cho S, Park JH, Pae AN, *et al.* (2012) Hypnotic effects and GABAergic mechanism of licorice (*Glycyrrhiza glabra*) ethanol extract and its major flavonoid constituent glabrol. *Bioorg Med Chem* **20**(11): 3493–3501.
46. Jin Z, Kim S, Cho S, *et al.* (2013) Potentiating effect of glabridin on GABAA receptor-mediated responses in dorsal raphe neurons. *Planta Med* **79**(15): 1408–1412.

47. Jang EY, Choe ES, Hwang M, *et al.* (2008) Isoliquiritigenin suppresses cocaine-induced extracellular dopamine release in rat brain through GABA(B) receptor. *Eur J Pharmacol* **587**(1–3): 124–128.
48. Ma F, Wang D, Zhang Y, *et al.* (2018) Characterisation of the mucilage polysaccharides from *Dioscorea opposita* Thunb. with enzymatic hydrolysis. *Food Chem* **245**: 13–21.
49. Zhang Y, Chao L, Ruan J, *et al.* (2016) Bioactive constituents from the rhizomes of *Dioscorea septemloba* Thunb. *Fitoterapia* **115**: 165–172.
50. Zeng M, Zhang L, Li M, *et al.* (2018) Estrogenic effects of the extracts from the Chinese yam (*Dioscorea opposita* Thunb.) and its effective compounds *in vitro* and *in vivo*. *Molecules* **23**(2): 11.
51. Wong KL, Lai YM, Li KW, *et al.* (2015) A novel, stable, estradiol-stimulating, osteogenic yam protein with potential for the treatment of menopausal syndrome. *Sci Rep* **5**: 10179.
52. Pearce ST, Jordan VC. (2004) The biological role of estrogen receptors alpha and beta in cancer. *Crit Rev Oncol Hematol* **50**(1): 3–22.
53. Lu J, Wong RN, Zhang L, *et al.* (2016) Comparative analysis of proteins with stimulating activity on ovarian estradiol biosynthesis from four different *Dioscorea* species *in vitro* using both phenotypic and target-based approaches: Implication for treating menopause. *Appl Biochem Biotechnol* **180**(1): 79–93.
54. He DY, Dai SM. (2011) Anti-inflammatory and immunomodulatory effects of *Paeonia lactiflora* Pall., a traditional chinese herbal medicine. *Front Pharmacol* **2**: 10.
55. Parker S, May B, Zhang C, *et al.* (2016) A pharmacological review of bioactive constituents of *Paeonia lactiflora* Pallas and *Paeonia veitchii* Lynch. *Phytother Res* **30**(9): 1445–1473.
56. Xu Y, Li X, Chen T, *et al.* (2019) *Radix Paeoniae Alba* increases serum estrogen level and up-regulates estrogen receptor expression in uterus and vagina of immature/ovariectomized mice. *Phytother Res* **33**(1): 117–129.
57. Mao QQ, Ip SP, Tsai SH, *et al.* (2008) Antidepressant-like effect of peony glycosides in mice. *J Ethnopharmacol* **119**(2): 272–275.
58. Song J, Hou X, Hu X, *et al.* (2015) Not only serotonergic system, but also dopaminergic system involved in albiflorin against chronic unpredictable mild stress-induced depression-like behavior in rats. *Chem Biol Interact* **242**: 211–217.
59. Sun P, Li Y, Wei S, *et al.* (2019) Pharmacological effects and chemical constituents of Bupleurum. *Mini Rev Med Chem* **19**(1): 34–55.

60. Yang F, Dong X, Yin X, *et al.* (2017) *Radix Bupleuri*: A review of traditional uses, botany, phytochemistry, pharmacology, and toxicology. *Biomed Res Int* **2017**: 7597596.
61. Wang P, Ren J, Tang J, *et al.* (2010) Estrogen-like activities of saikosaponin-d *in vitro*: A pilot study. *Eur J Pharmacol* **626**(2–3): 159–165.
62. Liao JF, Jan YM, Huang SY, *et al.* (1995) Evaluation with receptor binding assay on the water extracts of ten CNS-active Chinese herbal drugs. *Proc Natl Sci Counc Repub China B* **19**(3): 151–158.
63. Kwon S, Lee B, Kim M, *et al.* (2010) Antidepressant-like effect of the methanolic extract from *Bupleurum falcatum* in the tail suspension test. *Prog Neuropsychopharmacol Biol Psychiatry* **34**(2): 265–270.
64. Lee B, Yun HY, Shim I, *et al.* (2012) *Bupleurum falcatum* prevents depression and anxiety-like behaviors in rats exposed to repeated restraint stress. *J Microbiol Biotechnol* **22**(3): 422–430.
65. Chao WW, Lin BF. (2011) Bioactivities of major constituents isolated from *Angelica sinensis* (Danggui). *Chin Med* **6**: 29.
66. Wei WL, Zeng R, Gu CM, *et al.* (2016) *Angelica sinensis* in China: A review of botanical profile, ethnopharmacology, phytochemistry and chemical analysis. *J Ethnopharmacol* **190**: 116–141.
67. Circosta C, Pasquale RD, Palumbo DR, *et al.* (2006) Estrogenic activity of standardized extract of *Angelica sinensis. Phytother Res* **20**(8): 665–669.
68. Deng S, Chen SN, Yao P, *et al.* (2006) Serotonergic activity-guided phytochemical investigation of the roots of *Angelica sinensis. J Nat Prod* **69**(4): 536–541.
69. Dong Y, Feng ZL, Chen HB, *et al.* (2018) *Corni Fructus*: A review of chemical constituents and pharmacological activities. *Chin Med* **13**: 34.
70. Huang J, Zhang Y, Dong L, *et al.* (2018) Ethnopharmacology, phytochemistry, and pharmacology of *Cornus officinalis* Sieb. et Zucc. *J Ethnopharmacol* **213**: 280–301.
71. Shi R, Han Y, Yan Y, *et al.* (2019) Loganin exerts sedative and hypnotic effects via modulation of the serotonergic system and GABAergic neurons. *Front Pharmacol* **10**: 409.
72. Gao QH, Wu CS, Wang M. (2013) The jujube (*Ziziphus jujuba* Mill.) fruit: A review of current knowledge of fruit composition and health benefits. *J Agric Food Chem* **61**(14): 3351–3363.
73. Yang B, Yang H, Chen F, *et al.* (2013) Phytochemical analyses of *Ziziphus jujuba* Mill. var. spinosa seed by ultrahigh performance liquid chromatography-tandem mass spectrometry and gas chromatography-mass spectrometry. *Analyst* **138**(22): 6881–6888.

74. Liu J, Qiao W, Yang Y, *et al.* (2012) Antidepressant-like effect of the ethanolic extract from Suanzaorenhehuan Formula in mice models of depression. *J Ethnopharmacol* **141**(1): 257–264.
75. Liang Y, Yang X, Zhang X, *et al.* (2016) Antidepressant-like effect of the saponins part of ethanol extract from SHF. *J Ethnopharmacol* **191**: 307–314.
76. Wang Y, Huang M, Lu X, *et al.* (2017) *Ziziphi spinosae* lily powder suspension in the treatment of depression-like behaviors in rats. *BMC Complement Altern Med* **17**(1): 238.
77. Yang HY, Tan, JP, Chen CF. (1987) Central pharmacological effects of five Chinese herbs. *Chin Med J* **40**: 193–200.
78. Ma Y, Han H, Eun JS, *et al.* (2007) Sanjoinine A isolated from Zizyphi Spinosi Semen augments pentobarbital-induced sleeping behaviors through the modification of GABA-ergic systems. *Biol Pharm Bull* **30**(9): 1748–1753.
79. Han H, Ma Y, Eun JS, *et al.* (2009) Anxiolytic-like effects of sanjoinine A isolated from Zizyphi Spinosi Semen: Possible involvement of GABAergic transmission. *Pharmacol Biochem Behav* **92**(2): 206–213.
80. Ma Y, Han H, Nam SY, *et al.* (2008) Cyclopeptide alkaloid fraction from Zizyphi Spinosi Semen enhances pentobarbital-induced sleeping behaviors. *J Ethnopharmacol* **117**(2): 318–324.
81. Wang LE, Bai YJ, Shi XR, *et al.* (2008) Spinosin, a C-glycoside flavonoid from semen Zizhiphi Spinozae, potentiated pentobarbital-induced sleep via the serotonergic system. *Pharmacol Biochem Behav* **90**(3): 399–403.
82. Wang LE, Cui XY, Cui SY, *et al.* (2010) Potentiating effect of spinosin, a C-glycoside flavonoid of Semen Ziziphi spinosae, on pentobarbital-induced sleep may be related to postsynaptic 5-HT(1A) receptors. *Phytomedicine* **17**(6): 404–409.
83. Wang Y, Dan Y, Yang D, *et al.* (2014) The genus Anemarrhena Bunge: A review on ethnopharmacology, phytochemistry and pharmacology. *J Ethnopharmacol* **153**(1): 42–60.
84. Nian H, Qin LP, Chen WS, *et al.* (2006) Protective effect of steroidal saponins from rhizome of *Anemarrhena asphodeloides* on ovariectomy-induced bone loss in rats. *Acta Pharmacol Sin* **27**(6): 728–734.
85. Ren LX, Luo YF, Li X, *et al.* (2007) Antidepressant activity of sarsasapogenin from *Anemarrhena asphodeloides* Bunge (Liliaceae). *Pharmazie* **62**(1): 78–79.
86. Ren LX, Luo YF, Li X, *et al.* (2006) Antidepressant-like effects of sarsasapogenin from *Anemarrhena asphodeloides* Bunge (Liliaceae). *Biol Pharm Bull* **29**(11): 2304–2306.

87. Lu MZ, Zhang ZQ, Yi J, *et al.* (2010) Study on the effect and mechanisms of timosaponin B-II on antidepressant. *J Pharm Pract* **1**(4): 283–287.
88. Jiang W, Guo J, Xue R, *et al.* (2014) Anti-depressive activities and biotransformation of timosaponin B-III and its derivatives. *Nat Prod Res* **28**(18): 1446–1453.
89. Zhang Q, Guo F, Fu ZW, *et al.* (2016) Timosaponin derivative YY-23 acts as a non-competitive NMDA receptor antagonist and exerts a rapid antidepressant-like effect in mice. *Acta Pharmacol Sin* **37**(2): 166–176.
90. Franco OH, Chowdhury R, Troup J, *et al.* (2016) Use of plant-based therapies and menopausal symptoms: A systematic review and meta-analysis. *JAMA* **315**(23): 2554–2563.
91. Morito K, Hirose T, Kinjo J, *et al.* (2001) Interaction of phytoestrogens with estrogen receptors alpha and beta. *Biol Pharm Bull* **24**(4): 351–356.

7

Clinical Evidence for Acupuncture and Related Therapies

OVERVIEW

Acupuncture and related therapies are used frequently in clinical practice for menopausal symptoms and have been the subject of many clinical studies. This chapter presents a selection of acupuncture clinical studies. Among 97 such studies, the different interventions that have been tested for menopausal symptoms are described, Chinese medicine syndromes discussed and the efficacy and safety of these treatments reviewed. Acupuncture was the most frequently tested intervention and may be beneficial for improving sleep, psychological symptoms and global symptom severity.

Introduction

The term 'acupuncture' is used to describe a range of different techniques that stimulate acupuncture points to correct imbalances of energy and restore health. The most common technique in clinical practice is acupuncture, which involves the insertion of an acupuncture needle into specific acupuncture points. Other techniques include acupressure (application of pressure to acupuncture points), moxibustion (burning of a herb [*ai ye* 艾叶, *Artemesia vulgaris* L.] close to, or on, the skin to induce a warming sensation) and electroacupuncture (application of an electrical current to acupuncture needles whilst *in situ*). While acupuncture, acupressure and moxibustion have been used for millennia, other techniques such as electroacupuncture have emerged as new technologies in the last century. Many of these techniques are used in clinical practice to alleviate bothersome symptoms of menopause.

Previous Systematic Reviews

The comprehensive search identified eight systematic reviews (SRs) and meta-analyses published in Chinese and ten SRs published in English that evaluated the efficacy and safety of acupuncture and related therapies for menopause. Among the Chinese articles, two meta-analyses[1,2] compared acupuncture and related therapies, including manual acupuncture, electroacupuncture, moxibustion and ear acupressure, with pharmacotherapy. Results from one study reviewed 28 randomised controlled trials (RCTs) and showed acupuncture therapy was more effective than pharmacotherapy in reducing Kupperman Index (KI) score,[1] but the second SR of 19 RCTs revealed no difference between two comparators.[2]

In 2012, Cheng *et al.* (2018)[3] reviewed six RCTs and reported there was no statistical difference between electroacupuncture and hormone therapy (HT) in terms of KI score, but found fewer adverse events (AEs) in the electroacupuncture group. Lai *et al.* 2017[4] systematically reviewed the effectiveness and safety of manual acupuncture in 40 RCTs and revealed that manual acupuncture was superior to pharmacotherapy with a low frequency of AEs. Two meta-analyses[5,6] showed acupuncture and related therapies were more effective than pharmacotherapy in reducing Pittsburgh Sleep Quality Index (PSQI) score in menopausal women. Grading of Recommendations Assessment, Development and Evaluation (GRADE) assessment indicated 'very low' certainty evidence in one of the studies.[6] This SR also reported acupuncture was superior to sham acupuncture, and GRADE evaluation indicated 'low' certainty evidence. Two SRs revealed that there was no difference between acupuncture and pharmacotherapy in terms of Hamilton Rating Scale for Depression (HAM-D) score.[7,8]

Many of the SRs published in English focused on evaluating the effect of acupuncture on hot flushes. A Cochrane SR of 16 RCTs found acupuncture was superior to no treatment, not different to sham/placebo but was inferior to HT in reducing hot flushes.[9] Ee *et al.* (2017) came to similar conclusions in their updated review of the evidence.[10] Earlier SRs by Lee *et al.* (2009)[11] and Cho and Whang (2009)[12] also reached the same findings. The most recent SR on acupuncture for menopausal hot flushes concluded that acupuncture was superior to sham acupuncture in improving hot flushes.[13] In addition to searching the English- and Chinese-language databases, this SR also searched Korean-language databases.

Taylor-Swanson *et al.* (2015)[14] examined the efficacy of acupuncture, moxibustion or Chinese herbal medicine (CHM) on symptom clusters, that is, hot flushes combined with at least one other menopausal symptom of sleep, mood, sleep disturbances or pain. The authors concluded that acupuncture and moxibustion were beneficial for hot flushes based on narrative synthesis of the included studies.

The efficacy of acupuncture has also been tested for menopausal sleep disorders.[15] Diversity in the 12 RCTs prevented meta-analysis, with the authors stating that acupuncture improved sleep-related outcome measures. The effect of acupuncture on quality of life has been examined in two SRs.[16,17] Chiu *et al.* (2015)[16] concluded that, based on 12 RCTs, acupuncture reduced the frequency and severity of hot flushes, reduced scores on the psychological, somatic and urogenital subscales of the Menopause Rating Scale (MRS) and reduced scores on the vasomotor domain of the Menopause-specific Quality of Life Questionnaire (MENQOL). Li *et al.* (2018)[17] reached similar conclusions about the positive effect of acupuncture on menopause-related quality of life, albeit based on a smaller number of RCTs with 'low' certainty evidence.

An umbrella SR and meta-analysis published in 2018[18] concluded that acupuncture alone, or as an adjunct treatment, can reduce vasomotor symptoms and improve health-related quality of life. This conclusion was based on analysis of three SRs and four new RCTs. Furthermore, the authors concluded that there is no indication that acupuncture has the potential to cause significant harm.

Identification of Clinical Studies

The comprehensive search identified 49,278 potentially relevant citations in the nine databases (Fig. 7.1). Results were exported to reference management software and duplicates removed. The title and abstract for each remaining citation were reviewed, which resulted in more than 12,000 citations being excluded. After full-text review, 104 clinical studies were selected which were reported in 107 publications. Seven studies tested interventions not commonly practised outside of China; these were not analysed. Ninety-seven studies were reported in 100 publications. These included 79 RCTs, six controlled clinical trials (CCTs) and 12 non-controlled studies. Studies are indicated by the letter 'A' followed by a number. The references for included studies can be found at the end of the chapter.

Acupuncture

The majority of included studies tested acupuncture alone or combined with other acupuncture therapies. Seventy clinical studies of acupuncture included 57 RCTs (A1–A57), six non-randomised CCTs (A58–A63) and seven non-controlled studies (A64–A70).

Randomised Controlled Trials of Acupuncture

Fifty-seven RCTs, involving 5,049 women, met the inclusion criteria for this review (A1–A57). The majority were conducted in China, while six were conducted in the United States (A1–A6) and one study each was conducted in Norway (A7), Brazil (A8), Switzerland (A9), Turkey (A10) and Korea (A11). Three studies included three arms (A2, A4, A12). Only two of the three arms in one study met the inclusion criteria, and data for the third arm were excluded (A12). The studies by Avis *et al.* (A2) and Painovich *et al.* (A4) both compared acupuncture with no treatment and with sham acupuncture. One four-arm study included acupuncture, sham acupuncture, CHM and placebo CHM. The results for CHM have been included in Chapter 5 and only

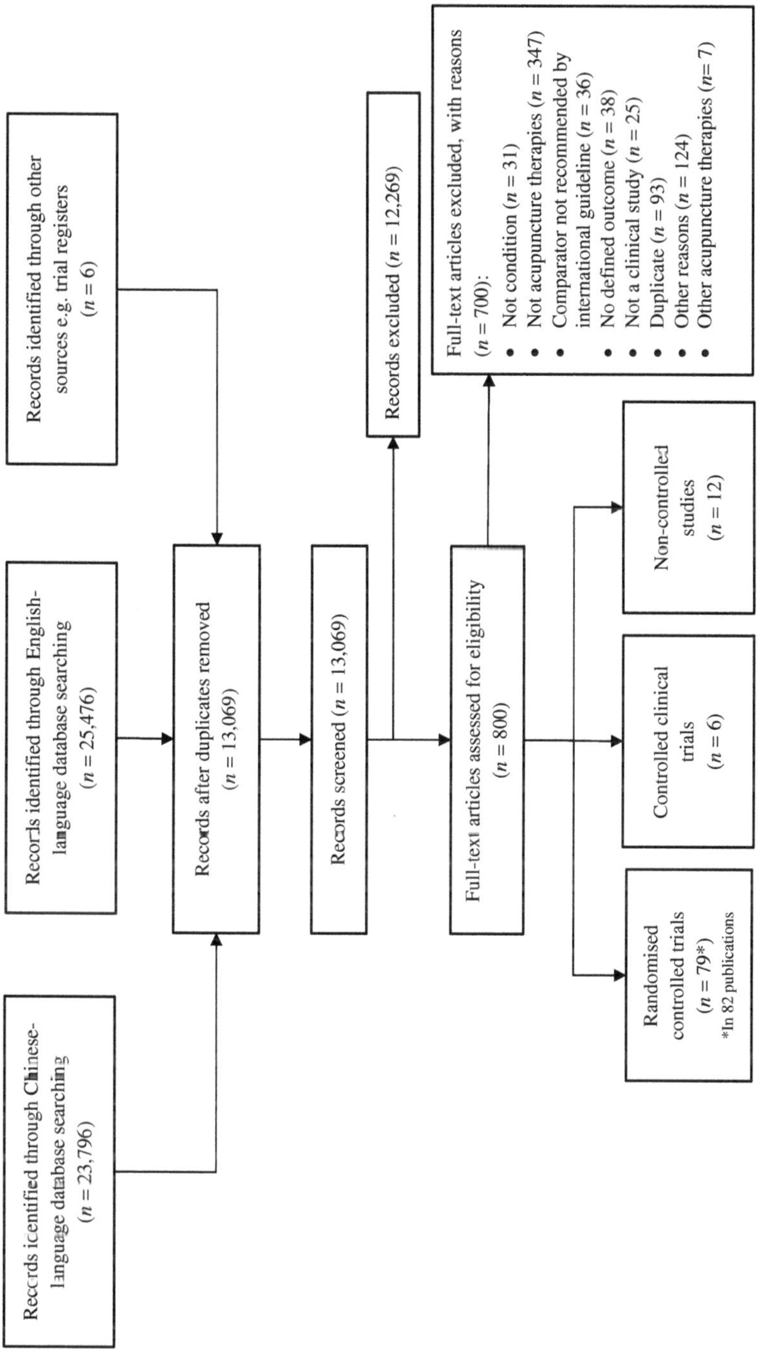

Fig. 7.1 Flowchart of study selection process: Acupuncture and related therapies.

the acupuncture and sham acupuncture arms are included in this analysis.

Many of the studies conducted in China included women with comorbidities. Sixteen studies (A13–A28) included women with depression, 15 studies (A29–A43) included women with insomnia, one study (A44) included women with anxiety, one study (A45) included women with loss of appetite and one study (A46) included depressed women with pain. Five studies (A5, A7, A9–A11) included postmenopausal women, one study (A47) included women who had had an ovariectomy, six studies (A1–A3, A6, A8, A48) included both perimenopausal and postmenopausal women, two studies (A4, A49) did not specify menopausal status and the remaining studies described women as perimenopausal.

Chinese medicine syndrome differentiation was reported in 17 studies (A1–A3, A5, A7, A9, A19, A29, A32, A36, A38, A42, A45, A48, A50–A52). Syndromes that described similar concepts were grouped for analysis. The most frequently reported syndromes were Kidney deficiency, including Kidney *yin* deficiency and Kidney *yin* and *yang* deficiency (five studies) and Kidney and Heart not communicating (five studies). Other frequently reported syndromes were Liver and Kidney *yin* deficiency (four studies), Spleen and Kidney *yang* deficiency (four studies), Kidney and Liver *yin* deficiency with Liver *yang* rising (three studies) and *qi* stagnation with Blood stasis (three studies).

Ten studies used acupuncture as integrative medicine (A5, A7, A13, A15, A17, A35, A36, A39, A41, A44), which included treatment with pharmacotherapy or diet/lifestyle advice. Other studies tested acupuncture alone, apart from five studies that combined acupuncture with other related techniques including electroacupuncture (A5), moxibustion (A33, A53) and ear acupressure (A44, A47).

Acupuncture points included a mix of meridian points and extra points. The most frequently used acupuncture point was SP6 *Sanyinjiao* 三阴交 (Table 7.1). Other commonly used acupuncture points included HT7 *Shenmen* 神门, LR3 *Taichong* 太冲 and CV4 *Guanyuan* 关元.

Table 7.1 Most Frequently Reported Points in Acupuncture Randomised Controlled Trials

Acupuncture Point	Frequency of Use
SP6 *Sanyinjiao* 三阴交	27
HT7 *Shenmen* 神门	21
LR3 *Taichong* 太冲	21
CV4 *Guanyuan* 关元	19
BL23 *Shenshu* 肾俞	17
PC6 *Neiguan* 内关	17
GV20 *Baihui* 百会	16
ST36 *Zusanli* 足三里	16
BL18 *Ganshu* 肝俞	15
KI3 *Taixi* 太溪	15
EX-HN1 *Sishencong* 四神聪	15

Duration of treatment ranged from 15 days (A54) to 12 months (A8) and the median treatment duration was six weeks. Thirteen studies (A1–A3, A5–A7, A9, A11, A21, A46–A48, A55) conducted follow-up assessment after treatment ceased. Follow-up duration ranged from four weeks (A11, A21, A46, A47, A55) to 12 months (A7). Twenty studies (A1, A3–A11, A14–A16, A21, A31, A38, A43, A47, A48, A51) reported loss to follow-up. Comparators included no treatment (A1, A4, A31), sham acupuncture (A2, A6, A8, A9, A11, A13, A49), placebo acupuncture (A3, A5, A10, A43, A48), HT (A12, A15, A18, A27, A47, A50–A57), antidepressants (A13, A14, A17, A19–A26, A28, A30, A44, A46), benzodiapezines (A29, A32–A42, A45), psychological treatment (A16) and self-care/lifestyle advice (A5, A7).

Risk of Bias

Studies were limited by potential sources of bias (Table 7.2). Thirty-three RCTs used appropriate methods to allocate women to study

Table 7.2 Risk of Bias of Randomised Controlled Trials: Acupuncture

Risk of Bias Domain	Low Risk *n* (%)	Unclear Risk *n* (%)	High Risk *n* (%)
Sequence generation	33 (57.9)	17 (29.8)	7 (12.3)
Allocation concealment	12 (21.1)	43 (75.4)	2 (3.5)
Blinding of participants	12 (21.1)	0 (0)	45 (78.9)
Blinding of personnel*	0 (0)	16 (28.1)	41 (71.9)
Blinding of outcome assessors	8 (14.0)	49 (86.0)	0 (0)
Incomplete outcome data	54 (94.7)	2 (3.5)	1 (1.8)
Selective outcome reporting	2 (3.5)	53 (93.0)	2 (3.5)

*Blinding of personnel (acupuncturists) is challenging in manual therapy studies.

groups and were judged 'low' risk of bias. Seven RCTs that allocated women according to visit order or alternate allocation were judged as 'high' risk. Twelve studies used central randomisation or sealed envelopes to conceal group allocation, posing 'low' risk of bias, while two studies used methods that were unlikely to conceal group allocation. Few studies blinded participants to group allocation, with 45 RCTs being judged as 'high' risk of bias. The majority of studies were judged 'high' risk of bias (41 of 57) due to a lack of blinding of personnel, although it is acknowledged that this is challenging in manual therapy studies.

Eight studies blinded outcome assessors to group allocation and were judged 'low' risk for this domain, while no such information was provided in the remaining studies. Most studies (54 RCTs) either had no missing data, used appropriate statistical methods to account for missing data, or were considered unlikely to impact on outcomes, and were judged as 'low' risk of bias. For two studies it was not possible to determine the impact of missing data on study results ('unclear' risk of bias) and missing data from one study was considered likely to impact on outcomes ('high' risk of bias). The trial protocols for two studies were available and papers reported all pre-specified outcomes; these were assessed as 'low' risk of bias. Differences were noted between outcomes specified in trial registration and those reported in the study reports for two RCTs, posing 'high' risk of bias.

Outcomes

Outcome measures used in included studies reflected the diversity in menopausal symptoms and the comorbidities of women included in the studies. Several studies reported results in a way that did not permit re-analysis and these results have not been included in the quantitative analyses described hereafter. None of the included studies assessed genitourinary symptoms of menopause.

Psychological symptoms were evaluated in 27 RCTs, most commonly with the HAM-D[19] or Hamilton Rating Scale for Anxiety (HAM-A).[20] Global symptom assessment was conducted in 23 RCTs, with most studies using the KI.[21] Twenty RCTs reported assessment of sleep symptoms, which were frequently measured using the PSQI.[22] Fewer studies assessed vasomotor symptoms (11 RCTs), health-related quality of life (7 RCTs) and musculoskeletal symptoms (one RCT). Safety was assessed in half of all studies (29 RCTs).

Vasomotor Symptoms

Eleven RCTs (A1–A5, A7–A9, A11, A47, A48) assessed vasomotor symptoms, most of which assessed daily hot flush frequency or severity. Results were analysed according to the comparison.

Acupuncture versus no treatment

A composite measure of hot flushes and night sweats was calculated by multiplying the number of vasomotor symptoms by severity (4-point scale, lower is better) (A1). In 209 postmenopausal women, acupuncture was more effective than no treatment in changing vasomotor symptom score from baseline to the end of treatment (mean difference [MD] −42.70 points [95% confidence intervals −45.28, −40.12]).

Acupuncture versus sham/placebo acupuncture

Four RCTs that compared acupuncture with sham or placebo acupuncture assessed daily hot flush frequency and/or severity.

Meta-analysis of two studies showed no difference between acupuncture and sham/placebo acupuncture in reducing the frequency of hot flushes at the end of treatment (two RCTs, 408 women, MD −1.06 flushes [−2.27, 0.15]; A8, A48). Follow-up assessments in one study (A48) showed no difference between acupuncture and sham acupuncture in hot flush frequency at three months (327 women, MD 0.41 flushes [−1.15, 1.97]) or at six months (327 women, MD 0.08 flushes [−1.51, 1.67]).

A third study (A3) that reported daily hot flush frequency was analysed separately as the study investigators used non-parametric tests in their analysis, suggesting data were not normally distributed. This study found no difference between groups in hot flush frequency at the end of treatment (29 women, MD −2.15 flushes [−5.07, 0.77]). At follow-up assessment after one month, the result favoured acupuncture (29 women, MD −2.48 flushes [−4.30, −0.66]).

Daily hot flush severity was reported in two studies (A3, A48). Studies were analysed individually for the reasons described above. In the study by Ee *et al.* (2016; A48), daily hot flush severity was not statistically different between groups at the end of treatment (327 women, MD 0.32 points [−2.97, 3.61]), at three months follow-up (327 women, MD 0.28 points [−3.14, 3.70]), or at six months follow-up (327 women, MD −0.17 points [−3.90, 3.56]). Similarly, in the smaller study by Nir *et al.* (A3), women who received acupuncture reported hot flush severity that was not statistically different to placebo acupuncture at the end of treatment (29 women, MD −0.36 points [−0.85, 0.13]) or at one month follow-up (29 women, MD −0.46 points [−0.95, 0.03]).

The change in hot flush frequency and severity was assessed weekly in the study by Nedeljkovic *et al.* (A9). Acupuncture resulted in a greater reduction in weekly hot flush frequency from baseline to the end of treatment than sham acupuncture (20 women, MD −24.00 flushes [−47.05, −0.95]), although the change was not statistically different at follow-up (20 women, MD −14.50 flushes [−44.59, 15.59]). Change in weekly hot flush severity was not different between acupuncture and sham acupuncture at end of treatment

(20 women, MD −45.20 points [−92.31, 1.91]), or at follow-up (20 women, MD −26.10 points [−82.29, 30.09]). Kim *et al.* (A11) used non-parametric tests to analyse weekly hot flush severity at end of treatment, and this study was analysed separately. Among the 49 women included in analysis, women who received acupuncture reported less severe hot flushes than women who received sham acupuncture (MD −11.33 points [−14.28, −8.38]).

Acupuncture plus ear acupressure versus hormone therapy

One small study assessed frequency and severity of daily hot flushes in 43 women who had undergone ovariectomy (A47). Women who received acupuncture plus ear acupressure reported more hot flushes per day than women who received tibolone at the end of treatment (MD 2.84 flushes [1.07, 4.61]) and at follow-up after four weeks (MD 2.11 flushes [1.18, 3.04]). There was no difference between groups in the severity of hot flushes at the end of treatment (MD 0.20 points [−0.40, 0.80]), but four weeks after treatment ceased, women who received acupuncture plus ear acupressure reported more severe hot flushes (MD 1.82 points [1.09, 2.54]).

Acupuncture plus self-care advice versus self-care advice alone

In one RCT (A7) that combined acupuncture with self-care advice, women in the treatment group reported a greater change in daily hot flushes (267 women, MD −2.10 flushes [−3.10, −1.10]) and less severe hot flushes (MD −1.40 points [−1.96, −0.84]) from baseline to the end of treatment, compared to women who received self-care advice alone. These effects were no longer statistically significant at six months follow-up (hot flush frequency: MD −0.30 flushes [−1.55, 0.95]; hot flush severity: MD −0.30 points [−0.94, 0.34]) or at 12 months follow-up (hot flush frequency: MD −0.20 flushes [−1.59, 1.19]; hot flush severity: MD 0.00 points [−0.68, 0.68]).

Acupuncture plus electroacupuncture plus self-care advice versus placebo acupuncture plus self-care advice

One RCT tested the effect of acupuncture, electroacupuncture and diet/lifestyle advice against placebo acupuncture plus diet/lifestyle advice (A5). This study showed no difference of the intervention in reducing the frequency of daily hot flushes (51 women, MD 0.10 flushes [−1.47, 1.67]).

Pittsburgh Sleep Quality Index

Fourteen RCTs (A1, A29–A32, A34–A39, A41–A43) used the PSQI to measure sleep symptoms.

Acupuncture versus no treatment

Two RCTs compared the effect of acupuncture and no treatment on the PSQI (A1, A31). Meta-analysis showed acupuncture was not statistically different to no treatment in PSQI scores at the end of treatment (274 women, MD −4.10 points [−9.48, 1.28], I^2 = 99%). Statistically considerable heterogeneity was detected that lowers confidence in the results.

Acupuncture versus placebo acupuncture

Acupuncture was compared with placebo acupuncture in one RCT that used the PSQI to measure sleep symptoms (A43). Women who received acupuncture scored 6.14 points lower at the end of treatment than women who received placebo acupuncture (74 women [−7.57, −4.71]), indicating greater improvements in sleep symptoms.

Acupuncture versus pharmacotherapy

Seven studies (A29, A30, A32, A34, A37, A38, A42) compared acupuncture with pharmacotherapy in 532 perimenopausal women with insomnia. Acupuncture was not statistically different

Table 7.3 Acupuncture versus Pharmacotherapy: Pittsburgh Sleep Quality Index

Group	No. of Studies (Participants)	Effect Size (MD [95% CI], I^2)	Included Studies
All studies	7 (532)	−1.87 [−3.94, 0.19], 96%	A29, A30, A32, A34, A37, A38, A42
Low RoB SG	5 (310)	−1.75 [−4.67, 1.17], 97%	A29, A30, A34, A37, A38
Treatment: ≤8 w	5 (310)	−1.75 [−4.67, 1.17], 97%	A29, A30, A34, A37, A38
Treatment: >8 w	2 (222)	−2.40 [−3.07, −1.74]*, 0%	A32, A42

*Statistically significant, see Chapter 4.
Abbreviations: CI, confidence interval; MD, mean difference; RoB, risk of bias; SG, sequence generation; w, weeks.

to pharmacotherapy in reducing PSQI scores at the end of treatment (MD −1.87 points [−3.94, 0.19], I^2 = 96%). Subgroup analyses were conducted to examine potential causes for statistical heterogeneity (Table 7.3). Statistical heterogeneity remained 'high' in studies that were assessed as 'low' risk of bias for sequence generation, all of which provided treatment for eight weeks or less. The subgroup with the least amount of statistical heterogeneity was treatment for more than eight weeks, which also showed a result that favoured acupuncture over pharmacotherapy. Due to the small number of studies included in this subgroup analysis, the results should be viewed with caution.

Acupuncture plus pharmacotherapy versus pharmacotherapy alone

Four RCTs (A35, A36, A39, A41) that used acupuncture as integrative medicine with pharmacotherapy assessed sleep using the PSQI. Meta-analysis of all four studies showed women who received the combination of acupuncture and pharmacotherapy scored 2.28 points lower on the PSQI than women who received

Table 7.4 Acupuncture Plus Pharmacotherapy versus Pharmacotherapy Alone: Pittsburgh Sleep Quality Index

Group	No. of Studies (Participants)	Effect Size (MD [95% CI], I^2)	Included Studies
All studies	4 (320)	−2.28 [−3.17, −1.40]*, 56%	A35, A36, A39, A41
Low RoB SG	2 (156)	−1.73 [−3.01, −0.44]*, 56%	A36, A41
Treatment: ≤8 w	2 (138)	−2.38 [−5.24, 0.48], 85%	A36, A39
Treatment: >8 w	2 (182)	−2.28 [−2.93, −1.63]*, 0%	A35, A41

*Statistically significant, see Chapter 4.
Abbreviations: CI, confidence interval; MD, mean difference; RoB, risk of bias; SG, sequence generation; w, weeks.

pharmacotherapy alone ([−3.17, −1.40], I^2 = 56%; Table 7.4). Statistical heterogeneity was reduced in subgroup analysis of two studies that provided treatment for more than eight weeks, although the number of women included in the analysis was small.

Insomnia Severity Index

In addition to using the PSQI to assess sleep symptoms, one study (A43) also used the Insomnia Severity Index.[23] Women who received acupuncture scored 7.89 points lower at the end of treatment than women who received placebo acupuncture (74 women, [−10.15, −5.63]).

Other Sleep Symptom Scales

Several other sleep symptom scales were used among the included studies. Avis *et al.* (A1) used the Patient-Reported Outcomes Measurement Information System (PROMIS) Sleep Disturbance scale[24] and found women who received acupuncture scored 4.27 points lower than women who received no treatment (209 women,

[−4.66, −3.88]). When acupuncture was used in combination with self-care advice, women who received this combination reported a greater increase in hours of sleep per night from baseline to the end of treatment, than women who received self-care advice alone (267 women, MD 0.28 hours [0.07, 0.49]; A7). One study (A33) used the Athens Insomnia Scale[25] to assess sleep symptoms. Among the 50 women included in the analysis, women who received acupuncture plus moxibustion reported lower scores, indicating better sleep, than women who received diazepam (MD −3.36 points [−3.73, −2.99]).

Hamilton Rating Scale for Depression

Eighteen studies (A13–A29, A46) assessed depressive symptoms using the HAM-D. Most of these studies compared acupuncture with pharmacotherapy.

Acupuncture versus pharmacotherapy

Fourteen studies (A14, A18–A29, A46) were included in meta-analysis for the outcome HAM-D. Analysis of all studies showed HAM-D scores to be 1.09 points lower among perimenopausal women who received acupuncture compared with those who received pharmacotherapy (1,236 women, [−2.15, −0.03], I^2 = 81%). Statistical heterogeneity was 'high', and subgroup analyses were conducted to identify potential sources (Table 7.5). Statistical heterogeneity was unable to be reduced to acceptable levels and each subgroup analysis showed no difference between acupuncture and pharmacotherapy. Confidence in the result is low due to unexplained statistical heterogeneity.

Acupuncture versus psychological treatment

One RCT of 68 women (A16) used the 24-item HAM-D to assess the role of acupuncture compared to psychological treatment. No statistical difference was found between the two groups (MD 1.70 points [−6.09, 9.49]).

Table 7.5 Acupuncture versus Pharmacotherapy: Hamilton Rating Scale for Depression

Group	No. of Studies (Participants)	Effect Size (MD [95% CI], I^2)	Included Studies
All studies	14 (1,236)	−1.09 [−2.15, −0.03]*, 81%	A14, A18–A29, A46
Low RoB SG	3 (358)	−0.79 [−2.71, 1.12], 72%	A19, A21, A46
Treatment: ≤ 8 w	11 (864)	−0.86 [−2.14, 0.42], 81%	A19–A26, A28, A29, A46
Treatment: > 8 w	3 (372)	−1.86 [−3.79, 0.06], 76%	A14, A18, A27
Antidepressants	12 (928)	−1.11 [−2.38, 0.17], 82%	A14, A19–A26, A28, A29, A46
Hormone therapy	2 (309)	−1.13 [−3.22, 0.95], 80%	A18, A27

*Statistically significant, see Chapter 4.
Abbreviations: CI, confidence interval; MD, mean difference; RoB, risk of bias; SG, sequence generation; w, weeks.

Acupuncture plus pharmacotherapy versus pharmacotherapy alone

Meta-analysis of two RCTs (A15, A17) showed the combination of acupuncture plus pharmacotherapy to be more effective than pharmacotherapy alone in reducing depressive symptoms on the HAM-D (162 perimenopausal women, MD −3.06 points [−5.08, −1.04], $I^2 = 0\%$).

Acupuncture plus pharmacotherapy versus sham acupuncture plus pharmacotherapy

Acupuncture was combined with fluoxetine in one study with 80 perimenopausal women (A13). Sham acupuncture plus fluoxetine were used in the control group. Analysis of HAM-D scores at the end of treatment found women who received acupuncture plus fluoxetine scored 2.67 points lower than women who received sham acupuncture plus fluoxetine ([−4.84, −0.50]).

Hamilton Rating Scale for Anxiety

Three studies (A28, A29, A44) assessed anxiety using the HAM-A. Meta-analysis was able to be conducted with studies that compared acupuncture with pharmacotherapy.

Acupuncture versus pharmacotherapy

Meta-analysis of two studies showed acupuncture resulted in lower HAM-A scores at the end of treatment than pharmacotherapy in 122 perimenopausal women (MD −2.57 points [−4.06, −1.08], $I^2 = 0\%$; A28, A29).

Acupuncture plus pharmacotherapy versus pharmacotherapy alone

One study of 30 perimenopausal women found no benefit of the combination of acupuncture and flupentixol/melitracen over flupentixol/melitracen alone (MD 1.20 points [−2.10, 4.50]; A44).

Beck Depression Inventory

Two studies (A5, A7) used the Beck Depression Inventory (BDI)[26] to assess depressive symptoms. Studies compared different interventions and comparators and were analysed separately.

Acupuncture versus self-care advice

One study (A7) compared acupuncture with self-care advice. Among 72 postmenopausal women, acupuncture was no more or less effective in reducing depressive symptoms on the BDI than self-care advice (MD −0.45 points [−3.17, 2.27]).

Acupuncture plus electroacupuncture plus lifestyle advice versus placebo acupuncture plus lifestyle advice

One study (A5) tested the combination of acupuncture, electroacupuncture and dietary/lifestyle advice for depressive symptoms. No benefit was seen in combining acupuncture with electroacupuncture and lifestyle advice compared to placebo acupuncture plus lifestyle advice (MD 0.20 points [−2.51, 2.91]).

Other Psychological Symptom Scales

Various other outcomes were used to assess psychological symptoms. Results are presented according to the comparison.

Acupuncture versus no treatment

One study involving 209 postmenopausal women (A1) used multiple outcome scales to measure psychological symptoms. Scores on the Perceived Stress Scale[27] were lower, indicating improved symptoms, in women who received acupuncture compared with those who received no treatment (209 women, MD −0.82 points [−0.98, −0.66]). Similarly, the same study found acupuncture to be superior to no treatment in improving outcomes on the Centre for Epidemiologic Studies Depression Scale[28] (MD −1.35 points [−1.59, −1.11]), the Generalized Anxiety Disorder 7-item scale[29] (MD −1.47 points [−1.78, −1.16]) and the PROMIS Anxiety[24] (MD −2.64 points [−3.06, −2.22]) and Depression[24] scales (MD −0.93 points [−1.31, −0.55]).

Acupuncture versus placebo acupuncture

One study (A48) assessed psychological symptoms using the Hospital Anxiety and Depression Scale.[30] Scores for the Anxiety and Depression components were analysed at the end of treatment and at two follow-up periods. Scores on the Anxiety subscale domain were not statistically different between women who received acupuncture and those who received placebo acupuncture at the end of treatment (327 women,

MD −0.22 points [−1.33, 0.89]), at 20 weeks follow-up (327 women, MD −0.11 points [−1.23, 1.01]) and at 32 weeks follow-up (327 women, MD 0.15 points [−1.00, 1.30]). Similar trends were seen on the Depression subscale domain: no differences were found between groups at the end of treatment (MD −0.23 points [−1.20, 0.74]), at 20 weeks follow-up (MD −0.09 points [−1.08, 0.90]) and at 32 weeks follow-up (MD 0.14 points [−0.85, 1.13]).

Acupuncture versus pharmacotherapy

One study (A45) used a self-rated health measurement scale to assess psychological symptoms. The scale uses a 10-point scale for 48 items, with lower scores meaning better outcomes. Perimenopausal women who received acupuncture scored lower on the scale than those who received diazepam (60 women, MD −24.05 points [−44.46, −3.64]).

Acupuncture plus electroacupuncture plus lifestyle advice versus placebo acupuncture plus lifestyle advice

Anxiety was assessed using the Beck Anxiety Scale[31] in one study with 51 postmenopausal women (A5). Women who received acupuncture, electroacupuncture and diet/lifestyle advice reported scores at the end of treatment that were not statistically different to women who received placebo acupuncture and diet/lifestyle advice (MD −0.10 points, [−3.43, 3.23]).

Bodily Pain

Bodily pain was assess using a 10 centimetre (cm) visual analogue scale (VAS) in one study of 60 perimenopausal women (A46). Bodily pain was not statistically different between women who received acupuncture and women who received flupentixol/melitracen at the end of treatment (MD −0.50 cm [−1.19, 0.19]), but was lower in women who received acupuncture at four weeks (MD −1.70 cm [−2.42, −0.98]).

Kupperman Index

Sixteen RCTs (A8, A12–A14, A24, A27, A29, A31, A38, A45, A50–A52, A54–A56) measured global symptom severity using the original or modified version of the KI.

Acupuncture versus no treatment

One study (A31) compared acupuncture with no treatment in 65 perimenopausal women. Women who received acupuncture scored 6.14 points lower on the KI at the end of treatment compared with women who received no treatment ([−9.57, −2.71]).

Acupuncture versus sham acupuncture

When acupuncture was compared with sham acupuncture in 81 menopausal women (A8), women who received acupuncture scored 23.29 points lower on the KI ([−26.98, −19.60]).

Acupuncture versus pharmacotherapy

The effect of acupuncture, compared to pharmacotherapy, on the KI was assessed in 13 RCTs (A12, A14, A24, A27, A29, A38, A45, A50–A52, A54–A56) involving 838 perimenopausal women. Some studies used the original version of the KI, while others made modifications that typically included assessing urinary symptoms and dyspareunia. Studies were analysed using standardised mean difference (SMD) to account for these modifications.

Compared with pharmacotherapy, acupuncture resulted in a lower score at the end of treatment (SMD −0.83 [−1.18, −0.47], $I^2 = 83\%$). Statistical heterogeneity was explored through subgroup analyses (Table 7.6). Subgroup analyses with studies that used appropriate methods of group allocation, various treatment durations and the different version of KI failed to explain statistical heterogeneity. The reason for heterogeneity may relate to other factors, such as comor-

Table 7.6 Acupuncture versus Pharmacotherapy: Kupperman Index

Group	No. of Studies (Participants)	Effect Size (MD/ SMD [95% CI], I²)	Included Studies
All studies	13 (838)	SMD −0.83 [−1.18, −0.47]*, 83%	A12, A14, A24, A27, A29, A38, A45, A50–A52, A54–A56
Low RoB SG	5 (366)	SMD −0.74 [−1.29, −0.19]*, 84%	A27, A29, A38, A45, A50
Treatment: ≤8 w	7 (412)	SMD −0.65 [−1.09, −0.21]*, 78%	A12, A24, A29, A38, A45, A54, A55
Treatment: >8 w	6 (426)	SMD −1.02 [−1.63, −0.42]*, 88%	A14, A27, A50, A51, A52, A56
KI	4 (304)	MD −0.58 [−0.82, −0.34]*, 91%	A14, A27, A52, A55
mKI	9 (534)	SMD −0.75 [−0.93, −0.57]*, 79%	A12, A24, A29, A38, A45, A50, A51, A54, A56

*Statistically significant, see Chapter 4.

Abbreviations: CI, confidence interval; KI, Kupperman Index; MD, mean difference; mKI, modified Kupperman Index; RoB, risk of bias; SG, sequence generation; SMD, standardised mean difference; w, weeks.

bidities or comparator type (HT versus other drug classes). Regardless, confidence in the result is lower due to unexplained statistical heterogeneity.

One study (A55) assessed KI four weeks after the end of treatment and found lower scores among perimenopausal women who received acupuncture compared to those who received tibolone (MD −4.13 points [−6.46, −1.80]).

Two studies (A51, A54) reported scores for the individual items of a modified KI. Meta-analysis showed benefits of acupuncture over HT for the items: paraesthesia, insomnia, nervousness, melancholia, weakness, headache, palpitations, formication and urinary symptoms (Table 7.7). Acupuncture was not statistically different to HT for the following items: vasomotor, vertigo, arthralgia and dyspareunia.

Table 7.7 Acupuncture versus Hormone Therapy: Modified Kupperman Index Item Scores

mKI Item	No. of Studies (Participants)	Effect Size (SMD [95% CI], I^2)	Included Studies
Vasomotor	2 (102)	−0.17 [−0.56, 0.22], 0%	A51, A54
Paraesthesia	2 (102)	−0.63 [−1.06, −0.19]*, 97%	A51, A54
Insomnia	2 (102)	−0.91 [−1.32, −0.50]*, 79%	A51, A54
Nervousness	2 (102)	−1.29 [−1.75, −0.82]*, 97%	A51, A54
Melancholia	2 (102)	−0.75 [−1.16, −0.35]*, 69%	A51, A54
Vertigo	2 (102)	−0.11 [−0.50, 0.28], 0%	A51, A54
Weakness	2 (102)	−0.91 [−1.33, −0.49]*, 89%	A51, A54
Arthralgia	2 (102)	−0.32 [−0.71, 0.07], 0%	A51, A54
Headache	2 (102)	−0.65 [−1.10, −0.21]*, 97%	A51, A54
Palpitations	2 (102)	−0.81 [−1.24, −0.38]*, 95%	A51, A54
Formication	2 (102)	−0.43 [−0.83, −0.02]*, 89%	A51, A54
Dyspareunia	2 (102)	−0.08 [−0.47, 0.31], 0%	A51, A54
Urinary symptoms	2 (102)	−0.70 [−1.18, −0.22]*, 98%	A51, A54

*Statistically significant, see Chapter 4.

Abbreviations: CI, confidence interval; mKI, modified Kupperman Index; SMD, standardised mean difference.

Acupuncture plus pharmacotherapy versus sham acupuncture plus pharmacotherapy

One study (A13) compared acupuncture plus fluoxetine with sham acupuncture plus fluoxetine. Among the 80 perimenopausal women, those who received acupuncture scored 10.03 points lower on the KI, compared to sham acupuncture plus fluoxetine ([−11.44, −8.62]).

Acupuncture plus moxibustion versus pharmacotherapy

When acupuncture was combined with moxibustion, women who received this treatment scored worse on the KI than women who received tibolone (90 women, MD 4.88 points [3.30, 6.46]; A53).

Greene Climacteric Scale

The Green Climacteric Scale (GCS)[32] was used to measure menopausal symptoms in two studies (A5, A16).

Acupuncture versus psychological treatment

One study (A16) that compared acupuncture with psychological treatment in 66 perimenopausal women found no difference between the two groups at the end of treatment (MD 3.70 points [−2.53, 9.93]).

Acupuncture plus electroacupuncture plus lifestyle advice versus placebo acupuncture plus lifestyle advice

The GCS was used to assess symptoms in 51 postmenopausal women (A5). At the end of treatment there was no difference between total GCS scores in women who received acupuncture, electroacupuncture and lifestyle advice and those who received placebo acupuncture plus lifestyle advice (MD 1.20 points [−4.87, 7.27]). Domain scores were also reported, with no difference between groups for the psychological domain (MD 0.00 points [−2.42, 2.42]), physical domain (MD 0.80 points [−0.94, 2.54]), vasomotor domain (MD 0.00 points [−0.94, 0.94]) and sexual domain (MD 0.00 points [−0.38, 0.38]).

Menopause Rating Scale

The MRS[33] was used in two studies to evaluate menopausal symptoms (A9, A10). One study (A10) reported total and domain scores at the end of treatment, while the other (A9) reported change from baseline to end of treatment and follow-up. Due to differences in scoring, studies were not pooled for analysis and the results are reported separately.

Acupuncture versus placebo acupuncture

In 53 postmenopausal women, acupuncture resulted in a mean total score 10.9 points lower than placebo acupuncture at the end of treatment ([−14.06, −7.74]; A10). Results also favoured acupuncture on the psychological domain (MD −4.20 points [−5.74, −2.66]) and somatic domain (MD −5.60 points [−6.79, −4.41]), while no difference between groups was seen on the urogenital domain (MD −1.20 points [−2.49, 0.09]).

Acupuncture versus sham acupuncture

In a small study of 20 postmenopausal women (A9), the change from baseline to end of treatment was greater among those who received acupuncture than those who received sham acupuncture at the end of treatment (MD −12.50 points [−16.83, −8.17]) and at 12 weeks follow-up (MD −4.70 points [−9.12, −0.28]). Domain scores were also reported. Women who received acupuncture reported greater improvements in symptoms on the psychological domain of the MRS at the end of treatment (MD −4.40 points [−6.81, −1.99]), but not at follow-up (MD −0.50 points [−3.41, 2.41]). Benefits were seen at the end of treatment and at follow-up on the somatic domain (end-of-treatment: MD −5.40 points [−7.71, −3.09]; follow-up: MD −2.70 points [−4.39, −1.01]) and urogenital domains (end-of-treatment: MD −2.70 points [−4.08, −1.32]; MD −1.50 points [−2.89, −0.11]).

Menopause-specific Quality of Life Questionnaire

Three studies (A3, A4, A48) assessed the impact of acupuncture using the MENQOL. Meta-analysis was conducted where possible.

Acupuncture versus no treatment

One study of 21 menopausal women (A4) that compared acupuncture with no treatment reported the change in total and domain scores for MENQOL. Change from baseline in the MENQOL total score was greater in women who received acupuncture than in women who received no treatment (MD −1.10 points [−1.97, −0.23]). Acupuncture was superior to no treatment in reducing scores on the psychosocial domain (MD −1.50 points [−2.81, −0.19]) and vasomotor domain (MD −1.80 points [−3.05, −0.55]), but was not statistically different to no treatment on the physical domain (MD −0.80 points [−1.88, 0.28]) and sexual domain (MD −0.60 points [−1.93, 0.73]).

Acupuncture versus sham/placebo acupuncture

The change from baseline to end-of-treatment in total MENQOL score was not statistically different between the two groups (24 women, MD 0.30 points [−0.70, 1.30]; A4). Three studies (A3, A4, A48), that compared acupuncture with sham/placebo acupuncture, reported domain scores of the MENQOL. One was a three-arm study that also compared acupuncture with no treatment (see above; A4). Results for the study by Nir *et al.* (A3) were reported separately due to differences in data.

Meta-analysis of domain scores showed no difference between sham/placebo acupuncture in scores for the physical domain (MD 0.09 points [−0.28, 0.47], $I^2 = 0\%$), psychosocial domain (MD 0.03 points [−0.37, 0.43], $I^2 = 0\%$), vasomotor domain (MD −0.05 points [−0.50, 0.39], $I^2 = 0\%$) and sexual domain (MD 0.01 points [−0.52, 0.54], $I^2 = 0\%$) (Table 7.8).

Table 7.8 Acupuncture versus Sham/Placebo Acupuncture: Menopause-specific Quality of Life Questionnaire

MENQOL Domain	No. of Studies (Participants)	Effect Size (MD [95% CI], I^2)	Included Studies
Physical	2 (351)	0.09 [−0.28, 0.47], 0%	A4, A48
Psychosocial	2 (351)	0.03 [−0.37, 0.43], 0%	A4, A48
Vasomotor	2 (351)	−0.05 [−0.50, 0.39], 0%	A4, A48
Sexual	2 (351)	0.01 [−0.52, 0.54], 0%	A4, A48

Abbreviations: CI, confidence interval; MD, mean difference; MENQOL, Menopause-specific Quality of Life questionnaire.

Ee *et al.* (2016; A48) conducted follow-up assessment at three and six months. Acupuncture was not superior to placebo acupuncture in scores on the physical domain (three months follow-up: MD 0.02 points [−0.38, 0.42]; six months follow-up: MD 0.18 points [−0.24, 0.60]), psychosocial domain (three months follow-up: MD 0.02 points [−0.42, 0.46]; six months follow-up: MD 0.06 points [−0.37, 0.49]), vasomotor domain (three months follow-up: MD 0.14 points [−0.34, 0.62]; six months follow-up: MD 0.09 points [−0.40, 0.58]) and sexual domain (three months follow-up: MD 0.13 points [−0.44, 0.70]; six months follow-up: MD 0.19 points [−0.39, 0.77]).

The study of 29 women by Nir *et al.* (A3) found no difference between women who received acupuncture and those who received placebo acupuncture on the physical domain at end of treatment (MD 0.05 points [−0.58, 0.68]) and at one month follow-up (MD −0.22 points [−0.98, 0.54]). No difference was found between groups on the psychosocial domain at end of treatment (MD −0.62 points [−1.51, 0.27]); however, at one month follow-up women who received acupuncture scored lower, indicating better health-related quality of life than women who received placebo acupuncture (MD −0.99 points [−1.88, −0.10]). On the vasomotor domain, acupuncture was not superior to placebo acupuncture in change from baseline to end of treatment (MD 0.24 points [−1.10, 1.58]) and from baseline to one month follow-up (MD −1.14 points [−2.40, 0.12]). Acupuncture was superior to placebo acupuncture in score changes on the sexual domain at end of treatment (MD −1.29 points [−2.25, −0.33]), but this effect was not sustained at one month follow-up (MD −0.50 points [−1.55, 0.55]).

Women's Health Questionnaire

Two studies (A1, A7) used the Women's Health Questionnaire (WHQ)[34] to examine health-related quality of life.

Acupuncture versus no treatment

One study (A1) compared acupuncture with no treatment in 209 postmenopausal women. Scores for each subscale of the WHQ were lower, indicating better quality of life, in women who received acupuncture compared to no treatment: depressed mood (MD −0.04 points [−0.05, −0.03]), somatic (MD −0.16 points [−0.17, −0.15]), anxiety/fears (MD −0.10 points [−0.12, −0.08]), vasomotor (MD −0.20 points [−0.22, −0.18]), sleep (MD −0.18 points [−0.20, −0.16]), sexual (MD −0.13 points [−0.15, −0.11]), memory/concentration (MD −0.19 points [−0.24, −0.14]) and attractiveness subscales (MD −0.06 points [−0.08, −0.04]).

Acupuncture versus placebo acupuncture

Borud *et al.* (2009; A7) also reported the change in subscale scores for all items of the WHQ apart from the sexual subscale. Among the 267 postmenopausal women, those who received acupuncture reported a greater change from baseline to end of treatment on the somatic (MD −0.07 points [−0.12, −0.02]), vasomotor (MD −0.24 points [−0.31, −0.17]) and sleep subscales (MD −0.13 points [−0.21, −0.05]). These benefits were not sustained at follow-up assessments (Table 7.9). There was no difference on the depressed mood, anxiety/fears, memory/concentration and attractiveness subscales of the WHQ at any of the assessment times.

Table 7.9 Acupuncture versus Placebo Acupuncture: Women's Health Questionnaire

WHQ Domain	Assessment	No. of Studies (Participants)	Effect Size MD [95% CI]	Included Studies
Depressed mood	EoT	1 (267)	−0.05 [−0.10, 0.00]	A7
	Follow-up 1	1 (267)	−0.02 [−0.07, 0.03]	A7
	Follow-up 2	1 (267)	−0.01 [−0.06, 0.04]	A7
Somatic	EoT	1 (267)	−0.07 [−0.12, −0.02]*	A7
	Follow-up 1	1 (267)	0.01 [−0.05, 0.07]	A7
	Follow-up 2	1 (267)	0.01 [−0.05, 0.07]	A7
Anxiety/fears	EoT	1 (267)	−0.04 [−0.10, 0.02]	A7
	Follow-up 1	1 (267)	0.01 [−0.05, 0.07]	A7
	Follow-up 2	1 (267)	0.01 [−0.05, 0.07]	A7

(*Continued*)

Table 7.9 (*Continued*)

WHQ Domain	Assessment	No. of Studies (Participants)	Effect Size MD [95% CI]	Included Studies
Vasomotor	EoT	1 (267)	−0.24 [−0.31, −0.17]*	A7
	Follow-up 1	1 (267)	−0.04 [−0.13, 0.05]	A7
	Follow-up 2	1 (267)	−0.04 [−0.14, 0.06]	A7
Sleep	EoT	1 (267)	−0.13 [−0.21, −0.05]*	A7
	Follow-up 1	1 (267)	0.00 [−0.08, 0.08]	A7
	Follow-up 2	1 (267)	0.00 [−0.08, 0.08]	A7
Memory/ concentration	EoT	1 (267)	−0.06 [−0.13, 0.01]	A7
	Follow-up 1	1 (267)	0.05 [−0.03, 0.13]	A7
	Follow up-2	1 (267)	0.01 [−0.07, 0.09]	A7
Attractiveness	EoT	1 (267)	−0.05 [−0.13, 0.03]	A7
	Follow-up 1	1 (267)	−0.06 [−0.15, 0.03]	A7
	Follow-up 2	1 (267)	−0.07 [−0.16, 0.02]	A7

*Statistically significant, see Chapter 4.

Abbreviations: CI, confidence interval; EoT, end of treatment; MD, mean difference; WHQ, Women's Health Questionnaire.

Hot Flash Related Daily Interference Scale

One study (A1) assessed the impact of vasomotor symptoms on health-related quality of life using the Hot Flash Related Daily Interference scale (HFRDI).[35] Among the 209 postmenopausal women, those who received acupuncture reported lower scores, indicating less interference, than women who received no treatment (MD −18.81 points [−19.99, −17.63]).

36-Item Short-Form Health Survey

The study by Avis *et al.* (A1) also evaluated the effect of acupuncture on health-related quality of life using the Medical Outcome Study 36-Item Short-Form Health Survey (SF-36).[36] Postmenopausal women who received acupuncture scored higher, indicating better quality of life, on the physical component summary score (209 women, MD 1.46 points [1.17, 1.75]) and the mental component summary score (209 women, MD 2.45 points [1.98, 2.92]) than women who received no treatment.

Frequently Reported Acupuncture Points in Meta-analyses Showing Favourable Effect: Acupuncture

Four meta-analyses showed favourable results for acupuncture: PSQI (Table 7.4), HAM-D (Table 7.5 and section 'Acupuncture plus Pharmacotherapy versus Pharmacotherapy Alone'), HAM-A (section 'Acupuncture versus Pharmacotherapy') and KI (Table 7.6). The points used in studies included in these meta-analyses were examined to identify acupuncture points with high frequency of use that may contribute to the therapeutic effect. Four acupuncture points were used in two studies where acupuncture improved sleep measured with the PSQI: EX-HN1 *Sishencong* 四神聪, LR3 *Taichong* 太冲, GV24 *Shenting* 神庭 and HT7 *Shenmen* 神门. Clinicians may consider using these points to improve sleep in menopausal women.

Among studies that contributed to improvements in psychological outcomes, the most frequently used acupuncture points were: BL18 *Ganshu* 肝俞 (seven studies), EX-HN1 *Sishencong* 四神聪 (seven studies), GV20 *Baihui* 百会 (seven studies), BL23 *Shenshu* 肾俞 (seven studies), SP6 *Sanyinjiao* 三阴交 (six studies), BL15 *Xinshu* 心俞 (six studies), GV24 *Shenting* 神庭 (five studies), ST36 *Zusanli* 足三里 (five studies), LR3 *Taichong* 太冲 (four studies), GB13 *Benshen* 本神 (four studies) and HT7 *Shenmen* 神门 (four studies). These acupuncture points may be beneficial for women who experience psychological symptoms during menopause.

In studies that were included in favourable meta-analysis for global symptom severity assessed using the KI, the most frequently used acupuncture points were: BL18 *Ganshu* 肝俞 (five studies), GV20 *Baihui* 百会 (four studies), BL23 *Shenshu* 肾俞 (four studies), CV4 *Guanyuan* 关元 (three studies), PC6 *Neiguan* 内关 (three studies), EX-HN1 *Sishencong* 四神聪 (three studies), LR3 *Taichong* 太冲 (three studies), BL15 *Xinshu* 心俞 (three studies) and BL20 *Pishu* 脾俞 (three studies). Many of these points were also found in positive meta-analyses for psychological symptoms. Clinicians can consider these points in accordance with Chinese medicine (CM) syndrome differentiation.

Assessment Using Grading of Recommendations Assessment, Development and Evaluation

The GRADE approach was used to summarise results for clinically important questions. The process used to select interventions, comparators and outcomes for evaluation has been described in Chapters 4 and 5. Acupuncture and electroacupuncture were considered to be important interventions for menopausal symptoms, and experts considered that comparison with sham/placebo acupuncture and with HT would provide valuable information to inform clinical practice.

Acupuncture versus sham/placebo acupuncture

Ten RCTs (A3, A4, A6, A8–A11, A43, A48, A49) that compared acupuncture with sham/placebo acupuncture reported on the pre-specified outcomes. Data from one study (A3) were excluded from the summary of findings as the data were not normally distributed. The certainty of evidence ranged from 'low' to 'moderate' (Table 7.10). Acupuncture was not significantly different to sham/placebo acupuncture in terms of daily hot flush frequency ('low' certainty evidence) and severity ('moderate' certainty evidence). 'Moderate' certainty evidence showed no difference between the two groups in scores on the PSQI and all four domains of the MENQOL.

Nine of the ten RCTs (A3, A6, A8–A11, A43, A48, A49) that compared acupuncture with sham/placebo acupuncture reported on safety. No serious AEs were reported. More AEs were reported with acupuncture (54 AEs) than with sham/placebo acupuncture (27 AEs). Adverse events with acupuncture included 26 cases of bleeding/bruising/ecchymoses, seven cases of discomfort, seven cases of pain, three cases of lipothymia, two cases of syncope/presyncope, two cases of worsening of symptoms, two cases of insomnia, one case of

Table 7.10 GRADE: Acupuncture versus Sham/Placebo Acupuncture

Outcome; Treatment Duration	No. of Studies (Participants)	Relative Effect (MD [95% CI])	Certainty of the Evidence (GRADE)
Daily HF frequency; 8 w–6 m	2 (408)	−1.06 [−2.27, 0.15]	⊕⊕◯◯ LOW[a,b]
Daily HF severity; 8 w	1 (327)	0.32 [−2.97, 3.61]	⊕⊕⊕◯ MODERATE[c]
PSQI; 3 w	1 (74)	−6.14 [−7.57, 4.71]	⊕⊕⊕◯ MODERATE[c]
MENQOL-Ph; 7 w–12 w	3 (380)	0.08 [−0.24, 0.40]	⊕⊕⊕◯ MODERATE[c]
MENQOL-Psychosoc; 7 w–12 w	3 (380)	−0.08 [−0.47, 0.30]	⊕⊕⊕◯ MODERATE[c]
MENQOL-V; 7 w–12 w	3 (380)	−0.02 [−0.45, 0.40]	⊕⊕⊕◯ MODERATE[c]
MENQOL-S; 7 w–12 w	3 (380)	−0.45 [−1.38, 0.49]	⊕⊕⊕◯ MODERATE[c]

Abbreviations: CI, confidence interval; GRADE, Grading of Recommendations, Assessment, Development and Evaluation; HF, hot flush; m, months; MD, mean difference; MENQOL, Menopause Quality of Life questionnaire; Ph, physical domain; Psychosoc, psychosocial domain; PSQI, Pittsburgh Sleep Quality Index; S, sexual domain; V, vasomotor domain; w, weeks.

Notes

[a]High risk of bias for incomplete outcome data.

[b]Studies show different effects with wide confidence intervals for one study.

[c]Small sample size.

Study references

Daily HF frequency: A0, A40.

Daily HF severity: A48.

PSQI: A43.

MENQOL: A3, A4, A48.

tingling around the acupuncture point, one case of swelling around the acupuncture point and itching of the whole arm, one case of feeling hot and skin sensitivity, one case of itchiness and one case of twitching. Adverse events with sham/placebo acupuncture included six cases of discomfort, four cases of worsening insomnia, three cases of pain, three cases of irritability/restlessness, two cases of insomnia, and one case each of syncope/presyncope, worsening of symptoms, nervousness, essential tremor, bleeding/bruising, low energy, resentment, gas and temporary rash with pruritus.

Acupuncture versus hormone therapy

Five RCTS (A18, A27, A54, A55, A57) compared acupuncture with HT and reported on pre-specified outcomes. 'Very low' certainty evidence showed acupuncture was not statistically different to HT (Table 7.11).

All five RCTs (A18, A27, A54, A55, A57) that compared acupuncture with HT reported on safety, with no serious AEs occurring. The number of AEs was lower among women who received acupuncture (10 AEs) than in those who received HT (163 AEs). Adverse events in the acupuncture groups included five cases of poor appetite, two cases of pain during acupuncture, and one case each of diarrhoea, bloating and insomnia. Adverse events in the HT groups included 21 cases of nausea and/or vomiting, 14 cases of breast pain, 13 cases of blurred vision, 12 cases of constipation, 11 cases of lethargy, 11 cases of tachycardia, ten cases of headache, nine cases of dizziness, nine cases of vaginal discharge, nine cases of oedema, eight cases of bloating, eight cases of weight gain, seven cases of diarrhoea, seven cases of dry mouth, five cases of loss of appetite, two cases of vaginal bleeding, two cases of nausea and chest tightness, two cases of change in blood pressure, two cases of excitement and one case of tremor.

Table 7.11 GRADE: Acupuncture versus Hormone Therapy

Outcome; Treatment Duration	No. of Studies (Participants)	Relative Effect (MD [95% CI]	Certainty of the Evidence (GRADE)
HAM-D; 3 m	2 (308)	−1.13 [−3.22, 0.95]	⊕◯◯◯ VERY LOW[a,b,c]

Abbreviations: CI, confidence interval; HAM-D, Hamilton Rating Scale for Depression; m, months; MD, mean difference.

Notes

[a]High risk of bias from lack of blinding.
[b]Unexplained statisticalheterogeneity.
[c]Small sample size.

Study references
HAM-D: A18, A27.

Controlled Clinical Trials of Acupuncture

Six non-randomised CCTs (A58–A63) tested acupuncture in 443 women. One study (A60) was conducted in Iran and the rest were conducted in China. Three studies (A58, A59, A63) included peri-menopausal women, one study (A61) included women with bilateral ovariectomy and two studies (A60, A62) described women as meno-pausal without specifying stage. Two studies (A63, A58) included women with depression.

Chinese medicine syndrome differentiation was used as an inclu-sion criterion in one study (A59). Women with Liver and Kidney *yin* deficiency, Kidney *yang* deficiency, and Heart and Liver disharmony received treatments tailored according to their syndrome diagnosis. Four studies (A58–A61) tested acupuncture alone, one (A63) com-bined acupuncture with moxibustion and one (A62) combined acupuncture with ear acupressure.

Acupuncture points PC6 *Neiguan* 内关 and SP6 *Sanyinjiao* 三阴交 were used in three studies each, while seven points were used in two studies: BL23 *Shenshu* 肾俞, CV4 *Guanyuan* 关元, CV6 *Qihai* 气海, GB20 *Fengchi* 风池, GV20 *Baihui* 百会, KI3 *Taixi* 太溪 and LI4 *Hegu* 合谷. Comparators included HT (A60–A62), antidepressants (A58, A63) and a combination of diazepam, oryzanol (rice bran oil) and vitamins B6 and E (A59). Treatment duration ranged from four weeks (A58) to 12 weeks (A61). One study (A60) described treatment of five weeks in the intervention group and 12 weeks in the comparator group; outcome data for this study were excluded from quantitative analysis. Follow-up assessment four weeks after the end of treatment was conducted in one study (A58).

Outcomes

The KI was used to assess global symptom severity in three studies (A59, A61, A62). Two studies (A58, A63) assessed the effect of acu-puncture on depressive symptoms using the HAM-D and one study (A61) evaluated vaginal symptoms using the Vaginal Maturation Index (VMI).

Vaginal Symptoms

One study (A61) assessed the role of acupuncture in improving VMI in 67 women with ovariectomy. Acupuncture was not statistically different to tibolone in the percentage of basal (MD −0.20% [−0.66, 0.26]), intermediate (MD −1.10% [−3.00, 0.80]) and superficial cells (MD 3.40% [−0.81, 7.61]).

Hamilton Rating Scale for Depression

Two studies used the HAM-D to assess depressive symptoms (A58, A63). As these studies used different interventions, meta-analysis was not possible. Results are presented according to comparison.

Acupuncture versus antidepressants

In 58 perimenopausal women with depression, acupuncture was not statistically different to flupentixol/melitracen after four weeks of treatment (MD −1.50 points [−3.35, 0.35]; A58). However, at follow-up four weeks after the end of treatment, women who received acupuncture scored 4.90 points lower than women who received flupentixol/melitracen ([−7.30, −2.50]).

Acupuncture plus moxibustion versus antidepressants

One study, of 40 perimenopausal women, showed depressive symptom scores to be 5.44 points lower in women who received acupuncture plus moxibustion compared to women who received fluoxetine ([−8.39, −2.49]; A63).

Kupperman Index

Three studies (A59, A61, A62) reported global symptom severity using a modified version of the KI. Meta-analysis was conducted using SMD with two studies (A59, A61) that compared acupuncture with pharmacotherapy.

Acupuncture versus pharmacotherapy

In two studies with 123 women, global symptom severity was lower among women who received acupuncture compared to women who received pharmacotherapy (SMD −2.44 [−3.89, −1.00], I^2 = 88%; A59, A61).

Acupuncture plus ear acupressure versus hormone therapy

One study (A62) compared the combination of acupuncture plus ear acupressure with oestriol in 56 menopausal women. Acupuncture plus ear acupressure therapy resulted in a mean score 10.92 points lower on the modified KI compared to oestriol ([−12.79, −9.05]).

Non-controlled Studies of Acupuncture

Seven (A64–A70) non-controlled studies, involving 356 women, tested acupuncture for menopausal symptoms. Three studies (A64, A65, A68) tested acupuncture alone, one study (A66) used warm needle acupuncture (application of moxibustion on top of inserted needles) and three studies (A67, A69, A70) combined manual acupuncture with ear acupressure. Acupuncture and ear acupressure were used as integrative medicine in one study (A67). Postmenopausal women were included in the study by Wright and Aickin (A70), while all other studies included perimenopausal women.

Three studies (A66–A68) described using CM syndrome differentiation, which included Spleen and Kidney *yang* deficiency (A66, A67), Liver *qi* stagnation, Liver stagnation and Spleen deficiency, Spleen and Kidney *yang* deficiency, Liver and Kidney *yin* deficiency, and *yin* and *yang* deficiency (A67). The third study did not describe which syndromes were seen.

Four studies (A64, A66–A68) provided treatment for three months, with other studies providing treatment for four weeks (A70), five weeks (A69) and 16 weeks (A65). The most frequently used acupuncture points included: SP6 *Sanyinjiao* 三阴交 (eight uses among the seven studies), CV6 *Qihai* 气海 and LR3 *Taichong* 太冲 (five studies each), CV4 *Guanyuan* 关元, GV20 *Baihui* 百会 and ST36 *Zusanli* 足三里 (four studies each) and HT7 *Shenmen* 神门, KI3 *Taixi* 太溪, LI4 *Hegu* 合谷and ST29 *Guilai* 归来 (three studies each).

Safety of Acupuncture

Thirty-three studies reported on safety of acupuncture. One case series (A70) and three CCTs (A59, A61, A63) reported that no AEs occurred during the study. Among the 29 RCTs that reported on safety (A1, A3, A5–A11, A13, A14, A18, A20–A22, A25–A27, A38, A43–A49, A54, A55, A57), four (A5, A6, A10, A47) reported that no AEs occurred during the study.

Twelve RCTs (A1, A3, A8, A18, A21, A25, A43, A46, A48, A49, A55, A57) that evaluated acupuncture therapies alone reported 73 AEs in the intervention groups. Adverse events included 23 cases of pain, discomfort, numbness/tingling, swelling, twitch and/or itch, 16 cases of bleeding/bruising, ten cases of ecchymoses, five cases of poor appetite, three cases of insomnia, three cases of lipothymia, two cases of syncope/presyncope, two cases of worsening of symptoms, two cases of change in stools, and one case each of diarrhoea, bloating, dizziness, tachycardia, feeling hot with skin sensitivity, palpitations and change in stools plus palpitations.

Four RCTs (A5, A7, A13, A44) that tested acupuncture therapies as integrative medicine reported 286 AEs, with one study (A5) reporting that no AEs occurred. Other AEs included 53 cases of tiredness, 27 cases of worsening hot flushes, 24 cases of increased appetite, 13 cases of dizziness, two cases of headache and dizziness, two cases of anorexia, and one case each of diarrhoea, abdominal pain and burnout. In addition, there were 86 cases of women feeling more relaxed and 76 cases of increased energy.

In women who received no treatment (A1) or self-care advice (A7), no AEs occurred. In ten studies (A3, A5, A6, A8–A11, A43, A48, A49) that used sham/placebo acupuncture as the comparator, no AEs were reported in the comparator groups in four studies (A5, A6, A8, A10). Adverse events included nine cases of pain/discomfort, six cases of insomnia, three cases of irritability/restlessness, and one case each of gas, rash and pruritis, resentment, low energy, bleeding/bruising, essential tremor, nervousness, worsening of symptoms and syncope/presyncope.

In 17 studies (A13, A14, A18, A20–A22, A25–A27, A38, A44–A47, A54, A55, A57) that used pharmacotherapy as the comparator, all but one (A47) reported the occurrence of AEs in the control groups. In total, 244 AEs were reported. Adverse events included 29 cases of nausea and/or vomiting, 18 cases of dry mouth, 14 cases of breast pain, 13 cases of constipation, 13 cases of lethargy, 13 cases of dizziness, 13 cases of blurred vision, 11 cases of tachycardia, ten cases of headache, nine cases of vaginal discharge, nine cases of dry mouth and bad breath, nine cases of oedema, eight cases of bloating, eight cases of nausea, vomiting, dry mouth, indigestion, diarrhoea, insomnia, headache or dizziness, seven cases of diarrhoea, six cases of insomnia and breast pain, six cases of weight gain, six cases of irritability, dreams and breast pain, five cases of nausea and dizziness, five cases of loss of appetite, four cases of drowsiness, dizziness, fatigue, constipation and rash, four cases of burnout, four cases of anorexia, four cases of excitement/agitation, two cases of loss of appetite and nausea, two cases of vaginal bleeding, two cases of nausea and chest tightness, two cases of weight change, two cases of change in blood pressure, and one case each of insomnia, restlessness, dry mouth and nausea, tachycardia, tremor and palpitations.

Electroacupuncture

Twelve clinical studies that met the inclusion criteria for this review tested electroacupuncture for menopausal symptoms. Ten were RCTs (A71–A80) and two were case series (A81, A82).

Randomised Controlled Trials of Electroacupuncture

Ten studies (A71–A80) involving 927 women examined the potential benefit of electroacupuncture for menopausal symptoms. Two studies (A78, A79) were conducted in Sweden and included five arms, and all others were conducted in China. Both Swedish studies (A78, A79) used the same design in postmenopausal women, which included two treatment arms of physical exercise and applied relaxation (these were excluded from this analysis), an acupuncture group and two control groups who received HT or a type of sham electroacupuncture. It was unclear whether these two reports were from the same study; however, as different outcome measures were reported, the assumption was made that they were different studies and both were included in this review.

Two studies (A73, A77) included women with depressive symptoms and one study (A76) included women with a menopausal affective disorder. Chinese medicine diagnosis was used as an inclusion criterion in one study (A75). Syndromes included Kidney *yin* deficiency, Kidney *yang* deficiency and both Kidney *yin* and *yang* deficiency. The most frequently used acupuncture point was SP6 *Sanyinjiao* 三阴交, which was used in nine studies (Table 7.12).

Treatment was provided for four weeks (A75, A76), six weeks (A77), eight weeks (A71–A73, A80) or 12 weeks/three months (A74, A78, A79). The median duration of treatment was eight weeks. Follow-up after the end of treatment was conducted at four weeks (A71), three months (A72), six months (A74, A78, A79) and 24 weeks (A80). Five studies (A72, A77–A80) reported loss to follow-up.

Three studies used electroacupuncture as integrative medicine with either HT (A74, A76) or amitriptyline (A77). Five studies (A71,

Table 7.12 Most Frequently Reported Points in Electroacupuncture Randomised Controlled Trials

Acupuncture Point	Frequency of Use
SP6 *Sanyinjiao* 三阴交	9
CV4 *Guanyuan* 关元	6
EX-CA1 *Zigong* 子宫	5
GV20 *Baihui* 百会	5
LR3 *Taichong* 太冲	5
ST25 *Tianshu* 天枢	5
LI4 *Hegu* 合谷	3
PC6 *Neiguan* 内关	3
EX-HN3 *Yintang* 印堂	3

A72, A78–A80) included sham/placebo acupuncture as a control group, four studies (A74–A76, A79) used HT and two studies (A73, A77) used antidepressants.

Risk of Bias

None of the studies were free of bias (Table 7.13). Four studies (A71, A72, A73, A80) used appropriate methods of sequence generation and were judged to pose 'low' risk of bias. Two studies (A75, A76) that allocated participants according to registration order were considered 'high' risk for sequence generation. Four studies used either central randomisation (A80) or sealed envelopes (A72, A78, A79) to conceal group allocation, posing 'low' risk of bias. Studies that used sham/placebo acupuncture as a comparator were considered to be at 'low' risk of bias, although one multiple-arm study (A79) that compared electroacupuncture with HT was considered 'high' risk of bias overall. Personnel were either unblinded or their awareness of group allocation was 'unclear'. Blinding of outcome assessors was 'unclear' in three studies (A78, A79, A80). The impact of missing data was 'unclear' in one study (A78), while all remaining studies either reported no missing data or used appropriate statistical methods to account for missing data. All outcomes described in one trial registration (A80) were reported in the trial paper, posing 'low' risk of bias.

Table 7.13 Risk of Bias of Randomised Controlled Trials: Electroacupuncture

Risk of Bias Domain	Low Risk *n* (%)	Unclear Risk *n* (%)	High Risk *n* (%)
Sequence generation	4 (40)	4 (40)	2 (20)
Allocation concealment	4 (40)	6 (60)	0 (0)
Blinding of participants	4 (40)	0 (0)	6 (60)
Blinding of personnel*	0 (0)	3 (30)	7 (70)
Blinding of outcome assessors	0 (0)	3 (30)	7 (70)
Incomplete outcome data	9 (90)	1 (10)	0 (0)
Selective outcome reporting	1 (10)	9 (90)	0 (0)

*Blinding of personnel (acupuncturists) is challenging in manual therapy studies.

Outcomes

Several studies reported data in a way that did not permit re-analysis and these data were excluded from description below. The most frequently reported outcome was KI, reported in four studies. Vasomotor and depressive symptoms using the HAM-D were reported in three studies each, while the MRS and MENQOL were reported in two studies each. Differences in interventions, comparators and outcome measures meant that few meta-analyses were able to be conducted.

Vasomotor Symptoms

Three studies reported vasomotor symptoms (A72, A79, A80). As meta-analysis was not possible, results for individual studies are reporting according to comparison.

Electroacupuncture versus sham/placebo acupuncture

In one study (A72) of 58 perimenopausal women, women who received electroacupuncture reported 5.82 fewer hot flushes at the end of treatment ([−9.17, −2.47]) and 4.65 fewer hot flushes at follow-up ([−7.68, −1.62]) compared to placebo acupuncture. Another study (A79) reported a composite measure of hot flush frequency and severity in 28 women. Hot flush scores were not statistically different between women who received electroacupuncture and those who received sham acupuncture at the end of treatment (MD −0.30 points [−3.60, 3.00]) or at follow-up (MD −0.30 points [−3.90, 3.30]).

Electroacupuncture versus sham electroacupuncture

Electroacupuncture was compared with sham electroacupuncture in 360 women (A80). A composite measure of daily hot flush frequency and severity was calculated by multiplying the number of flushes by flush severity (1–3; mild to severe). Women who received electroacupuncture reported a greater change from baseline than women who received sham electroacupuncture at the end of treatment (MD 1.10 points [0.05, 2.15]), at follow-up after 20 weeks (MD 1.20 points [0.22, 2.18]) and at follow-up after 32 weeks (MD 2.20 points [0.82, 3.58]).

Electroacupuncture versus hormone therapy

One study (A79) compared electroacupuncture to oestradiol. Women who received oestradiol reported lower scores on a composite measure of daily hot flush frequency and severity at the end of treatment (24 women, MD 2.70 points [0.53, 4.87]) and at follow-up (20 women, MD 2.50 points [0.24, 4.76]).

Hamilton Rating Scale for Depression

Three studies (A73, A76, A77) assessed depressive symptoms using the HAM-D.

Electroacupuncture versus antidepressants

One study (A73) of 42 women, evaluated the effect of electroacupuncture on depressive symptoms using the HAM-D. Women who received electroacupuncture reported scores 2.29 points lower on the HAM-D than women who received escitalopram ([−4.48, −0.10]).

Electroacupuncture plus pharmacotherapy versus pharmacotherapy

Meta-analysis of two studies showed lower scores at the end of treatment among women who received electroacupuncture plus pharmacotherapy, compared to pharmacotherapy (145 women, MD −5.95 points [−8.02, −3.89], $I^2 = 0\%$; A76, A77).

Kupperman Index

Four studies (A71, A74, A75, A79) used the original or a modified version of the KI to assess global symptom severity. Analysis was conducted according to comparisons.

Electroacupuncture versus sham acupuncture

Two studies (A71, A79) used a modified version of the KI to assess global symptom severity. Electroacupuncture resulted in lower KI scores than sham acupuncture at the end of treatment (78 women, SMD −1.10 [−1.58, −0.62], I^2 = 0%) and at follow-up (78 women, SMD −0.52 [−0.98, −0.07], I^2 = 0%). One study (A71) of 50 women also reported individual KI items. No benefit was seen between groups for any of the 13 items assessed: vasomotor (MD −1.12 points, [−3.14, 0.90]), paraesthesia (MD −0.72 points, [−1.71, 0.27]), insomnia (MD −0.56 points, [−1.68, 0.56]), nervousness (MD −0.32 points, [−1.38, 0.74]), melancholia (MD 0.12 points, [−0.43, 0.67]), vertigo (MD −0.28 points, [−0.84, 0.28]), weakness (MD −0.12 points, [−0.64, 0.40]), arthralgia (MD 0.16 points, [−0.34, 0.66]), headache (MD −0.20 points, [−0.73, 0.33]), palpitations (MD 0.00 points [−0.52, 0.52]), formication (MD −0.24 points [−0.79, 0.31]), dyspareunia (MD 0.32 points [−0.71, 1.35]) and urinary tract infections (MD 0.16 points [−0.39, 0.71]).

Electroacupuncture versus hormone therapy

Two studies (A75, A79) with 84 women measured global symptom severity using a modified version of the KI. There was no difference between electroacupuncture and HT at the end of treatment (SMD −0.06 [−1.54, 1.43], I^2 = 89%). Follow-up assessment in one study (A79) showed no difference between electroacupuncture and HT (MD 5.80 points [−0.52, 12.12]).

Electroacupuncture plus hormone therapy versus hormone therapy

One study (A74) used the original 11-item KI to assess global symptom severity. There was no difference between the combination of electroacupuncture plus HT compared to HT alone in KI score at end-of-treatment (MD 0.13 points [−3.52, 3.78]) or at six months follow-up (MD −1.36 points [−4.44, 1.72]).

Menopause Rating Scale

The MRS was used to measure menopausal symptoms in two studies (A72, A80). Meta-analysis of end-of-treatment scores showed no difference between electroacupuncture and sham/placebo acupuncture at the end of treatment (418 women, MD −2.96 points [−5.95, 0.03], I^2 = 76%) and at first follow-up (418 women, MD −1.01 points [−8.09, 6.06], I^2 = 95%). Change scores were greater among women who received electroacupuncture during follow-up at 32 weeks in one study (360 women, MD 2.70 points [1.05, 4.35]; A80).

Domain scores from one study showed greater change in symptoms with electroacupuncture on all domains at the end of treatment and at both follow-up assessments. On the psychological domain, change score with electroacupuncture was 0.70 points greater at the end of treatment ([0.10, 1.30]), 0.90 points greater at 20 weeks ([0.20, 1.60]) and 1.00 points greater at 32 weeks ([0.25, 1.75]). On the physical domain, change score with electroacupuncture was 0.70 points greater at the end of treatment ([0.13, 1.27]), 1.00 points greater at 20 weeks ([0.47, 1.53]) and 1.10 points greater at 32 weeks ([0.53, 1.67]). On the urogenital domain, change score with electroacupuncture was 0.50 points greater at the end of treatment ([0.17, 0.83]), 0.60 points greater at 20 weeks ([0.20, 1.00]) and 0.60 points greater at 32 weeks ([0.12, 1.08]).

Global Symptom Assessment

One study (A79) used a VAS to assess global symptom severity. When electroacupuncture was compared to sham acupuncture, there was no difference between groups in global symptom severity at the end of treatment (28 women, MD −0.10 points [−0.92, 0.72]) and at follow-up (28 women, MD −0.20 points [−1.77, 1.37]). In the same study, women who received HT reported lower global symptom severity than women who received electroacupuncture at the end of treatment (24 women, MD 0.90 points [0.05, 1.75]). No such benefit was seen at follow-up (24 women, MD 1.30 points [−0.02, 2.62]).

Menopause-specific Quality of Life Questionnaire

Two studies (A72, A80) reported on the impact of electroacupuncture on health-related quality of life. Both studies reported total scores and one study (A80) reported domain scores. Domain scores were calculated as a sum of the scores for each item, which differs from the typical method of score calculation.

There was no difference between groups at the end of treatment (418 women, MD −5.58 points [−27.79, 16.62], $I^2 = 96\%$), but at follow-up the result favoured electroacupuncture (418 women, MD 6.66 points [0.67, 12.66], $I^2 = 0\%$). This result was heavily weighted towards one study that reported change from baseline score (A80). A second follow-up assessment at 32 weeks in one study (A80) also showed a greater change with electroacupuncture (360 women, MD 8.40 points [1.75, 15.05]).

The study of 360 women by Liu *et al.* (A80) also reported domain scores. On the physical domain, change score was not different between groups at the end of treatment (MD 2.90 points [−0.45, 6.25]), but favoured electroacupuncture at 20 weeks follow-up (MD 4.00 points [0.47, 7.53]) and at 32 weeks follow-up (MD 4.30 points [0.67, 7.93]). Change scores on the psychosocial domain favoured electroacupuncture at the end of treatment (MD 1.70 points [0.22, 3.18]), at 20 weeks (MD 1.90 points [0.15, 3.65]) and at 32 weeks (MD 2.10 points [0.20, 4.00]). Electroacupuncture was not statistically different to sham acupuncture on the vasomotor domain at the end of treatment (MD 0.90 points [−0.10, 1.90]) or at 20 weeks (MD 1.00 points [−0.03, 2.03]), but favoured electroacupuncture at 32 weeks (MD 1.40 points [0.40, 2.40]). No differences were seen between groups on the sexual domain at end of treatment (MD 0.30 points [−0.15, 0.75]), at 20 weeks (MD 0.20 points [−0.35, 0.75]) and at 32 weeks (MD 0.50 points [−0.28, 1.28]).

Frequently Reported Acupuncture Points in Meta-analyses Showing Favourable Effect: Electroacupuncture

Meta-analyses showed the benefit of electroacupuncture over comparators for the outcomes HAM-D and KI. The acupuncture points of studies included in these meta-analyses were reviewed to identify those which may contribute to the favourable effects seen. In the two RCTs (A76, A77) included in meta-analysis for HAM-D there was no overlap in acupuncture points. The acupuncture point SP6 *Sanyinjiao* 三阴交 was common to both studies (A71, A79) included in meta-analysis, showing a positive effect of electroacupuncture on KI.

Assessment Using Grading of Recommendations Assessment, Development and Evaluation

Electroacupuncture was tested less frequently in RCTs than acupuncture. Summary-of-findings tables were prepared for electroacupuncture versus sham/placebo acupuncture and electroacupuncture versus HT.

Electroacupuncture versus sham/placebo acupuncture

Three RCTs (A72, A79, A80) that compared electroacupuncture with sham/placebo acupuncture reported on outcomes selected for summary-of-findings tables. 'Low' certainty evidence suggested a benefit of electroacupuncture over sham/placebo acupuncture for daily hot flush frequency, while 'moderate' certainty evidence favoured electroacupuncture in reducing daily hot flush severity (Table 7.14). 'Moderate' certainty evidence suggested electroacupuncture may improve scores on the psychosocial domain of the MENQOL, while no differences were found between groups on the other MENQOL domains.

Table 7.14 GRADE: Electroacupuncture versus Sham/Placebo Acupuncture

Outcome; Treatment Duration	No. of Studies (Participants)	Relative Effect (MD [95% CI])	Certainty of the Evidence (GRADE)
Daily HF frequency; 8 w	1 (58)	−5.82 [−9.17, −2.47]*	⊕⊕◯◯ LOW[a,b]
Daily HF severity; 12 w	1 (28)	−0.30 [−3.6, −3.0]*	⊕⊕⊕◯ MODERATE[b]
MENQOL-Ph; 8 w	1 (360)	2.9 [−0.45, 6.25]	⊕⊕⊕◯ MODERATE[b]

(*Continued*)

Table 7.14 (*Continued*)

Outcome; Treatment Duration	No. of Studies (Participants)	Relative Effect (MD [95% CI])	Certainty of the Evidence (GRADE)
MENQOL-Psychosoc; 8 w	1 (360)	1.7 [0.22, 3.18]*	⊕⊕⊕◯ MODERATE[b]
MENQOL-V; 8 w	1 (360)	0.9 [−0.1, 1.90]	⊕⊕⊕◯ MODERATE[b]
MENQOL-S; 8 w	1 (360)	0.3 [−0.15, 0.75]	⊕⊕⊕◯ MODERATE[b]

*Statistically significant result.

Abbreviations: CI, confidence interval; d, days; HF, hot flush; GRADE, Grading of Recommendations, Assessment, Development and Evaluation; MD, mean difference; MENQOL, Menopause Quality of Life questionnaire; Ph, physical domain; Psychosoc, psychosocial domain; S, sexual domain; V, vasomotor domain; w, weeks.

Notes

[a]High risk of bias from lack of blinding.

[b]Small sample size.

Study references

Daily HF frequency: A72.

Daily HF severity: A79.

MENQOL: A80.

Safety of electroacupuncture was reported in two RCTs (A79, A80), with one (A79) reporting no AEs. Treatment-related AEs reported in women who received acupuncture included four cases of severe needling pain, two cases of subcutaneous haematoma, and one case each of dizziness, fatigue and abdominal discomfort. Two cases of fatigue were related to sham/placebo acupuncture.

Electroacupuncture versus hormone therapy

Two RCTs (A75, A79) that compared electroacupuncture with HT reported on important clinical outcomes. 'Moderate' certainty evidence showed electroacupuncture increased scores on a composite measure of hot flush frequency and severity, indicating worse outcomes (Table 7.15). Both RCTs reported on safety, with no AEs occurring.

Table 7.15 GRADE: Electroacupuncture versus Hormone Therapy

Outcome; Treatment Duration	No. of Studies (Participants)	Relative Effect (MD [95% CI])	Certainty of the Evidence (GRADE)
Daily HF frequency and severity; 12 w	1 (24)	2.7 [0.53, 4.87]*	⊕⊕⊕◯ MODERATE[a]

*Statistically significant result.
Abbreviations: CI, confidence interval; GRADE, Grading of Recommendations, Assessment, Development and Evaluation; HF, hot flush; MD, mean difference; w, weeks.

Note
[a]Small sample size.

Study reference
Daily HF frequency and severity: A79.

Non-controlled Studies of Electroacupuncture

Two case series (A81, A82), involving 74 perimenopausal women, evaluated the role of electroacupuncture. One study (A81) of women with anxiety included only women with the CM syndrome of Liver and Kidney *yin* deficiency. Treatment was provided twice in four weeks (A81) or 20 times in 40 days (A82). Two acupuncture points were used in both studies: SP6 *Sanyinjiao* 三阴交 and LR3 *Taichong* 太冲. Other points included EX-HN3 *Yintang* 印堂, GV20 *Baihui* 百会, PC6 *Neiguan* 内关, CV4 *Guanyuan* 关元, SP10 *Xuehai* 血海, EX-CA1 *Zigong* 子宫 (uterus) and ear TF4 *Shenmen* 耳神门 . Neither study reported on safety.

Safety of Electroacupuncture

Safety of electroacupuncture was reported in four RCTs (A74, A75, A79, A80). Three of these stated that no AEs occurred. Adverse events associated with electroacupuncture in the fourth study (A80) included four cases of severe needling pain, two cases of subcutaneous haematoma, and one case each of fatigue, abdominal discomfort and dizziness. Two cases of fatigue related to treatment were reported in women who received sham electroacupuncture.

Moxibustion

Three studies that met the inclusion criteria assessed the role of moxibustion for menopausal symptoms. Two were RCTs (A83, A84) and one was a case series (A85).

Randomised Controlled Trials of Moxibustion

Moxibustion was evaluated in two RCTs (A83, A84) with 137 women. One study (A83) was conducted in China and compared moxibustion with HT after three months of treatment, while the second study (A84) was conducted in South Korea and compared two intervention groups that received moxibustion with no treatment after four weeks of treatment. Moxibustion groups were considered sufficiently similar that results were merged for analysis.

Neither study reported CM syndrome diagnosis. Both studies applied moxibustion to BL23 *Shenshu* 肾俞. Other acupuncture points used in the studies included: BL13 *Feishu* 肺俞, BL15 *Xinshu* 心俞, BL18 *Ganshu* 肝俞, BL20 *Pishu* 脾俞, CV4 *Guanyuan* 关元, CV6 *Qihai* 气海, SP6 *Sanyinjiao* 三阴交, ST36 *Zusanli* 足三里, CV12 *Zhongwan* 中脘 and GV4 *Mingmen* 命门.

A computer-generated random number table was used for group allocation in one study (A84), posing 'low' risk of bias. The other study allocated participants according to registration order, which was considered 'high' risk. Insufficient information was available about how group allocation was concealed and both studies were judged 'unclear' risk for allocation concealment. A lack of blinding of participants was considered to pose 'high' risk of bias in both studies. One study (A84) conducted outcome assessment blind to group allocation ('low' risk) and it was considered not feasible to blind personnel ('unclear' risk). The second study was judged 'high' risk due to a lack of blinding of personnel and 'unclear' risk of bias due to insufficient information about blinding of outcome assessors. One study reported a small number of withdrawals and due to the small sample size and use of subjective outcomes it was unclear whether this was likely to influence the results. No missing data was reported in the second study. No trial protocol or registration was identified for either study, posing 'unclear' risk of bias.

One study (A84) reported on vasomotor symptoms; however, data were not presented in a way that permitted re-analysis. In the second study, moxibustion resulted in lower global symptom severity using a modified KI compared to HT. This result was found at the end of treatment (MD −2.88 points [−4.18, −1.58]) and at follow-up (MD −4.82 points [−6.31, −3.33]).

Non-controlled Studies of Moxibustion

One case series (A85) involving 43 perimenopausal women used moxibustion. All women received moxibustion to CV8 *Shenque* 神阙 once daily for four weeks.

Safety of Moxibustion

One of the three included studies (A84) reported on safety of moxibustion. Adverse events in the intervention group included an unspecified number of cases of general fatigue, stomach upsets, exacerbation of symptoms and headaches due to moxa smoke.

Acupressure

The potential role for acupressure in managing menopausal symptoms was tested in three RCTs (A86–A88) conducted in Iran. Three hundred and fifteen postmenopausal women participated in the studies. Two studies were three-arm trials: one (A86) compared acupressure with no treatment and with sham acupressure, while the other (A87) included one treatment arm of acupressure and a second treatment arm of pilates. The results for the pilates arm were not included in this review. The third study (A88) combined acupressure with lifestyle advice.

None of the studies described the use of CM syndrome differentiation either as an inclusion criterion or to guide treatment. Treatment duration was either four weeks/one month (A86, A88) or six weeks (A87). The acupuncture point HT7 *Shenmen* 神门 was used in all studies. Other acupuncture points used for acupressure were SP6 *Sanyinjiao* 三阴交 (two studies), and GB20 *Fengchi* 风池, KI7 *Fuliu* 复溜 and EX-HN3 *Yintang* 印堂 (one study each).

All studies used appropriate methods for group allocation and were judged as 'low' risk of bias for sequence generation. None reported details of allocation concealment, posing 'unclear' risk. One study (A88) that used sham acupressure as the comparator was assessed as 'low' risk of bias for sequence generation, one study (A86) was assessed as 'high' risk of bias as not all groups were blind to group allocation and the third study (A87) was judged 'unclear' risk of bias due to insufficient information. One study (A87) was assessed as 'high' risk of bias for blinding of personnel as it was considered unlikely to be achieved. The remaining two studies were assessed as 'unclear' risk for this domain. Outcome assessors were blinded to group allocation in one study ('low' risk; A87) and was 'unclear' in the remaining studies.

Two studies were assessed as 'low' risk of bias as all outcome data were available (A87) or reasons for missing data were considered unlikely to be related to the outcome (A86). In the third study (A88) it was possible that missing data was related to the treatment effect and this may have biased results. One study (A86) reported all outcomes described in the trial registration ('low' risk), one study (A88) failed to report on all outcomes specified in the trial registration ('high' risk) and no trial protocol or registration was identified for the third study (A87) ('unclear' risk).

Outcomes

Outcomes reported in studies of acupressure included vasomotor, psychological and sleep symptoms.

Vasomotor Symptoms

One study (A88) reported vasomotor symptoms in 70 postmenopausal women. The combination of acupressure and lifestyle advice resulted in 2.97 fewer hot flushes per day ([−3.47, −2.47]) and less severe flushes (MD −4.41 points [−6.14, −2.68]) than sham acupressure plus lifestyle advice. Frequency of night sweats was also lower in the treatment group (MD −1.03 night sweats, [−1.45, −0.61]).

State-trait Anxiety

State-trait anxiety scores at the end of treatment were 10.95 points lower among women who received acupressure plus lifestyle advice compared to women who received sham acupressure plus lifestyle advice ([−16.12, −5.78]; A88).

Pittsburgh Sleep Quality Index

Two studies (A86, A87) assessed sleep quality using the PSQI. At the end of treatment, results for PSQI were lower, indicating better outcomes, in women who received acupressure compared to women who received no treatment (141 women, MD 5.92 points [−8.10, −3.74], $I^2 = 85\%$). Statistical heterogeneity was considerable and may be due to reporting of change scores in one study (A86). One study that compared acupressure with sham acupressure in 73 women found better outcomes at the end of treatment in women who received ear acupressure (MD −2.89 points [−4.15, −1.63]; A86).

Frequently Reported Acupuncture Points in Meta-analyses Showing Favourable Effect: Acupressure

The meta-analysis for PSQI showed a positive effect favouring acupressure. The acupuncture point HT7 *Shenmen* 神门 was the only point common to both studies included in the meta-analysis (A86, A87). This acupuncture point is frequently used to calm the mind and its use in studies to improve sleep symptoms reflects clinical practice.

Safety of Acupressure

None of the included RCTs reported on safety of acupressure. Given that the technique is non-invasive it is considered unlikely to cause AEs; however, this should be examined in future clinical trials.

Ear Acupressure

Seven studies tested the role of ear acupressure in women managing menopausal symptoms. Two were RCTs (A89, A90) and five were case series (A67, A69, A70, A91, A92).

Randomised Controlled Trials of Ear Acupressure

Two RCTs (A89, A90) examined potential benefits of ear acupressure in 150 menopausal women. In one study (A89), women with insomnia were included, while the other study included women with anxiety. Both studies were conducted in China, used ear acupressure in combination with pharmacotherapy and provided treatment for four weeks.

Neither study reported CM syndrome differentiation. The acupuncture point TF4 *Shenmen* 耳神门 was used in both studies. Other points included: CO18 *Neifenmi* 内分泌 (Endocrine), AH6 *Jiaogan* 交感 (Sympathetic), CO10 *Shen* 肾 (Kidney) and AT4 *Pizhixia* 皮质下 (Subcortex). Ear acupressure plus alprazolam was compared with sham acupressure and alprazolam (A90) in one study, while the second study compared ear acupressure plus eszopiclone with eszopiclone alone.

Both studies used random number tables to allocate women to study groups and were judged 'low' risk. Insufficient information was available to determine the method for allocation concealment ('unclear' risk of bias). Blinding of participants and outcome assessors posed 'low' risk in one study (A90), while for the same study blinding of personnel was considered not feasible. Participants and personnel were not blind in the second study ('high' risk) and it was not clear whether outcome assessors were blind to group allocation ('unclear' risk). In one study (A90) participants withdrew due to a lack of treatment effect and intention-to-treat analysis was not conducted ('unclear' risk). There was no missing data in the other study ('low' risk). No trial protocols or registrations were identified for either study and both were judged as 'unclear' risk for selective outcome reporting.

Outcomes

Outcomes reported in included studies related to sleep, anxiety, global symptom severity and health-related quality of life.

Spiegel Sleep Questionnaire

Sleep quality was assessed using the Spiegel Sleep Questionnaire[37] in one study of 100 women (A89). Ear acupressure combined with eszopiclone improved sleep quality compared to eszopiclone alone (MD −3.08 points [−4.30, −1.86]).

Hamilton Rating Scale for Anxiety

The effect of ear acupressure plus alprazolam on anxiety was compared with sham acupressure plus alprazolam in 44 women (A90). Ear acupressure as integrative medicine was no more effective than sham acupressure plus alprazolam in improving anxiety symptoms measured using the HAM-A (MD −3.00 points [−6.56, 0.56]).

Menopause Rating Scale

Ear acupressure plus alprazolam was not statistically different to sham acupressure and alprazolam on the MRS in 44 women (MD −1.80 points [−4.97, 1.37]; A90).

Clinical Global Improvement

No difference was seen between ear acupressure plus alprazolam and sham acupressure plus alprazolam in clinical global improvement for either severity (44 women, MD −0.40 points [−0.97, 0.17]; A90) or improvement (44 women, MD −0.60 points [−1.21, 0.01]; A90).

36-Item Short-Form Health Survey

The effect of the combination on health-related quality of life was assessed using the SF-36 in one study with 44 women (A90). No difference was found between ear acupressure plus alprazolam and sham acupressure plus alprazolam on physical function (MD 8.10 points [−2.93, 19.13]), role function — health (MD 0.00 points [−21.94, 21.94]), role function — emotion (MD −14.50 points [−36.22, 7.22]), bodily pain (MD 2.90 points [−7.42, 13.22]), general health perceptions (MD 6.40 points [−7.16, 19.96]), vitality (MD 3.90 points [−8.17, 15.97]), social function (MD 2.70 points [−7.36, 12.76]) or mental health (MD 0.90 points [−9.76, 11.56]).

Non-controlled Studies of Ear Acupressure

Ear acupressure was tested in five case series (A67, A69, A70, A91, A92,). Three studies (A67, A69, A70) combined ear acupressure with manual acupuncture and have been described in the 'Acupuncture' section of this chapter. The two studies (A91, A92) that tested ear acupressure alone included 88 perimenopausal women with insomnia. Both provided treatment for one month and neither described CM syndrome differentiation. Three acupuncture points were used in both studies: ear TF4 *Shenmen* 耳神门, AH6 *Jiaogan* 交感 (Sympathetic) and AT4 *Pizhixia* 皮质下 (Subcortex). Other acupuncture points included: LO4 *Chuiqian* 垂前 (anterior earlobe), AT3 *Zhen* 枕 (Occiput), CO18 *Neifenmi* 内分泌 (Endocrine) and CO12 *Gan* 肝 (Liver).

Safety of Ear Acupressure

Both RCTs reported on safety, while none of the case series reported on this outcome. Among women who received ear acupressure, AEs included four cases of dry mouth, four cases of liver and kidney damage, three cases of dizziness and two cases of palpitations. Adverse events among women who received eszopiclone included three cases of heart palpitations, two cases of liver and kidney damage and one case each of dry mouth and dizziness.

Laser Acupuncture

One Australian RCT (A93) examined the role of laser acupuncture for menopausal symptoms in 40 women. Perimenopausal and postmenopausal women were included. All women received the same treatment, which included laser acupuncture to SP6 *Sanyinjiao* 三阴交, LU9 *Taiyuan* 太渊, LR3 *Taichong* 太冲, CV6 *Qihai* 气海, LI4 *Hegu* 合谷, HT7 *Shenmen* 神门, PC6 *Neiguan* 内关, ear TF4 *Shenmen* 耳神门, CO18 *Neifenmi* 内分泌 (Endocrine) and AH6 *Jiaogan* 交感 (Sympathetic). Treatment was provided fortnightly for 12 weeks. Laser acupuncture was compared with sham laser acupuncture.

Insufficient information was provided about sequence generation and allocation concealment, and the study was assessed as 'unclear' risk of bias for these domains. Both participants and personnel were blind to group allocation ('low' risk), while it was unclear whether outcome assessors were blind to group allocation. The study was judged 'unclear' risk of bias for incomplete outcome data due to a lack of information and was judged 'unclear' risk of bias for selective outcome reporting as no trial protocol or trial registration was identified. The study reported on hot flushes and an investigator-developed method for assessing global symptom severity, but data were not presented in a way that permitted re-analysis. The study authors reported that no AEs occurred during the trial.

Koryo Hand Therapy

One RCT (A94), conducted in Korea, tested Koryo hand therapy in 50 postmenopausal women. Eligible women were those with between one and ten years of amenorrhoea. Koryo therapy involved moxibustion and hand pellets to points on the hand, with treatment provided for eight weeks. Treatment was compared with no treatment.

The study used appropriate methods for group allocation through use of a coin toss and used methods to prevent prediction of group allocation, posing 'low' risk of bias for sequence generation and allocation concealment. Participants were not blind to group allocation ('high' risk) and it was considered not feasible to blind personnel ('unclear' risk). The study was judged 'unclear' risk for blinding of outcome assessors due to a lack of information. The reasons and amount of missing data were not clearly reported and the study was assessed as 'unclear' risk for incomplete outcome data. Finally, no trial protocol or trial registration was identified and the study was judged as 'unclear' risk of bias for selective outcome reporting.

Global symptom severity was assessed using the Neugarten and Kraines scale.[38] Women who received Koryo hand therapy scored lower at the end of treatment than women who received no treatment (MD −7.00 points [−10.90, −3.10]). The study did not report on the safety of Koryo hand therapy.

Point Percussion Therapy

Three RCTs (A95–A97) evaluated point percussion therapy in 204 perimenopausal women. Women were recruited from inpatient departments of hospitals in China. One study (A95) included women with a sleep disorder who received treatment for four weeks, while the other studies included perimenopausal women who received treatment for three months. One study used CM diagnoses of Liver and Kidney *yin* deficiency, and Kidney *yang* deficiency, as both an inclusion criterion and to guide treatment. Two acupuncture points were used in multiple studies: SP6 *Sanyinjiao* 三阴交 and ST36 *Zusanli* 足三里.

All studies used adequate methods to generate randomisation sequence and had outcome data for all included women; all were judged 'low' risk for sequence generation and incomplete outcome data. Sequentially numbered envelopes were used in one study (A97), which was judged 'low' risk for allocation concealment. None of the studies blinded participants to group allocation ('high' risk) while one study (A97) blinded study personnel and outcome assessors to group allocation ('low' risk). Published trial protocols and trial registrations were not able to be identified for any of the studies and all were considered to pose 'unclear' risk of bias for selective outcome reporting.

Outcomes

Outcomes related to sleep quality, psychological symptoms and global symptom severity. Analysis was conducted according to comparison.

Pittsburgh Sleep Quality Index

One RCT (A95) of 84 women with sleep disorders found women who received point percussion therapy had lower scores, indicating better outcomes, on the PSQI compared to estazolam (MD −7.00 points [−10.90, −3.10]).

Zung's Self-rating Depression Scale

The study that measured sleep change on the PSQI also measured depressive symptoms using Zung's Self-rating Depression Scale (SDS)[39] (A95). Women who received point percussion therapy had a greater improvement in depressive symptoms than women who received estazolam (84 women, MD −9.29 points [−12.55, −6.03]).

Zung's Self-rating Anxiety Scale

Anxiety symptoms were assessed in 84 women using the Zung's Self-rating Anxiety Scale (SAS)[40] (A95). Anxiety scores were 4.99 points lower at the end of treatment in women who received point percussion therapy than women who received estazolam ([−8.38, −1.60]).

Kupperman Index

Meta-analysis was possible for two studies (A96, A97) involving 120 women that reported global symptom severity using a modified version of the KI. Women who received point percussion therapy reported lower scores at the end of treatment compared with women who received tibolone (SMD −0.65 [−1.02, −0.28], $I^2 = 0\%$).

One study (A97) of 60 women also reported individual item scores. Women who received point percussion therapy reported lower scores at the end of treatment than women who received tibolone for the following items: insomnia (MD −1.27 points [−1.80, −0.74]), nervousness (MD −0.33 points [−0.61, −0.05]), vertigo (MD −0.40 points [−0.69, −0.11]), arthralgia (MD −0.73 points [−1.02, −0.44]), headache (MD −0.27 points [−0.52, −0.02]), formication (MD −0.23 points [−0.42, −0.04]) and urinary tract infection (MD −0.80 points [−1.32, −0.28]). No difference was seen between groups for the following items: vasomotor (MD −0.13 points [−1.32, 1.06]), paraesthesia (MD 0.27 points [−0.24, 0.78]), melancholia (MD −0.06 points [−0.32, 0.20]), weakness (MD −0.13 points [−0.38, 0.12]), palpitations (MD −0.26 points [−0.55, 0.03]) and dyspareunia (MD −0.34 points [−1.19, 0.51]).

Safety of Point Percussion Therapy

Safety of point percussion therapy was reported in one study (A97). Adverse events in the treatment group included two cases of subcutaneous freckle, while AEs in women who received tibolone included four cases of weight gain, three cases of vaginal bleeding and two cases of headache.

Clinical Evidence for Commonly Used Acupuncture and Related Therapies

Three acupuncture interventions were recommended in clinical textbooks and guidelines that informed Chapter 2: acupuncture, moxibustion and ear acupuncture. Acupuncture was tested in 70 clinical studies: 57 RCTs, six CCTs and seven non-controlled studies. Among all acupuncture studies, the most frequently used acupuncture points were SP6 *Sanyinjiao* 三阴交 (38 studies), LR3 *Taichong* 太冲 (27 studies), CV4 *Guanyuan* 关元 (25 studies), HT7 *Shenmen* 神门 (25 studies), GV20 *Baihui* 百会 (22 studies), PC6 *Neiguan* 内关 (22 studies), BL23 *Shenshu* 肾俞 (21 studies), ST36 *Zusanli* 足三里 (21 studies) and KI3 *Taixi* 太溪 (20 studies). Many of these points are recommended in clinical textbooks and guidelines in Chapter 2.

The best evidence for the effect of acupuncture comes from meta-analyses of RCTs. Acupuncture was found to be superior to pharmacotherapy in improving sleep symptoms measured with the PSQI, psychological symptoms assessed with the HAM-D and HAM-A, and global symptom severity on the KI. While results favoured acupuncture, statistical heterogeneity lowers confidence in the results. Results for individual studies showed mixed benefits: some analyses favoured acupuncture, some showed no difference between acupuncture and no treatment, sham/placebo acupuncture or pharmacotherapy, and some showed results that favoured pharmacotherapy. These findings suggest acupuncture may have a role to play in management of menopausal symptoms, but further research is needed to examine what that role might be.

Moxibustion was tested in three clinical studies: two RCTs and one case series. The acupuncture point, BL23 *Shenshu* 肾俞 was used in both RCTs and is the only point used in multiple studies. This point was not recommended in clinical texts included in Chapter 2; instead, clinical guidelines recommend the use of GV4 *Mingmen* 命门, CV6 *Qihai* 气海 and CV4 *Guanyuan* 关元. All three points were used in one of the RCTs. Evidence from one RCT showed moxibustion improved global symptom severity measured with the KI. No studies meeting the inclusion criteria evaluated ear acupuncture alone. However, ear acupressure was tested in seven studies (two RCTs and five case series).

Summary of Acupuncture and Related Therapies Clinical Evidence

There have been many studies that have evaluated the role of acupuncture and related therapies for bothersome symptoms of menopause, and a selection of these have been presented in this chapter. The majority of studies have focused on acupuncture as the intervention and this appears to reflect clinical practice both in, and outside of, China.

The median duration of treatment for acupuncture RCTs, which comprised the majority of clinical studies (57 of 97 included studies, 58.7%), was six weeks. Treatment with electroacupuncture was slightly longer (median of eight weeks in ten RCTs) and treatment with ear acupressure was slightly shorter (mean of four weeks in two RCTs). In clinical practice acupuncture treatment is typically provided for between six and eight weeks. One possible reason for the shorter duration seen with ear acupressure relates to the intervention itself — acupuncture press studs are typically left in place for three days and patients are instructed to press the points for several minutes multiple times per day. More frequent stimulation may reduce the time required to see change in symptoms.

Syndromes described in clinical studies mostly related to Kidney deficiency, for example Kidney *yin* deficiency, Kidney *yang* deficiency and Kidney *yin* and *yang* deficiency. This aligns with the syndromes described in clinical textbooks and guidelines (see Chapter 2). Several studies described syndromes involving the Kidney and another *zang* 脏 organ such as the Liver, Heart or Spleen. Again, such combinations of syndromes are reported in clinical texts. This highlights the interrelationship between organs in CM.

Diversity in comparators, outcome measures and ways in which outcomes were assessed prevented pooling of results for meta-analysis for some outcomes, meaning that for these outcomes the best evidence comes from individual studies. This limits our ability to be certain about implementing such interventions in clinical practice. For other outcomes, it was considered appropriate to use statistical methods to account for differences in ways outcome measures were scored and/or assessed, for example through the use of SMD. While this can assist in identifying whether a difference between groups exists, it does not provide information about the absolute anticipated effect that may be expected with treatment and can make it more challenging to determine whether the potential gains are clinically important for patients.

Meta-analyses were able to be conducted for several outcomes, with the results suggesting acupuncture was more effective than pharmacotherapy in improving psychological symptoms assessed with the HAM-D and HAM-A and improving global symptom severity measured using the KI. Furthermore, acupuncture as an integrative medicine with pharmacotherapy was more effective than pharmacotherapy alone in improving sleep symptoms measured with the PSQI and depressive symptoms on the HAM-D. These results suggest acupuncture therapies may improve sleep and psychological symptoms and may also improve overall severity of symptoms.

Assessment of clinically important questions using the GRADE framework highlighted that the strength and quality of evidence ('certainty') ranged from 'low' to 'moderate' when acupuncture was compared with sham/placebo, with no difference between groups in daily hot flush frequency and severity, sleep symptoms assessed with the PSQI and on the four domains of MENQOL. 'Very low' certainty evidence showed no benefit of acupuncture over HT for depressive symptoms measured with the HAM-D. 'Low' certainty evidence found that electroacupuncture was more effective in reducing daily hot flush frequency than sham/placebo and 'moderate' certainty evidence showed electroacupuncture to be more effective in reducing severity of hot flushes. 'Moderate' certainty evidence provided mixed results on the MENQOL domains. Finally, 'moderate' certainty evidence found HT to be more effective than electroacupuncture in reducing frequency and severity of hot flushes.

While no difference was seen between groups for several clinically important outcomes, it is important to note that HT is effective at improving menopausal symptoms, so a result of 'no difference' may suggest acupuncture therapies as a useful alternative to pharmacotherapy. Confidence in several of these results was lowered due to statistical heterogeneity and the number of clinical studies included in assessments for each outcome was small. Overall, the findings from these assessments are insufficient to change clinical practice, particularly as questions about superiority of one acupuncture intervention over another, the duration of effect and the best duration of treatment remain unanswered by this review.

Acupuncture therapies were generally well tolerated and, in some cases, produced fewer AEs than pharmacotherapies. Known AEs associated with acupuncture include pain/numbness/itching at the site of needle insertion and bleeding/bruising, even when acupuncture is provided by an appropriately qualified, trained and experienced practitioner. Given this, acupuncture may be considered as an alternative treatment option for women who wish to avoid use of pharmacotherapy for menopausal symptoms.

The studies included in this review had similar characteristics as those described in Chapter 5. Acupuncture was the main intervention tested in clinical studies conducted outside of China and was frequently compared to sham or placebo acupuncture. Acupuncture was also tested in clinical studies conducted in China, but was more likely to be compared to pharmacotherapy. Studies conducted in China focused on sleep, psychological symptoms and global severity of symptoms, while studies conducted outside of China tended to focus on vasomotor symptoms, global severity of symptoms and health-related quality of life. As has been highlighted in Chapter 5, this may reflect a difference in the symptoms that cause the most bother to women according to geographic location. This has also been reported elsewhere.[41,42]

Most of the studies included in this review were from China and included perimenopausal women. Studies of the effect of acupuncture therapies in postmenopausal women were typically conducted outside of China. The menopausal status of women has been described for each analysis where possible. It is important to note that the findings from this review may not be applicable to women of different menopausal status or women in different countries, as the experience of menopause can vary according to these factors.

None of the studies included in this review assessed genitourinary symptoms of menopause and few assessed the potential benefits of health-related quality of life. Future research assessing these outcomes will provide additional evidence about the appropriateness of acupuncture therapies for managing menopause-related quality of life.

References

1. 曹徽良 王, 李赛群, 孙佳琪, 周有君, 章薇. (2015) 针刺治疗围绝经期综合征疗效系统评价. 针灸临床杂志 **31**(09): 60–64.
2. 张议元 熊, 杜元灏. (2011) 针灸与西药治疗更年期综合征疗效比较的系统评价. 辽宁中医杂志 **38**(03): 538–544.
3. 成晓玲 周, 黄伟, 吴桂玲, 陈霞, 郑易炜. (2018) 电针与激素替代疗法比较治疗围绝经期综合征系统评价. 中国中医药信息杂志 **25**(03): 107–111.
4. 赖斌 焦, 熊俊, 钟欢, 严鸿丽. (2017) 针刺与西药治疗围绝经期综合征的疗效比较系统评价. 江西中医药大学学报 **29**(02): 104–108+24.
5. 张光彩 陈, 符文彬, 吴倩, 伍亚男. (2016) 基于GRADE评级对针灸治疗围绝经期睡眠障碍的系统评价. 广州中医药大学学报 **33**(01): 126–131.
6. 张宁, 胡静, 王雁. (2012) 针灸治疗围绝经期睡眠障碍随机对照研究Meta评价. 中国中医药信息杂志 **19**(08): 24–26.
7. 李昭凤 吴, 符文彬, 陈嘉仪. (2014) 针灸治疗围绝经期抑郁障碍有效性和安全性的系统评价(英文). 中华中医药杂志 **29**(05): 1746–1752.
8. 黄叶飞 符, 吴泰相, 张光彩, 苏临荣, 陈远芳. (2011) 针灸治疗围绝经期抑郁症有效性和安全性的系统评价[J]. 中华中医药杂志 **26**(05): 908–914+1242.
9. Dodin S, Blanchet C, Marc I, *et al.* (2013) Acupuncture for menopausal hot flushes. *Cochrane Database Syst Rev* (7): Cd007410.
10. Ee C, French SD, Xue CC, *et al.* (2017) Acupuncture for menopausal hot flashes: Clinical evidence update and its relevance to decision making. *Menopause* **24**(8): 980–987.
11. Lee MS, Shin BC, Ernst E. (2009) Acupuncture for treating menopausal hot flushes: A systematic review. *Climacteric* **12**(1): 16–25.
12. Cho SH, Whang WW. (2009) Acupuncture for vasomotor menopausal symptoms: A systematic review. *Menopause* **16**(5): 1065–1073.
13. Nam E-Y, Park J-Y, Lee J-Y, *et al.* (2018) Traditional acupuncture for menopausal hot flashes: A systematic review and meta-analysis of randomized controlled trials. *Eur J Integr Med* **17**: 119–128.
14. Taylor-Swanson L, Thomas A, Ismail R, *et al.* (2015) Effects of traditional Chinese medicine on symptom clusters during the menopausal transition. *Climacteric* **18**(2): 142–156.
15. Bezerra AG, Pires GN, Andersen ML, *et al.* (2015) Acupuncture to treat sleep disorders in postmenopausal women: A systematic review. *Evid Based Complement Alternat Med* **2015**: 563236.
16. Chiu HY, Pan CH, Shyu YK, *et al.* (2015) Effects of acupuncture on menopause-related symptoms and quality of life in women in natural menopause: A meta-analysis of randomized controlled trials. *Menopause* **22**(2): 234–244.

17. Li W, Luo Y, Fu W, *et al.* (2018) Acupuncture may improve quality of life in menopausal women: A meta-analysis of randomized controlled trials. *Complement Med Res* **25**(3): 183–190.
18. Befus D, Coeytaux RR, Goldstein KM, *et al.* (2018) Management of menopause symptoms with acupuncture: An umbrella systematic review and meta-analysis. *J Altern Complement Med* **24**(4): 314–323.
19. Hamilton M. (1960) A rating scale for depression. *J Neurol Neurosurg Psychiatry* **23**: 56–62.
20. Hamilton M. (1959) The assessment of anxiety states by rating. *Br J Med Psychol* **32**(1): 50–55.
21. Kupperman HS, Wetchler BB, Blatt MH. (1959) Contemporary therapy of the menopausal syndrome. *J Am Med Assoc* **171**: 1627–1637.
22. Buysse DJ, Reynolds CF, 3rd, Monk TH, *et al.* (1989) The Pittsburgh Sleep Quality Index: A new instrument for psychiatric practice and research. *Psychiatry Res* **28**(2): 193–213.
23. Bastien CH, Vallieres A, Morin CM. (2001) Validation of the Insomnia Severity Index as an outcome measure for insomnia research. *Sleep Med* **2**(4): 297–307.
24. Buysse DJ, Yu L, Moul DE, *et al.* (2010) Development and validation of patient-reported outcome measures for sleep disturbance and sleeprelated impairments. *Sleep* **33**(6): 781–792.
25. Soldatos CR, Dikeos DG, Paparrigopoulos TJ. (2000) Athens Insomnia Scale: Validation of an instrument based on ICD-10 criteria. *J Psychosom Res* **48**(6): 555–560.
26. Beck AT, Ward CH, Mendelson M, *et al.* (1961) An inventory for measuring depression. *Arch Gen Psychiatry* **4**: 561–571.
27. Cohen S, Kamarck T, Mermelstein R. (1983) A global measure of perceived stress. *J Health Soc Behav* **24**: 385–396.
28. Radloff L. (1977) The CES-D Scale: A self-report depression scale for research in the general population. *Appl Psychol Meas* **1**(3): 385–401.
29. Spitzer RL, Kroenke K, Williams JBW, *et al.* (2006) A brief measure for assessing generalized anxiety disorder: The GAD-7. *JAMA Intern Med* **166**(10): 1092–1097.
30. Zigmond AS, Snaith RP. (1983) The hospital anxiety and depression scale. *Acta Psychiatr Scand* **67**(6): 361–370.
31. Beck AT, Epstein N, Brown G, *et al.* (1988) An inventory for measuring clinical anxiety: Psychometric properties. *J Consult Clin Psychol* **56**(6): 893–897.

32. Greene JG. (1976) A factor analytic study of climacteric symptoms. *J Psychosom Res* **20**(5): 425–430.
33. Heinemann LA, Potthoff P, Schneider HP. (2003) International versions of the Menopause Rating Scale (MRS). *Health Qual Life Outcomes* **1:** 28.
34. Hunter M. (1992) The Women's Health Questionnaire: A measure of mid-aged women's perceptions of their emotional and physical health. *Psychol Health* **7**: 45–54.
35. Carpenter JS. (2001) The Hot Flash Related Daily Interference Scale: A tool for assessing the impact of hot flashes on quality of life following breast cancer. *J Pain Symptom Manage* **22**(6): 979–989.
36. Ware JJ, Sherbourne C. (1992) The MOS 36-item short-form health survey (SF-36). I. Conceptual framework and item selection. *Med Care* **30**: 473–483.
37. Spiegel R. (1981) *Sleep and Sleepiness in Advanced Age*. M.T.P. Press, Lancaster, UK.
38. Neugarten BL, Kraines RJ. (1965) Menopausal symptoms in women of various ages. *Psychosom Med* **27**: 266–273.
39. Zung WW. (1965) A self-rating depression scale. *Arch Gen Psychiatry* **12**: 63–70.
40. Zung WW. (1971) A rating instrument for anxiety disorders. *Psychosomatics* **12**(6): 371–379.
41. Im EO, Ko Y, Chee W. (2014) Ethnic differences in the clusters of menopausal symptoms. *Health Care Women Int* **35**(5): 549–565.
42. Obermeyer CM, Reher D, Saliba M. (2007) Symptoms, menopause status, and country differences: A comparative analysis from DAMES. *Menopause* **14**(4): 788–797.

References for Included Acupuncture Therapies Clinical Studies

Study No.	References
A1	Avis NE, Coeytaux RR, Isom S, *et al.* (2016) Acupuncture in Menopause (AIM) study: A pragmatic, randomized controlled trial. *Menopause* **23**(6): 626–637.
A2	Avis NE, Legault C, Coeytaux RR, *et al.* (2008) A randomized, controlled pilot study of acupuncture treatment for menopausal hot flashes. *Menopause* **15**(6): 1070–1078.

(*Continued*)

(*Continued*)

Study No.	References
A3	Nir Y, Huang MI, Schnyer R, *et al.* (2007) Acupuncture for postmenopausal hot flashes. *Maturitas* **56**(4): 383–395.
A4	Painovich JM, Shufelt CL, Azziz R, *et al.* (2012) A pilot randomized, single-blind, placebo-controlled trial of traditional acupuncture for vasomotor symptoms and mechanistic pathways of menopause. *Menopause* **19**(1): 54–61.
A5	Venzke L, Calvert JF, Gilbertson B. (2010) A randomized trial of acupuncture for vasomotor symptoms in post-menopausal women. *Complement Ther Med* **18**(2): 59–66.
A6	Vincent A, Barton DL, Mandrekar JN, *et al.* (2007) Acupuncture for hot flashes: A randomized, sham-controlled clinical study. *Menopause* **14**(1): 45–52.
A7	Borud EK, Alraek T, White A, *et al.* (2009) The Acupuncture on Hot Flushes Among Menopausal Women (ACUFLASH) study, a randomized controlled trial. *Menopause* **16**(3): 484–493. Dormaenen A, Heimdal MR, Wang CEA, Grimsgaard AS. (2011) Depression in postmenopause: A study on a subsample of the Acupuncture on Hot Flushes Among Menopausal Women (ACUFLASH) study. *Menopause* **18**(5): 525–530.
A8	Castelo Branco De Luca A, Maggio da Fonseca A, *et al.* (2011) Acupuncture-ameliorated menopausal symptoms: Single-blind, placebo-controlled, randomized trial. *Climacteric* **14**(1): 140–145.
A9	Nedeljkovic M, Tian L, Ji P, *et al.* (2014) Effects of acupuncture and Chinese herbal medicine (Zhi Mu 14) on hot flushes and quality of life in postmenopausal women: Results of a four-arm randomized controlled pilot trial. *Menopause* **21**(1): 15–24.
A10	Sunay D, Ozdiken M, Arslan H, *et al.* (2011) The effect of acupuncture on postmenopausal symptoms and reproductive hormones: A sham controlled clinical trial. *Acupunct Med* **29**(1): 27–31.
A11	Kim DI, Roh JJ, Choi MS, *et al.* (2007) A clinical trial to assess the efficacy of acupuncture on hot flashes in postmenopausal women. *Korean J Orient Med* **28**(4): 74–85.
A12	许青云. (2006) 围绝经期综合征针灸疗效的观察. 右江医学 **34**(04): 377–378.
A13	张晓霞, 眭兰. (2017) 氟西汀联合调任安神法针刺或传统取穴法针刺对围绝经期抑郁症患者起效时间的影响. 实用临床医药杂志 **21**(17): 181–182.

(*Continued*)

Study No.	References
A14	李海波. (2015) 针刺治疗肾虚肝郁型围绝经期抑郁症的临床观察. 黑龙江中医药大学.
A15	徐丽华. (2015) 针灸疗法辅助治疗围绝经期抑郁症60例. 中国药业 **24**(24): 247–248.
A16	邱连利, 蒋花. (2014) 探讨针刺及心理健康辅导对围绝经期情志抑郁的影响. 西部中医药 **27**(11): 131–133.
A17	和婧伟. (2014) 针刺联合药物治疗女性更年期抑郁症 25 例临床观察. 中国针灸学会针灸临床分会.中国针灸学会临床分会 2014 年年会暨第二十一次全国针灸临床学术研讨会论文集. 中国针灸学会针灸临床分会: 中国针灸学会 **2014**: 3.
A18	张玉泉. (2013) 针刺辨证治疗围绝经期抑郁症94例临床研究. 内蒙古中医药 **32**(11): 41–42.
A19	邢凯. (2011) 醒神解郁针法治疗女性更年期抑郁症 120 例临床观察. 中国妇幼保健 **26**(34): 5373–5375.
A20	迟慧, 邹伟. (2011) 益肾调肝针刺法治疗围绝经期抑郁症 30 例. 针灸临床杂志 **27**(07): 4–7.
A21	王小云, 黎霄羽, 邓霭静, 薄智云. (2010) 腹针与西药治疗更年期妇女抑郁症疗效对比研究. 中国针灸 **30**(11): 913–917.
A22	马静. (2008) 针刺治疗围绝经期抑郁症的临床研究. 中国中西医结合学会精神疾病专业委员会.第九届全国中西医结合治疗精神疾病学术研讨会论文集. 中国中西医结合学会精神疾病专业委员会: 中国中西医结合学会, 1.
A23	强宝全. (2008) 针刺治疗女性更年期抑郁症30例. 陕西中医 **29**(07): 871–872.
A24	丁丽, 刘波. (2007) 补肾调肝 健脾宁心针法治疗围绝经期抑郁症的临床观察. 中华中医药学刊 **25**(05): 1066–1067.
A25	钱洁, 张捷, 裴音, 陈杰. (2007) 王氏五脏俞加膈俞治疗更年期抑郁症的临床观察. 北京中医 **26**(08): 491–492.
A26	周胜红. (2007) 针刺治疗女性更年期抑郁症 60 例. 中国组织工程研究与临床康复 **11**(39): 7817–7819.
A27	郑盛惠, 吴云天, 廖金蓉, 许明珠, 胡中妮, 陈露华. (2010) ‘四神针’久留针治疗围绝经期抑郁症临床研究. 辽宁中医杂志 **37**(04): 726–728.
A28	陈忠, 周胜红. (2010) 针刺治疗女性更年期抑郁症 30 例. 山东中医药大学学报 **34**(01): 44–45.

(*Continued*)

(***Continued***)

Study No.	References
A29	张巍, 皮燕, 陈婷, 王维维, 杨万芳, 王政研. (2017) 从肝论治针刺治疗围绝经期失眠的临床观察. 四川中医 **35**(09): 152–155.
A30	禹旭红. (2017) 腹针治疗围绝经期失眠临床效果评价. 内蒙古中医药 (07): 65–66.
A31	林文馨, 尹平, 徐世芬. (2017) 调任通督针刺法对围绝经期失眠的临床疗效评价. 上海针灸杂志 **36**(08): 900–904.
A32	杨继若, 许会英, 白晶梅, 等. (2017) 头针体针并用治疗围绝经期失眠症81例. 西部中医药 **30**(02): 4–6.
A33	薛文雄, 张金媛, 葛玲玲, 丁瑛骅, 蒋阳. (2017) 针刺联合雷火灸治疗更年期失眠疗效观察. 按摩与康复医学 **8**(03): 25–26.
A34	王延玉. (2017) 针灸治疗更年期失眠 28 例. 中国保健营养 (11): 386.
A35	刘唯群. (2017) 中医针灸辅助治疗妇女更年期失眠的效果分析. 中国医药指南 **15**(19): 188–189.
A36	朱山坡, 李朋朋, 朱学亮. (2016) 调督安神针法治疗围绝经期失眠疗效观察. 现代中西医结合杂志 **25**(26): 2885–2888.
A37	马伟丽. (2016) 针药结合治疗更年期失眠的作用及对患者血清FSH与E_2水平的影响. 中医药学报 **44**(02): 89–91.
A38	康珲. (2015) 头针丛刺治疗心胆气虚型围绝经期失眠症的临床观察. 黑龙江中医药大学.
A39	高乐, 牛红月. (2014) 盘龙刺治疗围绝经期失眠临床观察. 吉林中医药 **34**(01): 88–90.
A40	李亚男. (2014) 针刺下三皇治疗更年期失眠 120 例疗效观察. 中国实用医药 **9**(19): 244–246.
A41	徐淑稳, 茹秀丽, 黄丽霞, 李义飞, 张红真. (2014) 中医针灸辅助治疗妇女更年期失眠效果分析. 中国中医基础医学杂志 **20**(01): 106–108.
A42	纪峰. (2008) 交通心肾针刺法治疗更年期失眠症临床观察. 上海针灸杂志 **27**(12): 21–22.
A43	Fu C, Zhao N, Liu Z, *et al.* (2017) Acupuncture improves peri-menopausal insomnia: A randomized controlled trial. *Sleep* **40**(11).
A44	李龙芬, 杨毅红, 尹国良. (2013) 耳压、针刺配合黛力新治疗更年期焦虑症临床观察. 新中医 **45**(05): 124–126.
A45	口锁堂. (2014) 针刺与药物对比治疗更年期烦躁:随机对照研究. 中国针灸 **34**(05): 455–458.

(*Continued*)

Study No.	References
A46	王小云, 黎霄羽, 薄智云. (2012) 薄氏腹针治疗更年期妇女抑郁性疼痛的随机对照研究. 中国北京.
A47	Zhou J, Qu F, Sang XS, *et al.* (2011) Acupuncture and auricular acupressure in relieving menopausal hot flashes of bilaterally ovariectomized Chinese women: A randomized controlled trial. *Evid Based Complement Alternat Med* **2011**: 713274.
A48	Ee C, Xue C, Chondros P, *et al.* (2016) Acupuncture for menopausal hot flashes: A randomized trial. *Ann Intern Med* **164**(3): 146–154.
A49	Girão ÁC, Alves MDS, Souza AMA, *et al.* (2014) Acupuncture in the treatment of anxiety in climacteric: Additional therapy in mental health promotion. *J Nursing UFPE/Revista de Enfermagem UFPE* **8**(6): 1538–1544.
A50	陈伟, 刘东灵, 姜兴鹏. (2016) 回阳针法治疗脾肾阳虚型更年期综合症临床疗效观察. 中国中医基础医学杂志 **22**(03): 401–403.
A51	陈贞贞. (2014) 针刺五脏背俞穴治疗肝肾阴虚型围绝经期综合征的临床研究. 湖北中医药大学.
A52	林祥军. (2009) 调任固冲针法治疗围绝经期综合征的临床观察. 长春中医药大学.
A53	陈智平, 赵彩娇. (2016) 针灸治疗围绝经期临床研究. 亚太传统医药 **12**(16): 113–114.
A54	金弘. (2006) 针刺膀胱经五脏俞治疗围绝经期综合征的临床研究. 黑龙江中医药大学.
A55	黎霄羽, 王小云, 薄智云. (2012) 薄氏腹针治疗女性更年期综合征的临床疗效观察. 中国北京.
A56	宋晶. (2016) 针刺八脉交会穴治疗围绝经期综合征临床观察. 上海针灸杂志 **35**(04): 433–436.
A57	Zhou Q, Wang JX. (2009) Clinical observation on acupuncture for perimenopausal depression. *J Acupunct Tuina Sci* **7**: 200–202.
A58	张静. (2015) 腹针与西药治疗更年期妇女抑郁症疗效对比研究. 世界最新医学信息文摘 **15**(64): 145 146.
A59	文丽, 骆路明, 郭鸿科, 刘丽君. (2007) 针灸辨证论治治疗更年期综合征 130 例的临床观察. 现代医药卫生 **23**(11): 1690–1691.
A60	Mohammadyari F, Seyedmehdi SA, Mousavi F, Tabatabaei R. (2015) Comparison of two effective methods in postmenopausal hot flash therapy: Acupuncture versus hormone therapy. *Galen* **4**(2): 83–89.

(*Continued*)

(*Continued*)

Study No.	References
A61	Qu F, Zhou J, Nan R. (2007) Acupuncture for perimenopausal symptoms in women who underwent oophorectomy: A comparative study. *Forsch Komplementarmed* **17**: 25–32.
A62	Ji P, Ma RH, Wang ZX. (1998) Body acupuncture plus ear pressing in the treatment of menopausal syndrome. *Int J Clin Acupunct* **9**(4): 471–473.
A63	白艳甫, 杨帆. (2016) 针刺四关配合艾灸百会治疗围绝经期妇女抑郁症 20 例疗效观察. 云南中医中药杂志 **37**(04): 45–46.
A64	张豪斌, 景向红, 王莹莹, 等. (2018) 针刺治疗围绝经期综合征 30 例. 中国针灸 **38**(01): 55–58.
A65	王青, 董浩旭, 黄冬梅, 余长江. (2017) 低频电针治疗围绝经期综合征30例. 中国中医药现代远程教育 **15**(02): 123–125.
A66	柳浩, 刘天喜. (2014) 温针灸为主对更年期综合征及其伴发肥胖患者的疗效观察. 辽宁中医杂志 **41**(04): 777–779.
A67	任彬彬, 刘志诚, 徐斌. (2012) 针灸治疗女性肥胖伴发更年期综合征疗效观察. 中国针灸 **32**(10): 871–876.
A68	Dong HG, Ludicke F, Comte I, *et al.* (2001) An exploratory pilot study of acupuncture on the quality of life and reproductive hormone secretion in menopausal women. *J Altern Complement Med* **7**(6): 651–658.
A69	Grosam B. (2009) Perimenopause: An acupuncture research study (Part 1). *Int J Clin Acupunct* **18**(1): 13–18.
A70	Wright CL, Aickin M. (2011) Improvement of menopausal symptoms with acupuncture not reflected in changes to heart rate variability. *Acupunct Med* **29**: 32–39.
A71	肖贵容, 汪开洋, 吴群. (2017) 补肾调气针法治疗围绝经期综合征临床观察. 上海针灸杂志 **36**(02): 157–161.
A72	周晓媚. (2015) 电针与安慰针治疗围绝经期综合征的对照研究. 广州中医药大学.
A73	孙艳杰, 覃忠, 蒋成艳, 粟胜勇. (2015) 电针治疗围绝经期轻中度抑郁障碍的临床观察. 广西中医药大学学报 **18**(04): 13–15.
A74	尔兆娟, 陈学军, 苏红军, 张洪秀, 岳秀英, 王贯民. (2015) 静心电针法治疗围绝经期综合征临床研究. 国际妇产科学杂志 **42**(04): 441–444.
A75	丁一. (2014) 电针治疗围绝经期综合征的临床研究. 湖北中医药大学.
A76	刘桂玲, 柳霞, 张弘, 等. (2011) 电针联合选择性雌激素受体调节剂治疗绝经期情感障碍的临床观察. 北京中医药大学学报 **34**(10): 718–720.

(*Continued*)

Study No.	References
A77	郭雅明, 刘翠峰. (2005) 电针配合小剂量阿米替林治疗更年期抑郁疗效观察. 光明中医 **20**(02): 32–33.
A78	Sandberg M, Wijma K, Wyon Y, *et al.* (2002) Effects of electro-acupuncture on psychological distress in postmenopausal women. *Complement Ther Med* **10**(3): 161–169.
A79	Wyon Y, Wijma K, Nedstrand E, Hammar M. (2004) A comparison of acupuncture and oral estradiol treatment of vasomotor symptoms in postmenopausal women. *Climacteric* **7**(2): 153–164.
A80	Liu ZS, Ai YK, Wang WM, *et al.* Acupuncture for symptoms in menopause transition: A randomized controlled trial. *Am J Obstet Gynecol* **219**(4): 373.e1–373.e10.
A81	赵爽. (2017) '颐神调气'针刺法治疗更年期焦虑症肝肾阴虚型的研究. 北京中医药大学.
A82	王健, 米慧卿, 陆敏, 徐海波, 严啸薇, 朱月伟. (2011) 针刺干预围绝经期综合征最佳时机观察. 浙江中医杂志 **46**(06): 448–449.
A83	魏瑞仙, 巴艳东, 吕虎军. (2016) 艾灸背俞穴治疗围绝经期综合征疗效观察. 中国医学创新 **13**(27): 45–48.
A84	Park JE, Lee MS, Jung SY, *et al.* (2009) Moxibustion for treating menopausal hot flashes: A randomized clinical trial. *Menopause* **16**(4): 660–665.
A85	田艳鹏. (2014) 神阙穴隔盐灸治疗围绝经期综合征的临床疗效观察. 中国针灸学会.2014'针药并用及穴位用药学术研讨会、山东针灸学会2014年学术年会论文集. 中国针灸学会: 山东针灸学会 **2014**: 7.
A86	Abedian Z, Eskandari L, Ebrahimzadeh S. (2015) The effect of acupressure on sleep quality in menopausal women: A randomized control trial. *Iran J Med Sci* **40**(4): 328–334.
A87	Ahmadinezhad M, Kargar M, Vizeshfar F, Hadianfard MJ. (2017) Comparison of the effect of acupressure and pilates-based exercises on sleep quality of postmenopausal women: A randomized controlled trial. *Iran J Nurs Midwifery Res* **22**(2): 140–146.
A88	Armand M, Ozgoli G, Giti RH, Majd HA. (2017) Effect of acupressure on early complications of menopause in women referring to selected health care centers. *Iran J Nurs Midwifery Res* **22**(3): 237–242.
A89	褚春莉, 姜晓琳. (2015) 右佐匹克隆片结合耳穴贴压对绝经期女性失眠症的疗效. 中国实用神经疾病杂志 **18**(10): 112–113.

(*Continued*)

(*Continued*)

Study No.	References
A90	Kao CL, Chen CH, Lin WY, *et al.* (2012) Effect of auricular acupressure on peri- and early postmenopausal women with anxiety: A double-blinded, randomized, and controlled pilot study. *Evid Based Complement Alternat Med* **2012**: 567639.
A91	饶琴珠. (2017) 耳穴贴压疗法治疗围绝经期失眠的护理观察. 内蒙古中医药 **36**(04): 164–165.
A92	陈莹, 李红, 陈玉婷, 吕绍光. (2017) 耳穴贴压治疗围绝经期非器质性失眠肝郁证患者临床观察. 世界中西医结合杂志 **12**(02): 211–214.
A93	O'Brien KA, Varigos E, Black C, Komesaroff PA. (2010) Laser acupuncture does not improve menopausal symptoms. *Menopause* **17**(3): 636–641.
A94	Shin HS. (2010) Effects of Koryo hand therapy on serum hormones and menopausal symptoms in Korean women. *J Transcult Nurs* **21**(2): 134–142.
A95	岳波, 阚丽君, 谭玉惠. (2016) 循经点穴疗法对老年围绝经期妇女睡眠障碍患者睡眠质量与心理状态的影响. 辽宁中医杂志 **43**(11): 2370–2374.
A96	贾超, 林敏, 张静, 等. (2010) 点按疗法对围绝经期综合征患者改良 Kupperman 评分的影响. 中医杂志 **51**(05): 432–434.
A97	林敏. (2010) 点穴治疗围绝经期综合征的临床疗效观察. 广州中医药大学.

8

Clinical Evidence for Other Chinese Medicine Therapies

OVERVIEW

In addition to Chinese herbal medicine and acupuncture, practitioners may consider prescribing other Chinese medicine therapies for women with menopausal symptoms. Clinical studies have evaluated other therapies such as *qigong* 气功 and *taichi* 太极. Characteristics of studies, syndromes, and evaluation of efficacy and safety of such therapies are described in this chapter.

Introduction

Chinese herbal medicine (CHM) and acupuncture therapies are commonly used in clinical practice and have been evaluated in clinical studies (see Chapter 5 and Chapter 7). Other Chinese medicine (CM) therapies, such as *qigong* 气功 (Chinese physical and breathing exercises) and *tuina* 推拿 (Chinese massage therapy), are also used to treat disease and maintain health. Physical exercise is important for healthy ageing and clinical studies have evaluated the potential of *qigong* 气功 and *taichi* 太极 to assist women through the menopausal transition. This chapter describes the clinical evidence for other CM therapies for menopause.

Previous Systematic Reviews

One systematic review was identified that evaluated the impact of *taichi* 太极 on health-related quality of life in perimenopausal women.[1] Evidence from five randomised controlled trials (RCTs) showed *taichi* 太极 improved quality of life measured using the Medical Outcome Study 36-Item Short-Form Health Survey (SF-36). Specifically, improvements were seen on the bodily pain, general health, vitality and mental health domains. The review also found improvements in bone mineral density after *taichi* 太极.

Identification of Clinical Studies

A comprehensive search of nine electronic biomedical databases identified 49,278 potentially relevant citations (Fig. 8.1). After review of full texts, 19 studies that evaluated other CM therapies for menopause met the inclusion criteria for this review. Three studies evaluated interventions not commonly practised outside China, and these were excluded from further analysis. The findings from 16 clinical studies are described below. Six were RCTs, four were controlled clinical trials (CCTs) and six were non-controlled studies. Studies are indicated by the letter 'O' followed by a number and the references for studies can be found at the end of the chapter.

Qigong 气功

Seven studies examined the effects of *qigong* 气功 during menopause (O1–O7). Five were RCTs and two were CCTs. No non-controlled studies met the inclusion criteria for this review. Results from all seven studies were analysed and the safety of *qigong* 气功 was summarised.

Randomised Controlled Trials of *Qigong* 气功

Five RCTs (O1–O5) involving 561 perimenopausal women compared *qigong* 气功 with no treatment. Studies were conducted in the community in China, with the exception of one study (O3) that recruited participants through a Chinese hospital outpatient department. Two studies reported duration of menopausal symptoms, which ranged from 1.96 (O3) to 5.81 years (O1). The mean age of

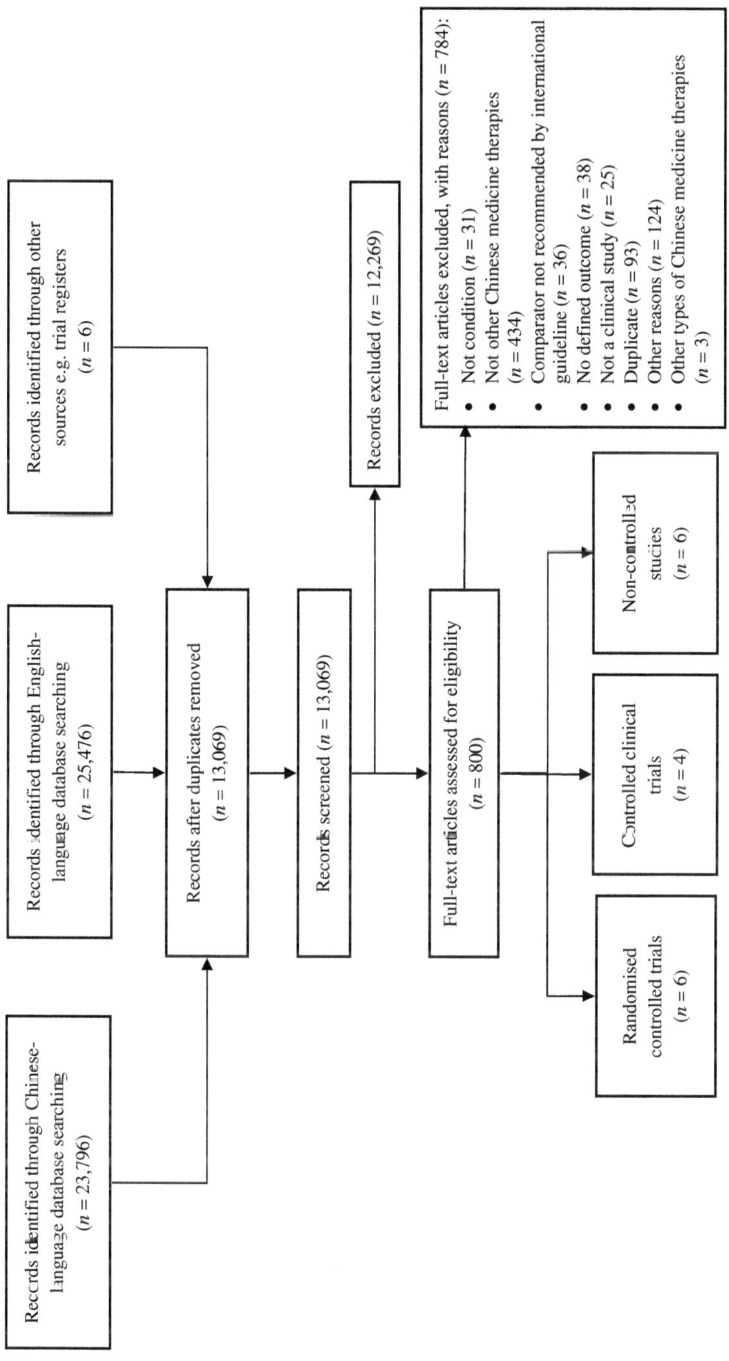

Fig. 8.1 Flowchart of study selection process: Other Chinese medicine therapies.

women was between 46.3 (O4) and 49.8 years (O2). Two studies (O4, O5) focused on menopausal women with depression.

None of the studies described using syndrome differentiation as an inclusion criterion or to guide treatment. All studies utilised a program of at least 12 weeks' duration, with two studies (O1, O4) evaluating a five-month/20-week program of *qigong* 气功. Three studies (O1, O2, O5) instructed participants to practise *qigong* 气功 daily. In the remaining two studies, women practised twice daily for six days per week (O3) or five times per week (O4). Fifteen of the 561 included participants were lost to follow-up.

Risk of Bias

Studies were assessed for risk of bias. One study (O5) did not specify the method used for group allocation and was assessed as 'unclear' risk. The remaining four studies were judged as 'low' risk as random number tables were used to allocate participants to groups. None of the studies described the method used to conceal group allocation and were judged as 'unclear' risk. Achieving blinding is difficult in physical therapy interventions and none of the studies reported blinding participants and personnel. All studies were assessed as 'high' risk for blinding of participants and personnel. No information was reported as to whether outcome assessors were blind to group allocation, posing 'unclear' risk of bias. All studies were judged as 'low' risk of bias for incomplete outcome data as there were either no missing data (O1, O2, O4, O5) or missing data was considered unlikely to impact on the results (O3). We were unable to identify published trial protocols or trial registrations for any of the studies and all were judged as 'unclear' risk for selective outcome reporting.

Outcomes

All studies evaluated the impact of *qigong* 气功 on global symptom severity using the Kupperman Index (KI).[2] Psychological symptoms were evaluated using the Center for Epidemiologic Studies Depression Scale (CES-D).[3] The CES-D is a 20-item scale, with each item rated from zero to three. Item scores are summed to provide a total score ranging from zero to 60. Higher scores indicate greater depressive symptoms. Health-related quality of life was evaluated in one study using the SF-36.[4] No study evaluated the effect of *qigong* 气功 on vasomotor symptoms, genitourinary symptoms, sexual dysfunction, sleep or musculoskeletal symptoms.

Center for Epidemiologic Studies Depression Scale

Meta-analysis was possible with the three studies (O2, O4, O5) that reported CES-D. *Qigong* 气功 resulted in scores 8.32 points lower than no treatment at the end of treatment (298 participants, [95% confidence intervals −9.47, −7.18, I^2 = 26%]).

Kupperman Index

Four studies (O2–O5) evaluated global symptom severity using the KI. One study (O3) modified the original outcome tool to replace formication with urinary symptoms. Due to the modification, results were analysed using standardised mean difference (SMD) (Table 8.1). There was no difference in KI scores between women who practised *qigong* 气功 and those who received no treatment (SMD −0.62

Table 8.1 *Qigong* 气功 versus No Treatment: Kupperman Index

Total Score	No. of Studies (Participants)	Effect Size (MD/SMD [95% CI], I^2)	Included Studies
EoT	4 (347)	SMD −0.62 [−2.09, 0.84], I^2 = 97%	O2–O5
Subgroup: low RoB SG	3 (247)	SMD −1.31 [−1.96, −0.66]*, I^2 = 80%	O2–O4
Subgroup: KI	3 (298)	MD −1.62 [−12.44, 9.20], I^2 = 99%	O2, O4, O5
Subgroup: modified KI	1 (49)	MD −5.35 [−7.56, −3.14]*	O3

*Statistically significant, see Chapter 4.
Abbreviations: CI, confidence interval; EoT, end of treatment; KI, Kupperman Index; MD, mean difference; RoB, risk of bias; SG, sequence generation; SMD, standardised mean difference.

[−2.09, 0.84], I^2 = 97). Statistical heterogeneity was considerable, so sensitivity analyses were conducted for studies judged as 'low' risk of bias for sequence generation. This resulted in a positive finding for *qigong* 气功; however, heterogeneity remained high. Further, statistical heterogeneity was 'high' for studies that used the KI in its original form. Our confidence in these results is limited.

Individual KI item scores were reported for 103 women included in the study by Hao *et al.* (2013; O1). *Qigong* 气功 was more effective than no treatment in improving vasomotor symptoms (mean difference [MD] −3.38 points [−4.56, −2.20]), vertigo (MD −0.41 points [−0.72, −0.10]), arthralgia (MD −0.28 points [−0.52, −0.04]) and palpitations (MD −0.24 points [−0.46, −0.02]). No benefit was seen in reducing paraesthesia (MD −0.49 points [−1.07, 0.09]), insomnia (MD −0.36 points [−1.02, 0.30]), nervousness (MD −0.57 points [−1.22, 0.08]), melancholia (MD −0.17 points [−0.54, 0.20]), weakness (MD −0.27 points [−0.58, 0.04]) or urinary symptoms (MD 0.10 points [−0.11, 0.31]).

36-Item Short-Form Health Survey

One study (O1) assessed health-related quality of life using the SF-36 in 103 women. *Qigong* 气功 resulted in higher scores, meaning better quality of life, for several SF-36 domains: physical function (MD 6.10 points [3.37, 8.83]), general health (MD 6.80 points [3.73, 9.87]) and vitality (MD 5.20 points [1.22, 9.18]). No difference was seen between women who practised *qigong* 气功 and those who received no treatment for the SF-36 domains role function health (MD 1.90 points [−2.80, 6.60]), role function emotion (MD 3.70 points [−3.87, 11.27]), bodily pain (MD 3.10 points [−2.10, 8.30]), social function (MD 1.10 points [−3.39, 5.59]) and mental function (MD 2.00 points [−5.90, 9.90]).

Controlled Clinical Trials of *Qigong* 气功

Two CCTs (O6, O7) evaluated *qigong* 气功 for menopause, both comparing *qigong* 气功 with no treatment. One hundred and forty-six women participated in the studies and two women were lost to follow-up (O7). One study (O6) was conducted in hospital outpatient departments in mainland China and the other was conducted in community clinics in Taiwan. The median of mean age was 48.8 years. Neither study described syndrome differentiation. *Qigong* 气功 was practised daily for 12 weeks in one study (O7) and on more than five days per week for six months in the second study. The outcomes evaluated included the Pittsburgh Sleep Quality Index (PSQI),[5] KI and the Greene Climacteric Scale (GCS).[6] One study evaluated psychological symptoms using the Symptom Checklist 90 (SCL-90).[7] No total scores were available and the data were excluded from further analysis.

Pittsburgh Sleep Quality Index

One study (O7) of 70 women evaluated the effect of *qigong* 气功 on sleep quality using the PSQI. *Qigong* 气功 improved sleep compared to no treatment, with women who practised *qigong* 气功 having scores 2.83 points lower than those who did not ([−3.50, −2.16]).

Kupperman Index

Both studies examined the effect of *qigong* 气功 on menopausal symptoms using the KI. In one study (O6), the KI was modified to include symptoms of dyspareunia and urinary symptoms. To account for this difference in the scales used, the results were analysed using SMD. There was no difference between groups in menopausal symptoms at the end of treatment (SMD −1.00 [−2.98, 0.98], $I^2 = 97\%$). Considerable statistical heterogeneity was detected; due to the small number of studies, this was unable to be explored in subgroup analyses.

Scores for individual items of the KI were reported by Zhong *et al.* (2009; O6). *Qigong* 气功 was not statistically different to no treatment in improving vasomotor symptoms (MD 0.09 points [−0.22, 0.40]), paraesthesia (MD 0.07 points [−0.16, 0.30]), insomnia (MD −0.10 points [−0.37, 0.17]), nervousness (MD 0.07 points [−0.25, 0.39]), melancholia (MD −0.02 points [−0.33, 0.29]), vertigo (MD −0.03 points [−0.33, 0.27]), weakness (MD −0.14 points [−0.39, 0.11]), arthralgia (MD 0.03 points [−0.24, 0.30]), headache (MD 0.03 points [−0.27, 0.33]), palpitations (MD 0.03 points [−0.28, 0.34]), formication (MD 0.06 points [−0.24, 0.36]), dyspareunia (MD −0.03 points [−0.34, 0.28]) and urinary symptoms (MD 0.02 points [−0.25, 0.29]).

Greene Climacteric Scale

One study (O7) of 70 women evaluated global symptom change using the GCS. In this study, *qigong* 气功 produced a greater improvement in symptoms than no treatment (MD −2.02 points [−2.60, −1.44]).

Safety of *Qigong* 气功

None of the seven studies that evaluated *qigong* 气功 in menopausal women reported on adverse events. The safety of *qigong* 气功 remains uncertain.

Chinese Medicine Psychological Treatment

Many women experience considerable psychological burden from menopause, and mind-body techniques are recommended for non-hormonal management in clinical practice guidelines.[8] Traditional CM psychological treatment has been evaluated in two clinical studies included in this review: one RCT (O8) and one CCT (O9).

Randomised Controlled Trials of Chinese Medicine Psychological Treatment

Chinese medicine psychological treatment was evaluated in the RCT by Yang *et al.* (2012; O8). The study was conducted in China and included four arms: CM psychological treatment, oral Chinese herbal medicine, the combination of CM psychological treatment and placebo. Only the CM psychological treatment and placebo arms are included in this chapter (see Chapter 5 and Chapter 9 for details of other treatment arms). Of the 424 women recruited to the trial, 104 were allocated to receive CM psychological intervention and 104 were allocated to receive oral placebo. Syndrome differentiation was used as an inclusion criterion and women with Kidney *yin* or *yang* deficiency were included.

Chinese medicine psychological treatment was provided for 12 weeks. Treatment involved one-on-one consultations for the first three steps and group therapy for the fourth step. Steps one to three involved: (1) Discussing psychological factors of menopause; (2) Inducing a strong sad emotion (thought to assist in addressing unhealthy feelings); and (3) Inducing happiness and laughter to balance the emotions. In the final step, 10–20 participants participated in a group discussion about prevention of symptoms and treatment of menopause.

Risk of bias was assessed. Participants were allocated according to a computer-generated randomisation schedule, with central randomisation used. This posed 'low' risk of bias for sequence generation and allocation concealment. Due to the nature of the intervention and comparator, achieving blinding was unlikely and the study was assessed as 'high' risk for blinding of participants and personnel. The outcome assessor was blind to group allocation and was judged 'low' risk. Reasons for drop-outs were described and intention-to-treat analysis was used to account for missing data. The study was judged 'low' risk for incomplete outcome assessment. No trial protocol or trial registration was able to be identified, posing 'unclear' risk.

Kupperman Index

Chinese medicine psychological treatment resulted in a KI score 0.56 points lower than placebo, indicating better outcomes, at the end of treatment ([−0.78, −0.34]). The clinical significance of this finding remains unclear, given that the KI score in both groups was below the clinically important level of 15 points.[9]

Menopause-specific Quality of Life Questionnaire

The impact of CM psychological treatment on health-related quality of life was assessed using the Menopause-specific Quality of Life Questionnaire (MENQOL).[10] Chinese medicine psychological treatment was no different to placebo in improving symptoms on the vasomotor domain (MD 0.90 points [−0.50, 2.30]), psychological domain (MD 0.90 points [−1.43, 3.23]), physical domain (MD 1.90 points [−2.40, 6.20]) and sexual symptoms domain (MD 0.60 points [−0.72, 1.92]).

Controlled Clinical Trials of Chinese Medicine Psychological Treatment

One CCT (O9) evaluated CM psychological treatment in perimenopausal women, which was compared with placebo. The study was conducted in China and recruited 201 women with menopausal symptoms for an average of two years. The median age of women was 50 years. Women received CM psychological treatment or oral placebo capsule for three months. The study did not report whether CM syndrome differentiation was used as an inclusion criterion or to guide treatment.

Kupperman Index

The KI scores at the end of treatment were not statistically different between women who received CM psychological treatment and those who received placebo (MD 0.00 points [−2.25, 2.25]; O6).

Safety of Chinese Medicine Psychological Treatment

One of the two studies (O8) reported on adverse events during the trial. No adverse events were reported in the intervention group. Adverse events among people who received placebo included one case each of sore throat, abdominal distension, deterioration of memory and nocturia.

Tuina 推拿

Six studies examined the role of *tuina* 推拿 for menopausal symptoms. This included one CCT (O10) and five non-controlled studies (O11–O15).

Controlled Clinical Trials of *Tuina* 推拿

One CCT (O10) evaluated *tuina* 推拿 in an outpatient hospital setting in China. Forty-eight perimenopausal women with insomnia were included, with symptoms present for at least four years on average. The median of mean age was 52 years. There was no description of CM syndrome differentiation. *Tuina* 推拿 was provided three times per week for five months and was compared with estazolam (hormone therapy). The study did not report on adverse events.

Pittsburgh Sleep Quality Index

The study evaluated the effect of *tuina* 推拿 on sleep using the PSQI. *Tuina* 推拿 resulted in a score 1.56 points lower than estazolam at the end of treatment ([−2.46, −0.66]).

Non-controlled Studies of *Tuina* 推拿

Five case series (O11–O15) met the inclusion criteria for this review. The effect of *tuina* 推拿 was evaluated in 242 menopausal women. The CM syndrome Kidney *yin* and *yang* deficiency was used as both an inclusion criterion and for treatment in one study (O15). *Tuina* 推拿 was applied to acupuncture points in four studies (O12–O15). There was considerable diversity in points, with 42 different acupuncture points described. The most frequently used point was CV12 *Zhongwan* 中脘, used in three studies. Other acupuncture points used in two studies each included SP6 *Sanyinjiao* 三阴交, CV13 *Shangwan* 上脘, CV10 *Xiawan* 下脘, PC6 *Neiguan* 内关, LI4 *Hegu* 合谷, LR3 *Taichong* 太冲, KI22 *Bulang* 步廊, KI24 *Lingxu* 灵墟, GV20 *Baihui* 百会, KI23 *Shenfeng* 神封, KI25 *Shencang* 神藏,

ST36 *Zusanli* 足三里 and GB20 *Fengchi* 风池. None of the studies reported adverse events.

Taichi 太极

Taichi 太极 was tested in 62 post-menopausal women in one case series (O16). Women participated in *taichi* 太极 three times per week for 12 weeks. The study did not describe using CM syndrome differentiation and the study did not report adverse events.

Clinical Evidence for Other Commonly Used Chinese Medicine Therapies

Clinical guidelines and textbooks described in Chapter 2 recommend CM psychological treatment for menopause. Psychological treatment has been evaluated in one RCT (O8) and one CCT (O9), with conflicting findings in relation to menopausal symptoms. In addition, Chinese menopause clinical guidelines recommend physical activity during the menopause transition.[11] *Qigong* 气功 appears to be a popular CM therapy for menopause, having been evaluated in seven clinical trials. *Qigong* 气功 may improve psychological wellbeing, but the evidence relating to menopausal symptoms is limited. A second physical intervention used in included studies was *taichi* 太极; however, the clinical evidence is insufficient to determine the potential role of *taichi* 太极 for menopause.

Summary of Other Chinese Medicine Clinical Evidence

The clinical evidence for other CM therapies is growing, and there is further research to be conducted. *Qigong* 气功 was the most frequently evaluated intervention, tested in seven clinical studies. *Qigong* 气功 reduced depression scores in a meta-analysis of CES-D but was not statistically different to no treatment in improving menopause symptoms on the KI. In one study, benefits were seen in improving some domains of the SF-36 but not for others. These findings appear to be consistent with those of the North-American Menopause Society,[8] which highlights general benefits of physical exercise in middle-aged women but no evidence for reducing vasomotor symptoms. The body of evidence is small and suffers from similar shortcomings as clinical studies of CHM and acupuncture. Further research will provide greater clarity about the role of *qigong* 气功 in the menopause transition.

Two CM physical exercises were tested in included studies: *qigong* 气功 and *taichi* 太极. None of the included studies reported on their safety. Many health benefits can be obtained from participating in regular physical exercise; however, menopausal women are at increased risk of fractures due to declining bone mineral density and oestrogen, and increased rates of bone turnover.[12] A review of the safety of *taichi* 太极 found adverse events were typically minor musculoskeletal aches and pains and unlikely to result in serious adverse events.[13] Nevertheless, menopausal women who wish to participate in *qigong* 气功 and *taichi* 太极 should take care to avoid injury to joints and the musculoskeletal system.

Psychological treatment is recommended in clinical guidelines and textbooks described in Chapter 2. Conflicting evidence was found in controlled trials. One RCT showed benefit in improving KI score compared to oral placebo, but no benefit in improving health-related quality of life assessed with MENQOL. Conversely, one CCT found no benefit of psychological treatment on KI. The evidence included in this review is insufficient. The RCT reported no adverse events with psychological treatment and such a practice may be safe when delivered by appropriately trained health professions.

Five non-controlled studies evaluated *tuina* 推拿, yet no controlled clinical trials of *tuina* 推拿 met the inclusion criteria for this review. Given the apparent interest in this technique, the lack of eligible controlled trials was surprising. The reasons for this are not clear but may relate to the absence of *tuina* 推拿 in key clinical textbooks and guidelines. Positive results found in preliminary studies, such as the case series included in this review, may lead to further later-phase clinical trials being conducted. This will provide further evidence for an intervention that is already being utilised in clinical practice.

References

1. Wang Y, Shan W, Li Q, *et al.* (2017) Tai chi exercise for the quality of life in a perimenopausal women organization: A systematic review. *Worldviews Evid Based Nurs* **14**(4): 294–305.
2. Kupperman HS, Wetchler BB, Blatt MH. (1959) Contemporary therapy of the menopausal syndrome. *J Am Med Assoc* **171**: 1627–1637.
3. Radloff L. (1977) The CES-D Scale: A self-report depression scale for research in the general population. *Appl Psychol Meas* **1**(3): 385–401.
4. Ware JJ, Sherbourne C. (1992) The MOS 36-item short-form health survey (SF-36). I. Conceptual framework and item selection. *Med Care* **30**: 473–483.
5. Buysse DJ, Reynolds CF, 3rd, Monk TH, *et al.* (1989) The Pittsburgh Sleep Quality Index: A new instrument for psychiatric practice and research. *Psychiatry Res* **28**(2): 193–213.
6. Greene JG. (1976) A factor analytic study of climacteric symptoms. *J Psychosom Res* **20**(5): 425–430.
7. Derogatis L. (1975) The SCL-90-R. Clinical Psychometric Research, Baltimore.
8. The North American Menopause Society. (2015) Nonhormonal management of menopause-associated vasomotor symptoms: 2015 position statement of The North American Menopause Society. *Menopause* **22**(11): 1155–1172.
9. Grant MD, Marbella A, Wang AT, *et al.* (2015) Menopausal Symptoms: Comparative Effectiveness of Therapies. Comparative Effectiveness Review No. 147. Agency for Healthcare Research and Quality, Rockville, MD. Available at: www.effectivehealthcare.ahrq.gov/reports/final.cfm.
10. Hilditch JR, Lewis J, Peter A, *et al.* (2008) A menopause-specific quality of life questionnaire: Development and psychometric properties. *Maturitas* **61**(1–2): 107–121.
11. 中华预防医学会妇女保健分会, 更年期保健学组. (2016) 更年期妇女保健指南 (2015年). 实用妇科内分泌杂志 **3**(2): 21–32.
12. The National Institute of Health and Care Excellence (NICE) Guideline. (2015) Menopause: Diagnosis and Management. Available from: https://www.nice.org.uk/guidance/ng23.

13. Wayne PM, Berkowitz DL, Litrownik DE, *et al.* (2014) What do we really know about the safety of *tai chi*?: A systematic review of adverse event reports in randomized trials. *Arch Phys Med Rehabil* **95**(12): 2470–2483.

References for Included Other Chinese Medicine Therapies Clinical Studies

Study No.	References
O1	郝晶, 窦娜, 马素慧, 等. (2013) 八段锦气功操对围绝经期妇女生活质量的影响. 中国老年学杂志 (21): 5266–5268.
O2	马素慧, 窦娜, 陈长香, 等. (2011) 步行与八段锦对围绝经期综合征伴抑郁症状的康复效果. 中国康复医学杂志 **26**(08): 738–741.
O3	龙于飞. (2011) 健身气功八段锦治疗肝肾阴虚型围绝经期综合征的临床研究. 南京中医药大学.
O4	马素慧, 窦娜, 陈长香, 等. (2011) 跳绳与八段锦健身操治疗围绝经期综合征合并抑郁症状患者的疗效对比. 中华物理医学与康复杂志 **33**(01): 49–51.
O5	马素慧, 窦娜, 陈长香, 等. (2010) 八段锦对围绝经期综合征及抑郁康复效果的研究. 中国全科医学 **36**(25): 2864–2865.
O6	钟志兵, 章文春, 张红, 等. (2009) 健身气功易筋经对更年期综合征妇女身心症状的影响. 中国民康医学 **21**(21): 2645–2647.
O7	Yeh SCJ, Chang MY. (2012) The effect of qigong on menopausal symptoms and quality of sleep for perimenopausal women: A preliminary observational study. *J Altern Complement Med* **18**(6): 567–575.
O8	Yang HY, Yang J, Wen Z. *et al.* (2012) Effect of combining therapy with traditional Chinese medicine-based psychotherapy and herbal medicines in women with menopausal syndrome: A randomized controlled clinical trial. *Evid Based Complement Alternat Med* **2012**: 354145
O9	成芳平, 王小云, 张春玲, 等. (2010) 中医情志疗法治疗绝经综合征的临床研究. 实用医学杂志 **26**(19): 3630–3632.
O10	高亮. (2016) 背腧穴擦法治疗更年期失眠临床观察. 浙江中西医结合杂志 **26**(05): 458–460.
O11	周小波, 马玉忠, 金涛, 等. (2009) 推拿补肾活血法治疗更年期综合征临床观察. 北京中医药 **28**(07): 526–527.
O12	贾超, 刘杰凯, 鲍治军, 等. (2017) 点穴疗法结合捏脊治疗女性更年期综合征44例临床观察. 新中医 **49**(02): 138–140.

(*Continued*)

(*Continued*)

Study No.	References
O13	杨金峰, 张春娇. (2014) 穴位按摩治疗妇女更年期综合征58例临床疗效分析. 中国妇幼保健 **29**(36): 6068–6070.
O14	李巧林, 贾超, 林敏, 张静, 袁学雅, 张秋玲. (2013) 点穴疗法对更年期综合征临床症状及性激素的影响. 按摩与康复医学 **4**(7): 6–8.
O15	贾梅. (2012) 应用点穴桉揉疗法治疗围绝经期失眠的临床观察. 黑龙江中医药大学.
O16	Barbat-Artigas S, Filion ME, Dupontgard S, *et al.* (2011) Effects of *tai chi* training in dynapenic and nondynapenic postmenopausal women. *Menopause* **18**(9): 974–979.

9

Clinical Evidence for Combination Therapies

OVERVIEW

Clinical practice of Chinese medicine often sees several therapy types used in combination, such as Chinese herbal medicine plus acupuncture. After assessment against inclusion criteria, 21 studies were selected for review. Sixteen randomised controlled trials, two controlled clinical trials and three non-controlled case series evaluated combinations of Chinese medicine therapies. The most common combination included Chinese herbal medicine with acupuncture therapies. Results showed benefits for some intervention combinations. As meta-analysis was not possible for most different combinations, there is insufficient evidence for various combinations of Chinese medicine therapies.

Introduction

Combination therapies are defined as two or more Chinese medicine (CM) interventions from different categories administered together, for example, Chinese herbal medicine (CHM) plus acupuncture, or CHM plus moxibustion. This approach is common in clinical practice. This chapter reviews the evidence from eligible clinical studies. Previous systematic reviews of combination therapies were not identified in the database searches.

Identification of Clinical Studies

Search of electronic databases identified 49,278 potentially relevant citations. After removal of duplicates, the title and abstracts of citations were read and more than 12,200 irrelevant citations were excluded (Fig. 9.1). The full texts of remaining articles were reviewed and two studies that used interventions not commonly practised outside of China (point application therapy and catgut embedding) were excluded. In total, 21 clinical studies that evaluated combinations of CHM therapy were included. Sixteen were randomised controlled trials (RCTs), two were controlled clinical trials (CCTs) and three were non-controlled case series. Studies are indicated by the letter 'C' followed by a number, and the references for studies can be found at the end of the chapter.

Randomised Controlled Trials of Combination Therapies

There were 16 RCTs (C1–C16) that evaluated combinations of CM therapies in menopausal women. All studies were conducted in China, recruiting 1,567 participants from hospital outpatient and inpatient departments. The majority of studies recruited participants in the perimenopausal stage and one study (C1) included women in various menopausal stages. One study (C2) did not specify the menopausal stage. One study of perimenopausal women used follicle-stimulating hormone (FSH) of greater than 10 international units (IU)/litre (L) as an inclusion criterion (C1). None of the studies used duration of amenorrhoea as an inclusion criterion, which raises questions about the reliability of the evidence.

Five RCTs (C1, C2, C7, C8, C15) focused on symptoms of menopause generally, while others evaluated specific symptoms: one RCT (C5) focused on anxiety disorder; four RCTs (C5, C6, C14, C16) focused on depression and six RCTs (C3, C4, C9–C12) focused on insomnia. All but three RCTs (C1, C2, C13) reported the duration of menopause. The mean duration of menopause/menopausal symptoms in the 13 RCTs was 11.43 months in the intervention group and

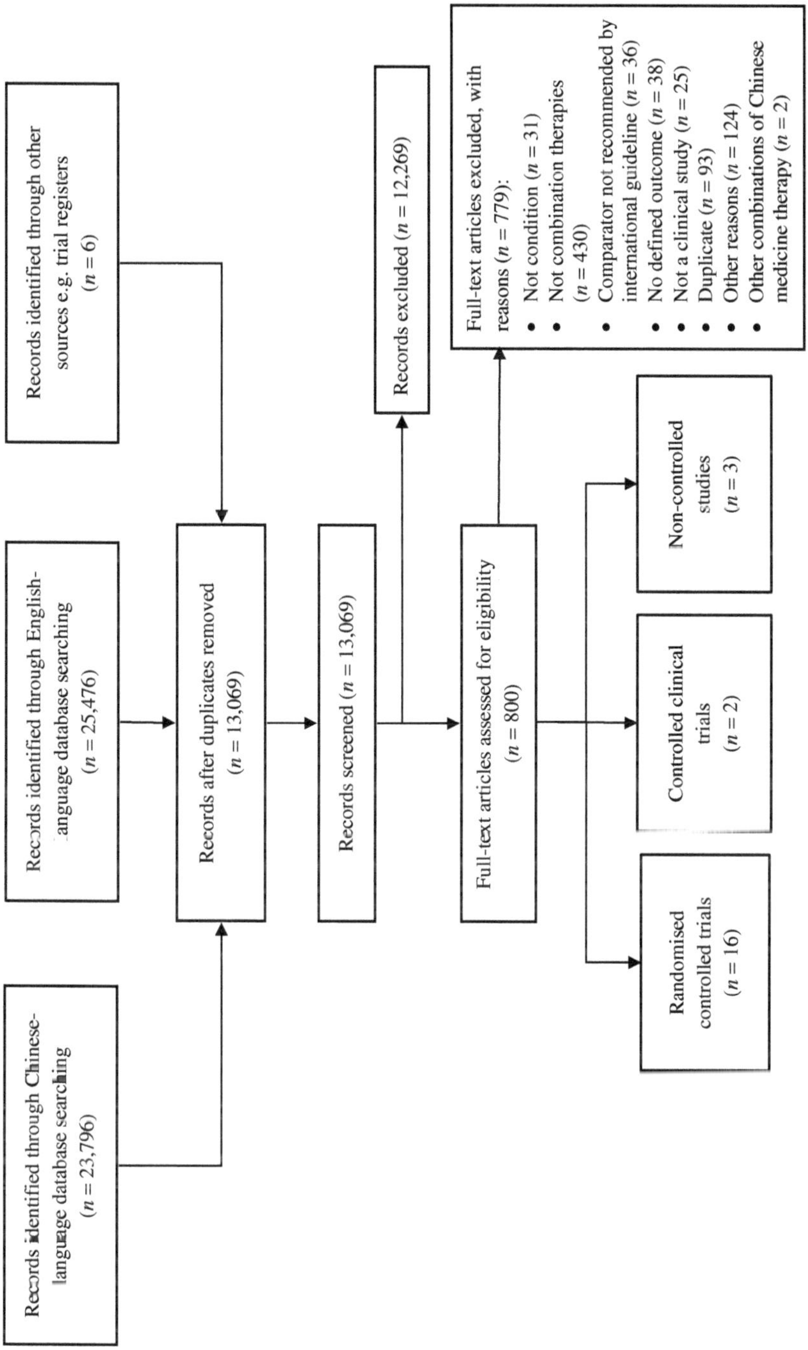

Fig. 9.1 Flowchart of study selection process: Combination therapies.

11.35 months in the control group. The mean age was 49.7 and 49.5 years in the intervention and control groups, respectively. The duration of treatment ranged from 14 days (C12) to three months (C6, C7). Four studies (C2, C4, C8, C16) reported follow-up assessment of participants after treatment had ceased, which varied in length from two (C4) to 12 weeks (C2).

Chinese medicine syndrome differentiation was used as an inclusion criterion in nine RCTs. Syndromes included Kidney *yin* deficiency (C2, C10, C15), Kidney *yang* deficiency (C2, C10), Kidney *yin* and *yang* deficiency (C10), Kidney deficiency and Liver stagnation (C4, C9, C13, C16), Kidney and Liver *yin* deficiency (C7), Kidney and Liver *yin* deficiency with hyperactive Liver *yang* (C1), Liver stagnation and Spleen deficiency (C4), and Heart and Spleen both deficient (C4).

There was diversity in the CM interventions used. These included CHM for oral use or as a foot bath, acupuncture, moxibustion, ear acupressure, cupping therapy, *tuina* 推拿, *qigong* 气功, music therapy and traditional CM (TCM)-based psychotherapy (Table 9.1). The most frequently evaluated combination was CHM plus acupuncture, used in five studies (C1, C8, C11–C13). Two studies combined CHM

Table 9.1 Summary of Interventions in Combination Therapies Randomised Controlled Trials

Combination Therapies	No. of Studies	Included Studies
CHM plus manual acupuncture	5	C1, C8, C11, C12,* C13
CHM plus ear acupressure	2	C10, C15
CHM plus TCM-based psychotherapy	2	C2, C16
CHM plus moxibustion	1	C6
CHM plus *Yijinjing qigong* 易筋经气功	1	C5
CHM plus *tuina* 推拿	1	C3
CHM foot bath plus music therapy	1	C9
Manual acupuncture plus music therapy	1	C7
Ear acupressure plus cupping	1	C4
CHM plus music therapy	1	C14*

*Integrated Chinese and conventional medicines.
Abbreviations: CHM, Chinese herbal medicine.

therapies with pharmacotherapy to manage symptoms of depression (C14) and insomnia (C12). One study (C2) compared combinations of CM with placebo. All other studies used pharmacotherapy as control, which included hormone therapy (HT), fluoxetine, estazolam, flupenthixol melitracen, diazepam and paroxetine.

Three studies used Chinese patent medicine: *Tian wang bu xin dan* 天王补心丹 (C5), *Kun bao wan* 坤宝丸 (C1), *Geng nian ning xin jiao nang* 更年宁心胶囊 and *Bu shen kou fu ye* 补肾口服液 (C2). Chinese herbal medicine decoction was used in 11 studies. There was no overlap in CHM formulas across studies. While not specified in the articles, the actions of these formulas are to nourish the Kidney and relieve the Liver. Frequently used herbs in these studies were *gan cao* 甘草 (seven studies), *chai hu* 柴胡 (six studies) and *bai shao* 白芍 (six studies) (Table 9.2). In studies that evaluated acupuncture

Table 9.2 Frequently Reported Herbs in Randomised Controlled Trials

Most Common Herbs	Scientific Name	Frequency of Use
Gan cao 甘草	*Glycyrrhiza* spp.	7
Chai hu 柴胡	*Bupleurum* spp.	6
Bai shao 白芍	*Paeonia lactiflora* Pall.	6
Dang gui 当归	*Angelica sinensis* (Oliv.) Diels	5
Shu di huang 熟地黄	*Rehmannia glutinosa* Libosch.	5
Shan yu rou 山茱萸	*Cornus officinalis* Sieb. et Zucc.	4
Fu ling 茯苓	*Poria cocos* (Schw.) Wolf	5
Ye jiao teng 首乌藤	*Polygonum multiflorum* Thunb.	3
Shan yao 山药	*Dioscorea opposita* Thunb.	3
Gou qi zi 枸杞子	*Lycium barbarum* L.	3
Mu dan pi 牡丹皮	*Paeonia suffruticosa* Andr	3
Bai he 百合	*Lilium* spp.	3
Tu si zi 菟丝子	*Cuscuta* spp.	3
Suan zao ren 酸枣仁	*Ziziphus jujuba* Mill. var. spinosa (Bunge) Hu ex H. F. Chou	3
Huang lian 黄连	*Coptis* spp.	3

Note: The use of some herbs may be restricted in some countries. Readers are advised to comply with relevant regulations.

therapies, there were a total of 35 acupuncture points used. The most frequently reported points were: BL23 *Shenshu* 肾俞 (eight studies), SP6 *Sanyinjiao* 三阴交 (seven studies), GV20 *Baihui* 百会 (six studies), HT7 *Shenmen* 神门 (six studies), BL18 *Ganshu* 肝俞 (six studies), BL15 *Xinshu* 心俞 (six studies) and ST36 *Zusanli* 足三里 (six studies).

Risk of Bias

All RCTs were reviewed to determine potential sources of bias (Table 9.3). Eight studies used either a random number table or computer software for sequence generation and were assessed as 'low' risk of bias. Fourteen studies were assessed as 'unclear' risk of bias for allocation concealment; one RCT was rated 'high' risk because randomisation assignments were placed in a visible table and one RCT was rated 'low' risk as central randomisation was used. Participants in the studies were unlikely to be blind due to the nature of the interventions and comparators and personnel were not blind to group allocation. The studies were judged to pose 'high' risk for blinding of participants and personnel. Two studies reported that outcome assessment was evaluated by a third party who was unaware of the interventions, and were judged as 'low' risk. Others did not describe whether outcome assessors were blind to group allocation and were judged as 'unclear' risk. For incomplete outcome data, the

Table 9.3 Risk of Bias of Randomised Controlled Trials: Combination Therapies

Risk of Bias Domain	Low Risk *n* (%)	Unclear Risk *n* (%)	High Risk *n* (%)
Sequence generation	8 (50)	8 (50)	0 (0)
Allocation concealment	1(6.25)	14 (87.5)	1 (6.3)
Blinding of participants	0 (0)	0 (0)	16 (100)
Blinding of personnel	0 (0)	0 (0)	16 (100)
Blinding of outcome assessors	2 (12.5)	14 (87.5)	0 (0)
Incomplete outcome data	15 (93.8)	1 (6.3)	0 (0)
Selective outcome reporting	0 (0)	16 (100)	0 (0)

reasons for drop-outs were not clearly described in one study that was assessed as 'unclear' risk of bias. All others were assessed as 'low' risk, as reasons for drop-out were reported and drop-out numbers were balanced between groups. None of the studies reported trial registration and published protocols were not able to be identified; all were assessed as 'unclear' risk for selective outcome reporting.

Outcomes

The clinical evidence for combination therapies from RCTs was grouped according to the pre-specified outcomes categories: vasomotor symptoms, genitourinary symptoms, sleep quality, psychological symptoms, musculoskeletal symptoms, global symptom severity scales and health-related quality of life. However, none of the included RCTs reported on vasomotor symptoms, genitourinary symptoms or musculoskeletal symptoms. Findings for sleep quality, psychological symptoms, global symptom severity scales and health-related quality of life are described below.

Pittsburgh Sleep Quality Index

Six RCTs (C3, C4, C9, C10, C12, C14) evaluated treatment effects on sleep quality using the Pittsburgh Sleep Quality Index (PSQI).[1] Treatment effects are presented below for each type of therapy. Due to diversity in combinations of intervention, results could not be pooled for meta-analysis.

Four studies compared CM combined therapies to the benzodiazepine estazolam. Positive benefits were seen in several studies. The combination of CHM plus *tuina* 推拿 (C3) reduced PSQI score by 5.29 points compared to estazolam (80 participants, [95% confidence intervals −6.51, −4.07]). Chinese herbal medicine foot bath plus music therapy (C9) was more effective than estazolam, reducing the mean score of PSQI by 4.72 points (79 participants, [−5.50, −3.94]). Ear acupressure plus cupping (C4) also significantly improved PSQI scores by 2.96 points, compared to estazolam (94 participants,

[−4.93, −0.99]). One RCT of 80 participants (C10) found CHM plus ear acupressure was not statistically different to estazolam (mean difference [MD] −0.38 points, [−1.50, 0.74]). The wide confidence intervals suggest CM combined therapies are unlikely to be of benefit in improving sleep quality.

One study (C12) reported CHM plus manual acupuncture as integrative medicine with diazepam, oryzanol and vitamin E, which was provided for 14 days to 92 women. The combination resulted in a PSQI score 3.25 points lower than in women who received diazepam, oryzanol and vitamin E alone ([−3.86, −2.64]). One RCT, of 100 women, found the combination of CHM, music therapy and paroxetine was more effective than paroxetine alone, reducing PSQI scores by 3.07 points ([−4.11, −2.03]; C14).

Psychological Symptoms

Seven RCTs evaluated treatment effects on psychological symptoms using the Self-rating Depression Scale (SDS),[2] Self-rating Anxiety Scale (SAS),[3] Hamilton Rating Scale for Depression (HAM-D)[4] or Hamilton Rating Scale for Anxiety (HAM-A).[5] Four studies (C6, C7, C8, C16) used multiple scales to evaluate different psychological symptoms. All studies evaluated different treatments and could not be pooled for meta-analysis.

Self-rating Depression Scale

Three studies compared combined therapies to HT to determine their effects on menopausal depression. One study of manual acupuncture plus music therapy (C7) showed no statistical difference in SDS scores compared with Climen® for 60 women (MD 2.60 points [−1.58, 6.78]). The combination of CHM plus TCM-based psychotherapy was evaluated in one study involving 54 women (C16). While combined therapies were not statistically different to tibolone in reducing SDS score after treatment (MD −1.08 points [−5.41, 3.25]), a significant improvement of 5.94 points was seen after one month of follow-up ([−10.61, −1.27]). Furthermore, SDS scores were reduced, indicating better outcomes, in 94 women who received CHM plus manual acupuncture (C8). After one month of follow-up, SDS scores were 5.08 points lower in people who received CHM plus manual acupuncture compared to HT with oestradiol valerate and cyproterone acetate ([−8.78, −2.82]).

Self-rating Anxiety Scale

Two RCTs determined the effects of CM combined therapies compared to HT on menopausal anxiety; both studies used the SAS. One study used manual acupuncture plus music therapy (C7). The combination was less effective than Climen® in reducing anxiety; the mean SAS score at the end of treatment was 8.17 points higher with manual therapy plus music therapy (60 participants, [3.93, 12.41]). The second study of CHM plus manual acupuncture was found to be more effective than HT with oestradiol valerate and cyproterone acetate (C8). The SAS scores were 6.80 points lower with combined CM therapies after one month follow-up ([−9.75, −3.85]).

Hamilton Rating Scale for Depression

Chinese herbal medicine plus moxibustion significantly reduced HAM-D scores by 7.83 points compared to Climen® and medroxyprogesterone acetate (60 participants, [−9.09, −6.57]; C6). Furthermore, the combination of CHM plus manual acupuncture also reduced HAM-D scores compared to fluoxetine (C13). The HAM-D scores were 7.33 points lower in women who received CHM plus acupuncture compared to women who received fluoxetine (60 participants, [−12.22, −2.44]). No such difference was seen in one RCT that compared manual acupuncture plus music therapy with Climen® in 60 women (MD −0.10 points, [−1.52, 1.32]; C7).

Hamilton Rating Scale for Anxiety

Four studies (C5, C6, C7, C14) measured anxiety using the HAM-A. Chinese herbal medicine plus moxibustion reduced HAM-A scores by

11.92 points more than Climen® and medroxyprogesterone acetate (60 participants, [−13.15, −10.69]; C6). When CHM was combined with *Yijinjing qigong* 易筋经气功, HAM-A scores were 3.10 points lower than flupentixol/melitracen at the end of treatment (100 participants, [−5.33, −0.87]; C5). Another study that compared CHM, music therapy and paroxetine with paroxetine alone found the combined therapy was more effective than paroxetine alone, reducing HAM-A scores by 8.5 points (100 participants, [−11.74, −5.26]; C14). The HAM-A scores were also significantly lower among people who received manual acupuncture plus music therapy (C7). At the end of treatment, HAM-A scores were 2.90 points lower in women who received manual acupuncture plus music therapy compared to Climen® ([−4.59, −1.21]).

Kupperman Index

Ten RCTs (C1, C2, C5–C8, C10, C11, C15, C16) evaluated treatment effects using the Kupperman Index (KI)[6] or a modified version of the Kupperman Index (mKI). Meta-analysis was able to be conducted with studies of CHM plus manual acupuncture and CHM plus ear acupressure (Table 9.4). In two studies (C1, C11) with 113 participants, CHM plus manual acupuncture was not statistically different to HT in reducing KI score (MD −1.61 points [−11.63, 8.41], I^2 = 93%). Meta-analysis of two RCTs comparing CHM plus ear acupressure to HT also failed to show statistically significant differences in mKI scores (140 participants, SMD −1.65 [−3.97, 0.66], I^2 = 97%; C10, C15).

Table 9.4 Combination Therapies versus Pharmacotherapy: Kupperman Index

Outcomes	Intervention	Comparator	No. of Studies (Participants)	Effect Size (MD/ SMD [95% CI], I^2)	Included Studies
KI	CHM plus manual acupuncture	Pharmacotherapy	2 (113)	MD −1.61 [−11.63, 8.41], 93%	C1, C11
mKI	CHM plus ear acupressure	Hormone therapy	2 (140)	SMD −1.65 [−3.97, 0.66], 97%	C10, C15

Abbreviations: CHM, Chinese herbal medicine; CI, confidence interval; KI, Kupperman Index; MD, mean difference; mKI, modified Kupperman Index; SMD, standardised mean difference.

Results from single studies showed some combinations of CM therapies were more effective than pharmacotherapy in improving KI scores after treatment and at follow-up. Studies that found such benefit at the end of treatment evaluated CHM plus *Yijinjing qigong* 易筋经气功 versus flupentixol/melitracen (100 participants, MD −7.50 points [−9.70, −5.30]; C5) and CHM plus moxibustion versus Climen® (60 participants, MD −7.91 points [−9.03, −6.79]; C6). At follow-up after one month, CHM plus manual acupuncture provided a greater reduction in KI score than HT with oestradiol valerate and cyproterone acetate (MD −6.80 points, [−9.63, −3.97]; C8).

Modified versions of the KI were used in three individual RCTs (C2, C7, C16) that were not able to be pooled for analysis. One study (C16) with 54 participants evaluated CHM plus TCM-based psychotherapy versus tibolone. The study found no statistically significant differences for mKI in the period after treatment (MD 0.51 points [−2.77, 3.79]) and follow-up (MD −2.60 points [−6.12, 0.92]). Another study (C2) also investigated CHM plus TCM-based psychotherapy, which was compared with placebo. The combination of CM therapies was more effective, reducing mKI scores by 1.43 points more than placebo ([−1.65, −1.21]). One study (C7), using manual acupuncture plus music therapy, showed a statistical difference in reducing mKI scores by 2.77 points compared to Climen® ([−5.34, 0.20]).

Menopause-specific Quality of Life Questionnaire

One RCT (C2) evaluated treatment effects using the Menopause-specific Quality of Life Questionnaire (MENQOL).[7] The study, involving 209 participants, reported scores of four domains: physical, psychological, vasomotor and sexual symptoms. The changes between baseline and end of treatment at 12 weeks showed no statistically significant difference between CHM plus TCM-based psychotherapy and placebo for three of the four domains. The mean difference between groups was 0.50 points for the physical domain ([−3.64, 4.64]), 1.60 points for the psychological domain ([−0.80, 4.00]) and 0.20 points for the sexual symptoms domain ([−1.05, 1.45]). However, women who received CHM plus TCM-based psychotherapy reported worse scores on the vasomotor domain than women who received placebo (MD 1.50 points [0.12, 2.88]).

Controlled Clinical Trials of Combination Therapies

Two studies (C17, C18) were identified as CCTs of combination therapies. Both studies were conducted in China, with 148 participants recruited from hospital inpatient and outpatient departments. All participants were in the perimenopausal period and neither study specified inclusion criteria relating to FSH and duration of amenorrhoea. One study (C17) focused on menopause symptoms generally, with a mean duration of nine months and the other (C18) focused on menopausal insomnia which had been present for 32.4 months on average. The CM syndrome of Liver stagnation was used as an inclusion criterion in one study (C17). The mean age was 48.7 and 48.8 years in the intervention and control groups, respectively. The duration of treatment with manual acupuncture plus herbal diet therapy was 60 days (C18) and the duration of treatment was 15 days with CHM plus manual acupuncture (C17). Neither study reported follow-up assessment at the end of treatment. Both studies compared combinations of CM therapies with HT, including Premarin® plus oryzanol (a rice bran oil product frequently used in China) (C17) and estazolam (C18).

Outcomes

The two CCTs (C17, C18) reported outcomes relating to sleep and global symptom improvement. Neither CCT evaluated the effects of combination of CM therapies on vasomotor symptoms, genitourinary symptoms, psychological symptoms, musculoskeletal symptoms and health-related quality of life.

Pittsburgh Sleep Quality Index

The PSQI was evaluated in one study (C18) of manual acupuncture plus herbal diet therapy. Treatment with combined CM therapies was not statistically different to estazolam in reducing PSQI scores for 66 participants (MD –0.29 points [–1.79, 1.21]).

Kupperman Index

One CCT (C17) of 82 participants reported on KI scores. Chinese herbal medicine plus manual acupuncture was more effective in reducing KI scores than Premarin® plus oryzanol, with KI score 5.28 points lower at the end of treatment ([–7.32, –3.24]).

Non-controlled Studies of Combination Therapies

Three non-controlled studies (C19–C21) met the inclusion criteria described in Chapter 4. One study (C20) was conducted in London, with participants recruited from the general population, another study (C21) recruited from hospital outpatient departments in China and the third (C19) was a case report from a private practice in the United States. A total of 160 participants in the perimenopausal or postmenopausal period were included.

One study (C21) of 42 participants assessed the effect of CHM plus acupuncture for perimenopausal people with Liver Blood deficiency and ascendant hyperactivity of Liver *yang*. The participants received oral CHM consisting of *dang gui* 当归, *suan zao ren* 酸枣仁, *bai shao* 白芍, *gan cao* 甘草, *sha shen* 沙参, *fu xiao mai* 浮小麦, *bai he* 百合 and *ju hua* 菊花 daily for 30 days. Acupuncture points included: BL15 *Xinshu* 心俞, BL17 *Geshu* 膈俞, BL18 *Ganshu* 肝俞, BL23 *Shenshu* 肾俞, LR3 *Taichong* 太冲 and KI3 *Taixi* 太溪. Acupuncture was applied once every other day for 15 days (one course of treatment). Participants received two courses, totalling 15 treatments.

One study (C20) of 117 participants used CHM and/or acupuncture along with dietary and lifestyle advice for London women suffering from menopausal symptoms. The details of the treatments were not specified. A maximum of 12 treatments over six months was allowed per patient. No adverse events or abnormalities in liver or kidney function were observed during the course of the study.

One case report (C19) evaluated the effectiveness of CHM plus acupuncture in the management of atrophic vaginitis and its accompanying symptoms. The case was a 54-year-old postmenopausal female with Kidney *yin* and Liver Blood deficiency and Liver *qi* stagnation who was treated for over three months. The patient received oral CHM using modified versions of the formula *Zhi bai di huang wan* 知柏地黄丸 and *Er zhi wan* 二至丸, once daily for three months. Body acupuncture points included: LR8 *Ququan* 曲泉, SP6 *Sanyinjiao* 三阴交, KI6 *Zhaohai* 照海, LR3 *Taichong* 太冲, PC6 *Neiguan* 内关, CV17 *Danzhong* 膻中, CV3 *Zhongji* 中极, CV4 *Guanyuan* 关元 and EX-HN3 *Yintang* 印堂. Ear acupuncture points included: TF4 *Shenmen* 神门, TF2 *Uterus* 子宫, CO10 *Kidney* 肾, CO12 *Liver* 肝 and CO15 *Heart* 心. Acupuncture was applied weekly for six weeks.

Clinical Evidence for Commonly Used Combination Therapies

Many combinations of CM therapies have been evaluated for menopausal symptoms. Clinical textbooks and guidelines described in Chapter 2 recommend a diversity of interventions, including CHM (oral or topical), acupuncture, moxibustion and ear acupressure, all of which were evaluated in clinical studies in this review. However, the majority of these interventions are recommended as individual treatments, with no recommendations in key textbooks/guidelines regarding combining these therapies.

Four studies have evaluated the combinations of CHM and acupuncture and two studies each have evaluated combinations of CHM and ear acupressure, and CHM and TCM-based psychotherapy. Combining CHM with acupuncture is common in clinical practice; this combination may be a promising area for future research. Many studies found positive results in improving menopausal symptoms. More evidence is needed that evaluates combinations of CHM therapies in order to inform clinical practice guidelines.

Safety of Combination Therapies

Five studies (C2, C4, C13, C16, C20) reported on adverse events, with one study (C20) reporting that no adverse events occurred. Fewer adverse events were reported in the treatment groups compared to the control groups (27 versus 105). Adverse events in the treatment groups included seven cases of fatigue, five cases of dizziness and headache, four cases of stomach ache, three cases of headache, two cases of skin rash, two cases of nausea and anorexia, and one case each of heart discomfort, oral ulcer, dizziness and cholecystitis. Adverse events in the control groups included 31 cases of fatigue, 28 cases of dizziness and headache, 22 cases of nausea and anorexia, five cases of nausea, headache, dizziness and fever, three cases of headache, two cases of dizziness, two cases of rash and itching, two cases of irregular vaginal bleeding, two cases of oedema, and one case each of sore throat, abdominal distension, memory deterioration, nocturia, heart discomfort, breast tenderness, weight gain and nausea. While fewer adverse events were seen with combination CM therapies than controls, there is insufficient evidence to describe the safety of specific combinations of CM therapies in people with menopausal symptoms.

Summary of Combination Therapies Evidence

This chapter evaluated the combination of two or more CM therapies used to manage menopausal symptoms. Among all included studies, CHM plus acupuncture was the most commonly used combination, followed by the combination of CHM plus ear acupressure and CHM plus TCM-based psychotherapy. Aside from one study that evaluated CHM as a topical treatment, CHM was administered orally and was the most commonly used therapy (18 of 21 studies, 85.7%). The CHM formulas the studies investigated were diverse with no overlap across studies. The most frequently used herbs were: *gan cao* 甘草, *chai hu* 柴胡, *bai shao* 白芍, *dang gui* 当归, *shu di* 熟地, *shan yu rou* 山萸肉, *fu ling* 茯苓, *ye jiao teng* 夜交藤 and *shan yao* 山药. Based on the actions of these herbs, the key aim of CHM treatment was to nourish the Kidney and relieve the Liver. Acupuncture therapy (including acupressure) was also used commonly, tested in two thirds of included studies (14 of 21). The most frequently reported points were: BL23 *Shenshu* 肾俞, SP6 *Sanyinjiao* 三阴交, GV20 *Baihui* 百会, HT7 *Shenmen* 神门, BL18 *Ganshu* 肝俞, BL15 *Xinshu* 心俞 and ST36 *Zusanli* 足三里. Studies used different combinations of herbs and acupuncture points and no clear conclusion about the best combination could be drawn from the current research.

Diversity was seen in the CM combination therapies and comparators that were used for menopausal symptoms and only two meta-analyses were able to be performed for global symptom scales (original or mKI). Meta-analysis showed no benefit of CHM plus manual acupuncture, and CHM plus ear acupressure in reducing KI or mKI scores. Results from other single studies showed benefit for reducing KI or mKI scores, such as CHM plus manual acupuncture, CHM plus moxibustion, CHM plus *Yijinjing qigong* 易筋经气功 and CHM plus music therapy. The KI score with CHM plus TCM-based psychotherapy was not statistically different to HT in the period both after treatment and follow-up. However, CHM plus TCM-based psychotherapy was more effective in reducing global symptoms (mKI) than placebo after treatment.

For menopausal sleep quality, most included studies showed greater effect with combination therapies than pharmacotherapy, including CHM foot bath plus music therapy, CHM plus ear acupressure and CHM plus *tuina* 推拿. For psychological symptoms, CHM plus manual acupuncture, CHM plus moxibustion, CHM plus *Yijinjing qigong* 易筋经气功 and CHM plus music therapy were superior to pharmacotherapy (HT or selective serotonin reuptake inhibitors) in reducing scores of various scales for psychological symptoms. However, manual acupuncture plus music therapy showed similar effects to those of Climen® for psychological symptoms. Furthermore, CHM plus TCM-based psychotherapy was not statistically different to HT at the end of treatment, but was more effective at follow-up, which suggests it could provide long-term improvement for psychological symptoms.

This review of clinical studies did not include studies comparing two or more CM therapies to one of them (for example, CHM plus acupuncture versus acupuncture alone). As such, it is unclear whether combining CM therapies is more beneficial than the use of CM interventions individually.

Based on the limited available evidence, CM combination therapies appear to be safe for the management of menopausal symptoms. Results from current research do not provide strong enough evidence to make specific recommendations for clinical practice. Further research is needed to evaluate CM combination therapies for menopausal symptoms. Based on the evidence of individual CM therapies (see Chapters 5, 7 and 8) and the evidence of combination therapies, practitioners should consider their use on an individual basis.

References

1. Buysse DJ, Reynolds CF, 3rd, Monk TH, *et al.* (1989) The Pittsburgh Sleep Quality Index: A new instrument for psychiatric practice and research. *Psychiatry Res* **28**(2): 193–213.
2. Zung WW. (1965) A self-rating depression scale. *Arch Gen Psychiatry* **12**: 63–70.
3. Zung WW. (1971) A rating instrument for anxiety disorders. *Psychosomatics* **12**(6): 371–379.
4. Hamilton M. (1960) A rating scale for depression. *J Neurol Neurosurg Psychiatry* **23**: 56–62.
5. Hamilton M. (1959) The assessment of anxiety states by rating. *Br J Med Psychol* **32**(1): 50–55.
6. Kupperman HS, Wetchler BB, Blatt MH. (1959) Contemporary therapy of the menopausal syndrome. *J Am Med Assoc* **171**: 1627–1637.
7. Hilditch JR, Lewis J, Peter A, *et al.* (2008) A menopause-specific quality of life questionnaire: Development and psychometric properties. *Maturitas* **61**(1–2): 107–121.

References for Included Combination Therapies Clinical Studies

Study No.	References
C1	Azizi H, Liu YF, Du L, *et al.* (2011) Menopause-related symptoms: Traditional Chinese medicine versus hormone therapy. *Altern Ther Health Med* **17**(4): 48–53.
C2	Yang HY, Yang J, Wen Z, *et al.* (2012) Effect of combining therapy with traditional Chinese medicine-based psychotherapy and herbal medicines in women with menopausal syndrome: A randomized controlled clinical trial. *Evid Based Complement Alternat Med* **2012**: 354145
C3	钱立锋, 赵青. (2017) 柴胡加龙骨牡蛎汤联合引阳人阴推拿治疗更年期失眠 40 例. 浙江中医杂志 **52**(6): 413.
C4	王博, 谢俊, 吴松. (2017) 耳穴压丸联合背部循经走罐治疗围绝经期失眠症的临床观察术. 针灸临床杂志 **33**(3): 22–25.
C5	王宁, 敖学艳, 杨俊. (2017) 浅析中医和'易筋经'锻炼同时应用于围绝经期女性焦虑症的效用. 心理医生 **23**(30): 300–301.
C6	蓝群英. (2017) 养心滋肾法配合艾灸治疗围绝经期抑郁症的临床研究. 中国中医药现代远程教育 **15**(11): 96–98.
C7	凌娴 (2017). 针刺结合乐疗治疗女性更年期综合征的临床观察. 云南中医学院硕士学位论文.
C8	李静. (2016) 中药汤剂联合针灸疗法治疗更年期综合征的临床观察. 医药前沿 **6**(18): 337–338.
C9	朱松姝, 曹岐新, 王群. (2016) 中药足浴联合背景音乐治疗肾虚肝郁型围绝经期综合征失眠 40 例. 浙江中医杂志 **51**(2): 119.
C10	李建煌. (2014) 二仙汤加减配合耳穴贴压治疗更年期失眠症的疗效观察. 广州中医药大学硕士学位论文.
C11	马润兴. (2014) 针灸联合宁神汤治疗女性更年期失眠 39 例. 河南中医 **34**(9): 1825–1826.
C12	郑舟霞. (2013) 针刺结合黄连阿胶汤辅助治疗更年期失眠临床观察. 新中医 **45**(8): 153–154.
C13	朱慧玲. (2013) 针药结合治疗肝郁肾虚型围绝经期抑郁症的临床观察. 黑龙江中医药大学硕士学位论文.
C14	郑希德. (2012) 帕罗西汀, 逍遥散结合音乐疗法治疗女性更年期抑郁症的疗效分析. 中国现代医生 **50**(9): 51–52, 55.

(*Continued*)

Study No.	References
C15	钟宏量, 蒙珊, 杜艳. (2009) 中药内服加耳穴贴压治疗肾阴虚型围绝经期综合征疗效观察. 广西中医药 **32**(1): 13–14.
C16	杨洪艳, 王小云, 许英温, *et al.* (2011) 中医心身同治方案治疗绝经综合征抑郁症状的随机对照研究术. 广东医学 **32**(16): 2209–2211.
C17	王志. (2015) 逍遥丸结合针刺治疗围绝经期综合征肝郁型临床疗效观察. 慢性病学杂志 **16**(4): 465–467.
C18	姚新, 孟晴, 刘兴山. (2016) 药膳配合针刺对妇女围绝经期失眠症的实验研究. 吉林医学 **37**(12): 3016–3017.
C19	Cahill K. (2012) The treatment of postmenopausal atrophic vaginitis and dyspareunia with acupuncture and Chinese herbs: A case study. *J Chin Med* **99**: 33–36.
C20	Scheid V, Tuffrey V, Weijburg T, *et al.* (2015) Chinese medicine treatment for menopausal symptoms in the UK health service: Is a clinical trial warranted? *Maturitas* **80**(2): 179–186.
C21	孙正军. (2006) 针药结合治疗妇女更年期综合征42例. 针灸临床杂志 **22**(8): 18–19.

10

Summary and Conclusions

OVERVIEW

Menopausal symptoms can cause significant bother to women and impact their quality of life. Hormone therapy may be offered to women with no contraindications and is effective in providing symptom relief. Not all women obtain adequate symptom relief with hormone therapy and some women may look to complementary and alternative medicines such as Chinese medicine for additional support. This chapter provides a 'whole-evidence' analysis of Chinese medicine treatments for menopausal symptoms. Evidence from classical and contemporary literature and clinical studies are compared. The implications for clinical practice and future research are described.

Introduction

The end of a woman's reproductive life can be marked by many physical and emotional changes that can last for months or years. Physical changes include vasomotor symptoms of hot flushes and night sweats, sleep disturbance, genitourinary symptoms such as vaginal atrophy, dysuria, recurrent urinary tract infections and musculoskeletal aches and pains. Psychological symptoms include irritability, anxiety and depression. These symptoms can reduce quality of life[1,2] and result in lost productivity.[2]

Hormone therapy (HT) is the most effective treatment for vasomotor and genitourinary symptoms.[3,4] After consideration of the short and long-term risks and benefits, HT can be considered for women with bothersome symptoms who do not have a history of contraindications.[4] Other non-hormonal treatments, such as selective serotonin reuptake inhibitors, are also effective for vasomotor symptoms.[5,6] Women who do not achieve adequate relief from symptoms with pharmacotherapy may wish to try complementary and alternative medicines (CAM), although evidence for many CAM therapies is lacking.[5] Complementary and alternative medicine use is known to be high among menopausal women.[7] Chinese medicine (CM) may have a role to play in providing relief from menopausal symptoms.

This book includes a 'whole-evidence' analysis in investigating CM for the management of menopausal symptoms. Chinese herbal medicine (CHM), acupuncture therapies and CM psychotherapy have been recommended in clinical guidelines and textbooks (Chapter 2). Analysis of the classical literature highlighted the use of CHM formulations and acupuncture for symptoms of menopause in past eras (Chapter 3). Findings from meta-analyses of clinical studies revealed some promising effects of CHM, acupuncture, electroacupuncture, point percussion therapy and *qigong* 气功 for menopausal symptoms.

Chinese Medicine Syndrome Differentiation

Syndrome differentiation, according to each individual's clinical presentation, is a cornerstone of CM treatment. The CM syndromes described in Chapter 2 include Kidney *yin* deficiency 肾阴虚, Kidney *yang* deficiency 肾阳虚, Kidney *yin* and *yang* deficiency 肾阴阳俱虚, Kidney deficiency with Liver stagnation 肾虚肝郁, and Heart and Kidney disharmony 心肾不交. The attribution of menopausal symptoms to Kidney deficiency appears to be the result of efforts to standardise CM education in the 1960s.[8]

A passage from one of the earliest and most well-known classical texts, the *Huang Di Nei Jing Su Wen* 黄帝内经素问 (c. 762 AD), describes decline of *qi*, Blood, *yin, yang, jing* 精 and *tian gui* 天癸 that begins in the fifth seven-year cycle (age 35) and culminates with the exhaustion of Kidneys, *tian gui* 天癸, and the *Ren* 任 and *Chong* 冲 vessels in the seventh seven-year cycle (age 49). This passage describes ageing generally. Citations from classical literature that were considered as possible cases of menopause were described in Chapter 3. Citations described the pathogenesis of menopausal symptoms. A deficiency of Stomach *qi* resulted in decreased production of *jin ye* 津液 (body fluids), which contributed to a deficiency of Blood. Heart deficiency and Lung dryness were also described, which is not surprising given that the term *zang zao* 脏躁 ('restless organs') has been used for psychological symptoms of menopause.[9,10]

Many studies described CM syndromes. In Chapter 5, 86 of the 281 (30.6%) included CHM studies described using CM syndrome, either as an inclusion criterion or to guide treatment. All syndromes listed in Chapter 2 were found in CHM clinical studies (some with slight differences in terminology). The most common syndromes were Kidney *yin* deficiency, Kidney *yin* deficiency with Liver stagnation, and *yin* deficiency with fire/heat. Twenty-six of the 97 acupuncture therapy studies in Chapter 7 reported syndromes used for selecting participants or for treatment. The most common of these were Kidney deficiency, Kidney *yin* deficiency, Kidney *yin* and *yang* deficiency, and Kidney and Heart not communicating. The combination of Kidney deficiency with Liver stagnation was not mentioned in any of the acupuncture studies, although several listed Liver and Kidney *yin* deficiency, or Liver *qi* stagnation alone.

Syndromes were infrequently mentioned in studies of other CM therapies: two of the 17 studies (11.8%) included syndromes of Kidney *yin* and *yang* deficiency and dampness-heat. This was not surprising, as the types of interventions included in this chapter are not dependent on a specific syndrome diagnosis. The analysis of syndromes from different sources of evidence highlights the change in perceptions of menopause pathogenesis and syndromes over time. The historical view of menopausal symptoms, as the result of a natural decline of Stomach *qi*, *jin ye* 津液 and Blood, and involvement of the Heart and Lung, has been replaced with a focus on Kidney deficiency in contemporary literature. The syndromes found in clinical studies reflect those in contemporary textbooks. This was an expected finding given that academics conducting acupuncture research have been educated within a contemporary CM framework.

Chinese Herbal Medicine

This section summarises the evidence from Chapters 2, 3, 5 and 9. Chinese herbal medicine treatments provide important treatment options for the management of the range of symptoms women experience during menopause. Key clinical textbooks and practice guidelines that informed content in Chapter 2 describe CHM traditional formulas and commercially manufactured products that can be considered based on syndrome differentiation. Treatments are for oral use.

The importance of oral CHM was also highlighted in treatment citations from classical CM texts (Chapter 3). The earliest use of CHM for menopause symptoms was from the book *Jin Gui Yao Lue Fang Lun* 金匮要略方论 (c. 206 AD). Chinese herbal medicine was described in 288 of the 291 treatment citations. The vast majority of citations referred to oral-use CHM, with 53 different formulas described. The most frequently cited formulas were *Gan mai da zao tang* 甘麦大枣汤 and *Bai he zhi mu tang* 百合知母汤. A small number of citations described topical treatments that could be used for menopausal symptoms (22 citations). All topical treatments involved the use of the herb *bai he* 百合, which was prepared in water and used as a skin wash.

Interest in CHM has continued, with many treatments being tested in clinical studies. The emphasis on oral CHM treatments was evident in Chapter 5, with 277 of the 281 clinical studies testing oral CHM. Topical CHM was tested in four clinical studies, and one study tested the combination of oral and topical CHM. Two hundred and twenty-four studies used CHM alone and 60 combined CHM with guideline-recommended conventional treatments. Several studies included multiple treatment arms testing CHM alone and as integrative medicine.

Results for randomised controlled trials (RCTs) and controlled clinical trials (CCT) were analysed for each of the pre-specified outcomes. Meta-analysis showed oral CHM to be superior to placebo in reducing daily hot flush frequency and severity (although results were heavily influenced by one study), improving the quality of sleep when assessed using the Pittsburgh Sleep Quality Index (PSQI)[11] and improving global symptom severity on the original or modified version of the Kupperman Index (KI)[12] and Menopause Rating Scale (MRS).[13] Oral CHM was not superior to placebo in improving health-related quality of life (HRQoL).

Benefits were seen in meta-analyses when oral CHM was compared with guideline-recommended pharmacotherapy treatments. Oral CHM improved sleep quality on the PSQI, Athens Insomnia Scale (AIS)[14] and Self-rating Sleep Scale;[15] symptoms of depression on the Hamilton Rating Scale for Depression (HAM-D);[16] anxiety symptoms on the Hamilton Rating Scale for Anxiety (HAM-A);[17] global symptom severity on the KI and some domains of the Medical Outcome Study 36-Item Short-Form Health Survey (SF-36).[18] When oral CHM was combined with guideline-recommended treatments, meta-analyses showed benefits of the combination in improving sleep quality on the PSQI, anxiety on Zung's Self-rating Anxiety Scale,[19] depressive symptoms on the HAM-D and global symptoms on the KI. Few benefits over pharmacotherapy were seen in improving HRQoL. Statistical heterogeneity was detected in many of these results, which limits our confidence in the results.

Due to the small number of studies of topical CHM, meta-analysis was not possible. Results from individual studies showed improvements on the PSQI, on vaginal symptoms and cytology. The combination of oral and topical CHM improved global symptom severity on the KI at the end of treatment in one study.[20]

Experts in menopause and CM were consulted to identify important clinical questions. Assessment of the strength and quality of evidence was conducted using the Grading of Recommendations Assessment, Development and Evaluation (GRADE) framework. For several important comparisons there were either no studies of that comparison or there were no studies that reported on outcomes considered important for clinical practice. The GRADE assessments were conducted for four comparisons: (1) Oral CHM versus placebo; (2) Oral CHM versus HT; (3) The formula *Er xian tang* 二仙汤 versus placebo; and (4) *Kun tai jiao nang* 坤泰胶囊 versus HT.

When oral CHM was compared with placebo, 'moderate' certainty evidence showed benefit of oral CHM in reducing daily hot flush frequency and severity (Chapter 5, Table 5.30). No difference was seen between groups on the four domains of the Greene Climacteric Scale (GCS; 'low' to 'moderate' certainty evidence).[21] 'Low' certainty evidence favoured oral CHM on the PSQI, while 'moderate' certainty evidence favoured placebo in reducing depressive symptoms on the HAM-D. 'Low' certainty evidence showed no difference between oral CHM and placebo on the four domains of the Menopause-specific Quality of Life questionnaire (MENQOL).[22]

'Moderate' certainty evidence from one study showed no difference between oral CHM and HT in daily hot flush frequency at the end of treatment, while oral CHM was superior to HT in reducing daily hot flush severity (Chapter 5, Table 5.31). 'Low' certainty evidence showed oral CHM to be superior to HT in scores on the psychological, physical and vasomotor domains of the GCS. 'Very low' certainty evidence showed no difference between oral CHM and HT on the HAM-D, while 'low' certainty evidence found no difference between groups on the four domains of MENQOL.

'Moderate' certainty evidence from one study showed benefit of *Er xian tang* 二仙汤 over placebo in reducing daily hot flush frequency and improving scores on the physical, psychosocial and vasomotor domains of MENQOL (Chapter 5, Table 5.32). No difference between groups was seen in reducing hot flush severity or on the sexual domain of the MENQOL. Finally, 'low' certainty evidence showed no benefit of *Kun tai jiao nang* 坤泰胶囊 over HT on all four domains of the MENQOL (Chapter 5, Table 5.33).

Despite being perceived as natural and therefore safe, CHM may cause side effects. Fewer adverse events were reported in women who received oral CHM than in those who were allocated to comparator groups. Adverse events were generally mild in nature and were similar to those seen in comparator groups.

Chinese Herbal Medicine Formulas in Key Clinical Guidelines and Textbooks, Classical Literature and Clinical Studies

The CHM formulas recommended in clinical textbooks and guidelines, those described in classical literature and those that have been tested in clinical studies are diverse. In order to identify consistency in practice over time, CHM formulas used in these three sources of evidence were analysed. Table 10.1 summarises the traditional CHM formulas described in clinical guidelines and textbooks (Chapter 2), classical literature (Chapter 3) and clinical studies (Chapter 5 and 9), while Table 10.2 summarises the evidence for manufactured products. The CHM treatments that have been used in multiple RCTs have also been included in these tables.

Table 10.1 Summary of Chinese Herbal Medicine Traditional Formulas

Formula Name	Clinical Guidelines and Textbooks	Classical Literature (No. of Citations)	Clinical Studies (Chapter 5)			Combination Therapies (Chapter 9)
			RCTs (No. of Studies)	CCTs (No. of Studies)	Non-controlled Studies (No. of Studies)	
Er xian tang 二仙汤	Yes	0	8	0	0	1
Tian wang bu xin dan 天王补心丹	Yes	0	0	0	0	1
Yi guan jian 一贯煎	Yes	0	0	0	1	0
You gui wan 右归丸	Yes	0	0	0	0	0
Zuo gui wan 左归丸 plus *Er zhi wan* 二至丸	Yes	0	0	0	0	0
Chai hu long gu mu li tang 柴胡龙骨牡蛎汤	No	0	2	0	0	0
Diao chong an shen tang 调冲安神汤	No	0	2	0	0	0
Dan zhi xiao yao wan/san 丹栀逍遥丸/散	No	0	2	1	1	1
Gan mai da zao tang 甘麦大枣汤	No	63	6	2	0	0
Gui pi tang 归脾汤	No	1	3	0	0	0
Qing xin zi shen tang 清心滋肾汤	No	0	3	0	0	0

(*Continued*)

Table 10.1 (*Continued*)

Formula Name	Clinical Guidelines and Textbooks	Classical Literature (No. of Citations)	Clinical Studies (Chapter 5) RCTs (No. of Studies)	CCTs (No. of Studies)	Non-controlled Studies (No. of Studies)	Combination Therapies (Chapter 9)
Suan zao ren tang 酸枣仁汤	No	1	8	1	0	0
Xiao yao wan/san 逍遥丸/散	No	0	9	1	0	1
Xue fu zhi yu tang 血府逐瘀汤	No	0	2	0	0	0
Zhi bai di huang wan 知柏地黄丸	No	0	3	3	1	1
Zi shui qing gan yin 滋水清肝饮	No	0	4	0	2	0

Abbreviations: CCTs, controlled clinical trials; RCTs, randomised controlled trials.

Table 10.2 Summary of Chinese Herbal Medicine Manufactured Products

Formula Name	Clinical Guidelines and Textbooks	Classical Literature (No. of Citations)	Clinical Studies (Chapter 5) RCTs (No. of Studies)	CCTs (No. of Studies)	Non-controlled Studies (No. of Studies)	Combination Therapies (Chapter 9)
Liu wei di huang wan 六味地黄丸	Yes	2	6	0	0	0
Kun bao wan 坤宝丸	Yes	0	2	0	0	0
Geng nian an 更年安	Yes	0	0	0	0	0
Long feng bao jiao nang 龙凤宝胶囊	Yes	0	0	0	0	0
Kun tai jiao nang 坤泰胶囊	Yes	0	10	0	0	0
Nü zhen ke li 女珍颗粒	Yes	0	0	0	0	0
Geng nian ning xin ke li 更年宁心颗粒	No	0	2	0	0	0
Shu gan jie yu jiao nang 疏肝解郁胶囊	No	0	5	1	0	0
Wu ling jiao nang 乌灵胶囊	No	0	3	0	0	0

Abbreviations: CCTs, controlled clinical trials; RCTs, randomised controlled trials.

Analysis of formulas was based on the formula name, not based on herb ingredients. It is possible that formulas with the same, or similar, herb ingredients but with different formula names were included in analyses. As such, it is possible that the number of uses of formulas shown in Tables 10.1 and 10.2 is an underestimate of the frequency of use.

None of the five traditional formulas recommended in clinical textbooks and guidelines were found in classical literature, while three of the five formulas have been tested in clinical studies (Table 10.1). No evidence from clinical studies was identified for *You gui wan* 右归丸, or for the combination of *Zuo gui wan* 左归丸 plus *Er zhi wan* 二至丸, although *Zuo gui wan* 左归丸 was used alone in three RCTs. The formula *Er xian tang* 二仙汤 was tested in nine clinical studies, including one in which it was combined with ear acupressure (see Chapter 9),[23] and it has also been the topic of one published systematic review by Chen *et al.* (2008).[24]

Tian wang bu xin dan 天王补心丹 was used as a combination therapy in one RCT included in Chapter 9, where it was combined with *Yijinjing qigong* 易筋经气功 exercise.[25] Despite being recommended in clinical textbooks and guidelines, only one non-controlled study of *Yi guan jian* 一贯煎 met the eligibility criteria for inclusion in this review. It is possible that evidence from studies not included in this review supports their use in clinical practice.

Three formulas that were not included in the textbooks and guidelines reviewed for Chapter 2 were found in classical literature and were tested in clinical studies: *Gan mai da zao tang* 甘麦大枣汤, *Gui pi tang* 归脾汤 and *Suan zao ren tang* 酸枣仁汤. *Gan mai da zao tang* 甘麦大枣汤 was the most frequently cited formula in classical literature, with 63 citations describing its use for menopausal symptoms, particularly psychological symptoms. *Gan mai da zao tang* 甘麦大枣汤 was as effective as pharmacotherapy in reducing depressive symptoms on the HAM-D (see Chapter 5). Meta-analysis of the evidence for *Gui pi tang* 归脾汤 and *Suan zao ren tang* 酸枣仁汤 was not possible due to differences in comparisons, outcomes and study designs.

Many other formulas that have not been recommended in textbooks and guidelines reviewed for Chapter 2 have been tested in clinical studies, including those listed in Table 10.1. The diversity in formulas may reflect the diversity in symptoms reported by women during menopause. This analysis highlights several formulas for which there is consistent use over time, as well as emerging formulas that may provide relief for women experiencing bothersome symptoms during the menopausal transition.

Table 10.2 summarises the manufactured CHM products that have been found in contemporary and classical literature, and that have been tested in clinical studies. One formula that has been recommended in clinical textbooks and guidelines in Chapter 2, was found in classical literature and has been tested in clinical studies: *Liu wei di huang wan* 六味地黄丸. One classical literature citation described *Liu wei di huang wan* 六味地黄丸 alone, while the second combined *Liu wei di huang wan* 六味地黄丸 with *Gui pi tang* 归脾汤. *Liu wei di huang wan* 六味地黄丸 is used to tonify the Kidney and Kidney *yin* and is recommended in guidelines for Kidney *yin* deficiency.

Two manufactured products that are recommended in clinical textbooks and guidelines in Chapter 2 have been tested in clinical studies: *Kun bao wan* 坤宝丸 and *Kun tai jiao nang* 坤泰胶囊 capsules. *Kun bao wan* 坤宝丸 enriches the Liver and Kidney and nourishes Blood and is recommended for Kidney *yin* deficiency. *Kun tai jiao nang* 坤泰胶囊 was the most frequently tested oral CHM in RCTs and has been evaluated in three previously published systematic reviews.[26–28] This formula is used to harmonise the Heart and Kidney. The popularity of *Kun tai jiao nang* 坤泰胶囊 capsules may relate to the convenience of using capsules compared to preparing a traditional decoction, or to the comparative ease with which manufactured products can be tested in clinical studies. Despite this, analysis in this review found limited evidence to support its use in clinical practice (see Chapter 5, Table 5.44).

Three formulas that were recommended in textbooks were neither found in classical literature, nor were tested in clinical studies: *Geng nian an* 更年安, *Long feng bao jiao nang* 龙凤宝胶囊 and *Nü zhen ke li* 女珍颗粒. Despite not being used in included clinical studies, it is possible that evidence exists to support the use of these manufactured products that was not included in this review.

Acupuncture and Related Therapies

This section summarises the evidence from Chapters 2, 3, 7 and 9. Acupuncture therapies are an important treatment choice for bothersome menopausal symptoms. Three acupuncture therapies have been recommended in clinical practice guidelines and textbooks that informed the content in Chapter 2: acupuncture, ear acupuncture and moxibustion. Acupuncture has a long history of use for symptoms of menopause; the earliest use of acupuncture for middle-aged women was in a text from 1565.

Fewer studies evaluated acupuncture therapies compared to CHM. However, the number of studies that evaluated acupuncture was not insignificant; 97 clinical studies met the criteria for inclusion in Chapter 7 and the majority of these were RCTs. Studies conducted in China tended to compare acupuncture therapies with pharmacotherapy, such as HT or treatments for comorbidities, in perimenopausal women. Studies conducted outside of China often evaluated efficacy, compared with no treatment, sham or placebo acupuncture in menopausal women including postmenopausal women.

Diversity was seen in interventions, comparators and outcome measures which prevented pooling of results on several occasions. Manual acupuncture was the most frequently tested intervention (71 of 97 studies, 73.2%), followed by electroacupuncture (12 of 97 studies, 12.4%). Other interventions included moxibustion, acupressure, ear acupressure, laser acupuncture, Koryo hand therapy and point percussion therapy, although these were evaluated in fewer than ten studies (see Chapter 7 for more details).

Meta-analyses were conducted where possible. Benefits were seen when acupuncture therapies were used alone, or as integrative medicine, with pharmacotherapy. Findings from meta-analyses suggested that acupuncture was more effective than pharmacotherapy in reducing psychological symptoms measured using the HAM-D and HAM-A. Acupuncture was also more effective than pharmacotherapy in reducing global symptom severity assessed using the KI. When acupuncture was combined with pharmacotherapy as integrative medicine, greater improvements were seen in sleep symptoms measured with the PSQI and in depressive symptoms measured using the HAM-D. Acupuncture appeared to be beneficial for improving sleep and psychological symptoms in menopausal women.

Assessment of the strength and quality of evidence was conducted using the GRADE framework for two interventions (acupuncture and electroacupuncture) and two comparators (sham/placebo acupuncture and HT). 'Low' to 'moderate' certainty evidence showed no difference between acupuncture and sham/placebo acupuncture in hot flush frequency and severity, sleep score on the PSQI, and the four domains of the MENQOL (Chapter 7, Table 7.10). No benefit was seen for acupuncture compared with HT for depressive symptoms using the HAM-D ('very low' certainty evidence; Chapter 7, Table 7.11).

Electroacupuncture was more effective in reducing hot flush frequency ('low' certainty evidence) and was more effective at reducing hot flush severity ('moderate' certainty evidence) than sham/placebo acupuncture (Chapter 7, Table 7.14). 'Moderate' certainty evidence showed benefit with electroacupuncture on the psychosocial domain of the MENQOL, but no difference between electroacupuncture and sham/placebo acupuncture on other MENQOL domains. The GRADE assessment showed 'moderate' certainty evidence that electroacupuncture was superior to HT in reducing a composite measure of hot flush frequency and severity (Chapter 7, Table 7.15).

Individual studies showed mixed and variable results. For some treatments recommended in clinical textbooks and guidelines, such as ear acupuncture, there was little evidence from included studies to support their use in clinical practice. Some treatments that are not described in clinical textbooks showed promising results and may be worthy of further research attention, for example, electroacupuncture. Acupuncture therapies appeared to be well tolerated in menopausal women, although RCTs and CCTs may not be the best study design to assess such outcomes — long-term surveillance studies are better suited to assess the safety profile of CM therapies.

Acupuncture Therapies in Key Clinical Guidelines and Textbooks, Classical Literature and Clinical Studies

Analysis was conducted to identify consistency of use of the different acupuncture therapies across the various sources of evidence. Treatments that are recommended in clinical textbooks and guidelines included in Chapter 2, and those tested in multiple RCTs, are described in Table 10.3. Acupuncture was the only intervention found in textbooks and clinical guidelines, in classical literature and in included clinical studies of acupuncture therapies alone and in combination with other CM treatments. Moxibustion has been recommended in contemporary clinical guidelines and textbooks and was tested in several RCTs and non-controlled studies. The evidence for acupuncture and, to a lesser extent, moxibustion, shows some promise in improving some menopausal symptoms but is currently insufficient to make recommendations for clinical practice.

Table 10.3 Summary of Acupuncture and Related Therapies

Intervention	Clinical Guidelines and Textbooks (Chapter 2)	Classical Literature (Chapter 3) (No. of Citations)	Clinical Studies (Chapter 7)* RCTs (No. of Studies)	CCTs (No. of Studies)	Non-controlled Studies (No. of Studies)	Combination Therapies (Chapter 9)
Acupuncture	Yes	3	57	6	7	11
Ear acupuncture	Yes	0	0	0	0	1
Moxibustion	Yes	0	4	0	1	1
Electroacupuncture	No	0	10	0	2	0
Acupressure	No	0	3	0	0	0
Ear acupressure	No	0	4	1	5	3
Point percussion therapy	No	0	3	0	0	0

*Some studies used more than one intervention (e.g., acupuncture plus moxibustion). These are counted separately in this table.
Abbreviations: CCTs, controlled clinical trials; RCTs, randomised controlled trials.

Ear acupuncture is a somewhat recent development in CM, originating in the 1950s.[29] Despite being recommended in clinical guidelines and textbooks, ear acupuncture was not evaluated in any clinical studies that met the eligibility criteria for inclusion in this review. This was an interesting finding, considering that ear acupressure was tested in several clinical studies. One could argue that ear acupuncture, as an invasive procedure, requires more careful monitoring to minimise the risk of infection when retained for up to three days. Additional monitoring would require additional resources, subsequently increasing the costs to conduct such a trial. Conversely, ear acupressure using seeds or magnets that do not penetrate the skin can be managed more easily by study participants at home. This may explain the appearance of ear acupressure and absence of ear acupuncture in clinical studies.

Several other interventions that have not been recommended in clinical guidelines and textbooks have been tested in multiple studies. Electroacupuncture was evaluated in 12 clinical studies, most of which were conducted in China. Some promising results in individual studies were seen with electroacupuncture for improving vasomotor symptoms, depressive symptoms and global symptom severity.

Point percussion therapy, a technique involving finger percussion, pinching, pressing and clapping on acupuncture points or meridians, is less commonly used compared with acupuncture and was tested in three RCTs. Results from single studies showed some benefit in improving sleep quality, psychological symptoms and global symptom severity compared to pharmacotherapy. If further research confirms this treatment to be beneficial for improving menopausal symptoms, it could be taught to patients and/or their carers to be administered at home, thereby reducing the burden on the health care system.

In addition to identifying the interventions used in each source of evidence, analysis was also undertaken to identify the acupuncture points which have a history of use and those that are frequently tested in clinical studies. Points recommended in clinical guidelines and textbooks for each intervention are described in Table 10.4 and the

Table 10.4 Summary of Acupuncture Points

Intervention	Clinical Guidelines and Textbooks (Chapter 2)	Classical Literature (Chapter 3) (No. of Citations)	Clinical Studies (Chapter 7)*			Combination Therapies (Chapter 9)*
			RCTs (No. of Studies)	CCTs (No. of Studies)	Non-controlled Studies (No. of Studies)	
Acupuncture						
KI3 *Taixi* 太溪	Yes	0	15	2	3	4
LR3 *Taichong* 太冲	Yes	0	21	1	5	5
CV4 *Guanyuan* 关元	Yes	0	19	2	4	4
SP6 *Sanyinjiao* 三阴交	Yes	0	27	3	8	7
BL15 *Xinshu* 心俞	Yes	0	14	0	0	5
BL18 *Ganshu* 肝俞	Yes	0	15	1	1	5
BL23 *Shenshu* 肾俞	Yes	0	17	2	2	6
Moxibustion						
GV4 *Mingmen* 命门	Yes	0	1	0	0	0
CV6 *Qihai* 气海	Yes	0	1	0	0	0
CV4 *Guanyuan* 关元	Yes	0	1	0	0	0
Ear acupuncture/acupressure						
TF2 *Zigong* (Uterus) 子宫	Yes	0	0	1	2	1
TF2 *Luanchao* (Ovary) 卵巢	Yes	0	0	0	0	0
CO18 *Neifenmi* (Endocrine) 内分泌	Yes	0	3	1	2	0
TF4 *Shenmen* 神门	Yes	0	4	1	4	1
AH6 *Jiaogan* (Sympathetic) 交感	Yes	0	3	0	3	0

(*Continued*)

Table 10.4 (*Continued*)

Intervention	Clinical Guidelines and Textbooks (Chapter 2)	Classical Literature (Chapter 3) (No. of Citations)	Clinical Studies (Chapter 7)* RCTs (No. of Studies)	CCTs (No. of Studies)	Non-controlled Studies (No. of Studies)	Combination Therapies (Chapter 9)*
AT4 *Pizhixia* (Subcortex) 皮质下	Yes	0	3	0	2	0
CO15 *Xin* (Heart) 心	Yes	0	2	1	1	1
CO12 *Gan* (Liver) 肝	Yes	0	2	1	2	1
CO10 *Shen* (Kidney) 肾	Yes	0	2	1	1	1

*Some studies used more than one intervention (e.g. acupuncture plus moxibustion). These are counted separately in this table.
Abbreviations: CCTs, controlled clinical trials; RCTs, randomised controlled trials.

number of uses of each point by the corresponding intervention is stated. None of the acupuncture points that are recommended in clinical texts and guidelines were found in the classical literature.

Points used for acupuncture were found more frequently in clinical studies purely due to acupuncture being used in over three quarters of all studies (Table 10.4). An interesting finding emerges when reviewing the total number of uses for each point across all acupuncture clinical studies. The acupuncture point SP6 *Sanyinjiao* 三阴交 was the most frequently used point in acupuncture clinical studies, used in 45 clinical studies. The second most frequently used point was LR3 *Taichong* 太冲 (32 studies). The acupuncture point SP6 *Sanyinjiao* 三阴交 is used to invigorate Blood, calm the *shen* 神, tonify the Stomach and Spleen and resolve dampness, while LR3 *Taichong* 太冲 has actions that nourish Liver Blood and *yin*, promote free flow of *qi*, subdue Liver *yang* and regulate menstruation.[30] Neither of these points directly benefit the Kidney, which is the main organ dysfunction described in syndromes included in Chapter 2. The high frequency of use of these two points may relate to the large number of studies that included menopausal women with insomnia, depression or anxiety.

When one looks further, the next most frequently used points are: CV4 *Guanyuan* 关元 (29 studies), BL23 *Shenshu* 肾俞 (27 studies) and KI3 *Taixi* 太溪 (24 studies). All three of these points tonify and nourish the Kidney and Kidney *yin*, and benefit *jing* 精. These points appear to address more directly the syndromes described in contemporary textbooks and guidelines and are typically used in clinical practice.

While none of the studies tested ear acupuncture, several examined ear acupressure. Due to the similarity in these two techniques, analysis of the points used in ear acupressure was undertaken. Key points for ear acupressure were TF4 *Shenmen* 神门 (used in ten studies), CO18 *Neifenmi* (Endocrine) 内分泌, AH6 *Jiaogan* (Sympathetic) 交感 and CO12 *Gan* (Liver) 肝 (used in six studies each). Practitioners wishing to use ear acupressure, so that women can continue to stimulate the points after leaving the consulting room, may wish to consider using these acupuncture points if appropriate for syndrome differentiation.

Other Chinese Medicine Therapies

This section summarises the evidence from Chapters 2, 3, 8 and 9. Clinical textbooks and guidelines recommend the use of CM psychotherapy for management of menopausal symptoms. Chinese medicine psychotherapy focuses on emotions as part of the five-phase theory, and treatment can be combined with CHM according to syndrome differentiation. No instances of CM psychotherapy were found in the classical literature, which may suggest this form of treatment is a more recent development in the history of CM.

Compared with CHM and acupuncture therapies, few studies tested CM psychotherapy. Results from one RCT[31] showed CM psychotherapy could reduce global symptom severity on the KI compared to placebo, but was not different to placebo in improving MENQOL scores at the end of treatment. One CCT[32] found no difference in KI scores at the end of treatment between women who received CM psychotherapy and those who received placebo. No adverse events were reported by women who received CM psychotherapy in the RCT. Information about the safety of this intervention is limited but it is considered unlikely to cause significant harm.

Whilst not recommended in clinical guidelines, *qigong* 气功 has been tested in five RCTs, two CCTs, and combined with CHM in one RCT. Meta-analysis showed women who practiced *qigong* 气功 scored lower on the Center for Epidemiologic Studies Depression Scale[33] and KI at the end of treatment, indicating better outcomes. Better quality of life measured using the SF-36 was reported in one study.[34] None of the studies of *qigong* 气功 reported on safety. Although evidence is currently insufficient as to whether exercise is an effective treatment for menopausal symptoms,[5] it seems possible that a low impact, gentle exercise like *qigong* 气功 may be beneficial. The risk of osteoporotic fracture increases during menopause,[35] so women wishing to participate in *qigong* 气功 exercise should consult their physician prior to commencing an exercise program.

Other Chinese Medicine Therapies in Key Clinical Guidelines and Textbooks, Classical Literature and Clinical Studies

Chinese medicine psychotherapy has been recommended in clinical textbooks and guidelines and in four clinical studies, two of which combined CM psychotherapy with other CM interventions (Table 10.5). Despite not being recommended in clinical guidelines,

Table 10.5 Summary of Other Chinese Medicine Therapies

Intervention	Clinical Guidelines and Textbooks (Chapter 2)	Classical Literature (Chapter 3) (No. of Citations)	Clinical Studies (Chapter 8)			Combination Therapies (Chapter 9)
			RCTs (No. of Studies)	CCTs (No. of Studies)	Non-controlled Studies (No. of Studies)	
Chinese medicine psychotherapy	Yes	No	1	1	0	2
Qigong 气功	No	No	5	2	0	1

Abbreviations: CCTs, controlled clinical trials; RCTs, randomised controlled trials.

there is a small body of research examining the role of *qigong* 气功 for menopausal symptoms. Results for meta-analysis and individual studies suggest some benefit; the safety of this intervention needs further attention.

Limitations of Evidence

Every effort has been made to ensure the accuracy of the content included in this book. Information about the CM syndromes and treatments used for menopause were sourced from highly authoritative CM textbooks and clinical practice guidelines. It was not possible to include information from every available source and it is possible that other sources may describe different CM syndromes, CHM formulas, acupuncture therapies and other CM therapies that can be used for menopausal symptoms. The contents in Chapter 2 should not be considered as exhaustive and CM clinicians should use their clinical experience and knowledge in caring for menopausal women.

Classical Literature

The electronic database that was utilised for evaluation of the classical literature, the *Zhong Hua Yi Dian* (ZHYD) 中华医典, is one of the largest collections of classical literature texts and is considered to be a representative collection.[36,37] Searching the classical literature to identify citations that were possible cases of menopause presented several challenges. Menopause can present as any number of symptoms, several of which may be associated with natural ageing. Vasomotor symptoms may be a defining feature of the menopausal transition for contemporary women, but it is not clear whether this was a prominent feature of menopause for Chinese women in past eras. Furthermore, many of the symptoms that present during the menopausal transition can occur at other stages of life and in other disease states. Therefore, a search strategy was needed that captured the key symptoms of menopause in women of menopausal age.

Eighteen search terms and combinations of search terms were selected after review of CM dictionaries, textbooks and guidelines, and pilot searches were conducted to test their accuracy. The terms *zang zao* 脏躁/脏燥 and *bai he bing* 百合病 are the CM diagnoses that are most likely to relate to menopause. However, CM historians assert that *zang zao* 脏躁/脏燥 describes a type of nutritive *qi* deficiency, while *bai he bing* 百合病 refers to excess heat (Li (1989), cited in Scheid (2008)).[38] Despite the different views on the meaning of these terms, both nutritive *qi* deficiency and excess heat may be the causes of several menopausal symptoms, such as sleep disturbance and mood changes.

The remaining terms were either searched for alone (e.g., *chao re* 潮热 [hot flushes]), or were combined with *fu ren* 妇人 (woman). Due to restrictions in the database, it is possible that searches for combinations of terms may have failed to identify some potentially relevant citations where both terms were not found in close proximity. Chinese language has changed over time and it is possible that terms were overlooked that may have identified relevant information which may alter the findings.

Inclusion criteria were developed to select citations that described key symptoms in ageing women or in the content of amenorrhoea. Additional criteria were developed to identify citations that were considered most like menopause. Citations were reviewed by an experienced CM gynaecologist and care was taken in applying inclusion and exclusion criteria. While due care was taken, it is possible that another gynaecologist may read the same citation and reach a different conclusion about the likelihood of relating to menopause. Finally, any modification in search terms and/or inclusion criteria is likely to alter the findings.

Analysis of CHM treatments was conducted to identify those that were frequently used. Analysis was based on the formula name only, that is, there was no consideration of the similarity of herb ingredients. The CHM formulas are typically modified by adding, removing or substituting one or multiple herb ingredients and it is challenging to identify the core formula from a herb list. The frequency of formulas described in Chapter 3 may be an over- or under-estimation of the actual frequency of the formula in the data set.

Clinical Studies

A comprehensive search was conducted in five English-language and four Chinese-language general and specialist biomedical databases, and of four clinical trial registers to identify clinical studies of CM therapies for menopausal symptoms. The databases selected provide broad breadth and scope of indexed journals, but do not include all published journals. Selection of studies was limited to those published in languages with which the research team had expertise. The Korean and Japanese language databases are likely to include herbal medicine and acupuncture studies that may meet the eligibility criteria. Inclusion of results from such studies may alter the findings of outcome analysis.

Nearly 50,000 (49,278) potentially relevant citations were identified through database searches. Titles and abstracts of citations were reviewed by researchers to exclude those that were obviously irrelevant to the topic and to locate the full text for those that were potentially eligible. It is possible that human error may have resulted in inadvertent exclusion of potentially relevant citations. Data were extracted in duplicate and/or were verified by a second researcher to ensure accuracy of data. Again, it is possible that misunderstandings of the data may have resulted in errors during the extraction process.

Potential sources of bias were assessed to summarise the quality of individual studies and GRADE assessment was used to summarise the strength and certainty of evidence for clinically important questions. These assessments followed the guidance provided by the Cochrane Collaboration and the GRADE Working Group. Both approaches are ultimately a judgement that is subjective, and judgements between different reviewers may vary according to their interpretation of the guidance and their training in using these approaches. Agreement was reached through discussion for both risk of bias and GRADE assessment.

Diversity was seen in the interventions tested and comparators used. Analysis of outcome results was conducted according to these comparisons, taking into account the menopausal status of women where possible. In some cases, this prevented pooling of results from multiple studies for meta-analysis and for some outcomes the best available evidence comes from individual studies. This reduces certainty when implementing CM interventions in clinical practice. When meta-analysis was possible, statistical heterogeneity was 'high' for many analyses. Subgroup and sensitivity analyses failed to identify the reasons for this, which lowers confidence in the results.

For outcomes such as the MENQOL, some studies used scoring methods that differed from those described by the developer. For other outcomes, such as the KI, modified versions were used that added or removed some items from the original version. Given that these were still measuring the same concept, results were analysed using standardised mean difference. This allows us to identify whether a difference exists between groups, however, it does not allow us to estimate the absolute difference that may be expected. This limits our ability to determine whether changes found are clinically important for patients.

Experimental Studies

Chapter 6 provides an overview of a small selection of experimental studies that have evaluated potential mechanisms of some common herbs. The search to identify relevant studies was conducted in the English language biomedical database PubMed. Additional studies that further elucidate the mechanisms of key herbs may have not been identified or may have been published in languages other than English. The chapter should be considered as a guide only and not a comprehensive review of all available literature.

Implications for Practice

The CM syndromes relevant to menopause described in Chapter 2 all relate to the concept of Kidney deficiency. As highlighted, the classical literature presents a different view of the pathogenesis of menopausal symptoms. In light of this difference, it was not surprising that the formulas recommended in contemporary textbooks and guidelines were not identified in classical literature. The most frequently used formula in classical literature was *Gan mai da zao tang* 甘麦大枣汤, a formula recommended in contemporary texts and guidelines for depression.[39–41]

Few clinical studies were included that evaluated the CHM formulas recommended in textbooks and guidelines, and many tested other formulas. Actions of other formulas included tonifying the Spleen and Heart (*Gui pi tang* 归脾汤), nourishing the Liver Blood and calming the *shen* 神 (*Suan zao ren tang* 酸枣仁汤), clearing *qi* stagnation (*Xiao yao wan/san* 逍遥丸/散) and clearing heat while nourishing *yin* (*Zhi bai di huang wan* 知柏地黄丸). The diversity in these formulas support the assertion by Avis *et al.* (2001) that there is no typical 'menopause syndrome'.[42] Clinicians may consider Kidney deficiency as a 'starting point' for diagnosis and develop their diagnosis and treatment plan based on the symptoms that are the most bothersome for each individual patient.

Evidence for CHM formulas has been analysed as part of the overall pool of studies. Additional analyses have been conducted, where possible, to determine the evidence for particular formulas that were tested in multiple studies and which reported the same outcomes. As a result, it is not clear whether treatments other than those recommended in contemporary literature offer greater, or less, benefit than those that have been recommended in contemporary literature.

Benefits were seen in meta-analyses of CHM, some acupuncture treatments and other CM therapies in improving sleep and depressive symptoms and global symptom severity. Many of the meta-analyses had considerable statistical heterogeneity and the certainty of evidence was from 'very low' to 'moderate' quality studies. This reduces our confidence in results and CM clinicians may find different results for individuals when applying these interventions in clinical practice.

Natural groupings were seen in studies of CHM and acupuncture according to the location where the study was conducted. Studies that reported sleep and psychological symptoms were frequently from studies of Chinese perimenopausal women. Thus, findings may not be transferable to postmenopausal women from Australia, for example. Furthermore, it has been noted that the symptoms women experience during menopause differ according to ethnicity.[43,44] Clinicians should advise patients of these limitations when discussing the evidence to allow women to make informed choices about their use of CM therapies.

Meta-analysis showed improvements in several outcomes with oral CHM and acupuncture; however, methodological shortcomings limit the certainty of the evidence. When meta-analyses indicated a superior effect with CHM alone or as integrative medicine, analysis was undertaken to identify the herbs that may have contributed to the effect. Some of the most frequently used herbs in studies included in meta-analyses favouring CHM were: *bai shao* 白芍, *chai hu* 柴胡, *dang gui* 当归, *fu ling* 茯苓, *gan cao* 甘草, *shan yao* 山药, *shan zhu yu* 山茱萸, *shu di huang* 熟地黄, *suan zao ren* 酸枣仁 and *zhi mu* 知母. Many of these herbs have demonstrated actions that regulate hormones, are antidepressive, antiosteoporotic or hypnotic (see Chapter 6). Understanding the biological activity of key herbs can assist clinicians in making modifications to formulas that address bothersome symptoms for menopausal women.

Implications for Research

Many systematic reviews have evaluated CM interventions for menopausal symptoms and a common recommendation is for more research. It is clear that further research is needed to provide more conclusive evidence of the effects of CM therapies. Efforts are currently underway to develop a core set of outcome measures for menopause research.[45] When this is available, it will increase the ability to synthesise studies in meta-analysis, allow for estimation of the anticipated absolute effects of treatment and permit clinicians to identify whether changes due to treatment are clinically meaningful for patients.

Once the core outcome set is established, it will take time to implement. In the interim, researchers are encouraged to use validated versions of outcome scales (noting that the KI has never been properly validated[46]) and to follow the recommended scoring methods. This will increase the ability to pool results for meta-analysis that permits an estimate of the anticipated absolute effects, thereby increasing the possibility of translating research findings into clinical practice. Studies need to be adequately powered with longer treatment duration that matches the long-term nature of the menopause transition. Incorporating CM syndrome diagnosis into trial design will also facilitate translation of research outcomes.

Menopausal symptoms can have a significant impact on HRQoL. Analyses showed that CM therapies may improve quality of life for menopausal women, but few studies assessed this outcome. In addition to using symptom-specific outcome measures, researchers should consider the use of validated HRQoL measures that are specific to menopause.

In many studies and for many risk-of-bias domains, there was insufficient information provided to make a judgement about the potential for bias. Particular attention to using appropriate methods for sequence generation and allocation concealment will reduce bias and increase reliability of results. Registering clinical trials in the available registers increases transparency in trial report, and trials should ensure they meet the reporting requirements of the Consolidated Standards of Reporting Trials (CONSORT)[47] and the available extensions for herbal medicine,[48] acupuncture[49] and moxibustion.[50] Publication of study protocols and adequate reporting increase the possibility of study replication to confirm benefits.

In clinical trials, blinding of participants and personnel to group allocation is considered important to reduce performance bias. Many of the studies conducted outside of China used sham/placebo in order to achieve this. Studies that were conducted in China tended to compare CM therapies with conventional medical treatments, making blinding of participants and personnel more challenging and unlikely to have occurred. Armstrong (2012)[51] has argued that the 'gold standard' design of a double-blind RCT no longer meets the needs of clinicians and policy makers. Pragmatic studies that reflect clinical practice can allow for greater translation of research findings into clinical practice, increasing value of research funding.

Safety was reported in clinical studies and was often limited solely to the number and nature of adverse events. Few studies assigned causality, making it difficult to assess the safety profile of CM treatments. Study designs, other than RCTs, are better suited to evaluating the potential risks of treatments. Such studies should be conducted for CM treatments when, and if, effectiveness is established.

Testing complex interventions like CHM formulas is important to understand their efficacy and effectiveness. Herbs used in studies that demonstrate positive effects can also provide promising avenues for drug discovery. Phytoestrogens from plants have been examined as potential treatments for menopause due to their oestrogenic effects. Experimental studies have shown that some of the key herbs used in RCTs of CHM for menopause have actions to regulate hormones, are antidepressive and are hypnotic, and these herbs may warrant further investigation as potential treatments for menopause.

Herb ingredients and their composition can vary according to factors associated with growth (in the case of plants). Because of this, authentication of CHM formulas and herb ingredients is a key part of the quality assurance process that should be reported in clinical trials. Quantification of the amount of active constituents will contribute to improved reporting and greater understanding of which constituents may be having relevant biological actions.

References

1. Sun N, Xing J, Li L, *et al.* (2018) Impact of menopause on quality of life in community-based women in China: 1 year follow-up. *Arch Psychiatr Nurs* **32**(2): 224–228.
2. Whiteley J, DiBonaventura M, Wagner JS, *et al.* (2013) The impact of menopausal symptoms on quality of life, productivity, and economic outcomes. *J Womens Health (Larchmt)* **22**(11): 983–990.

3. The North American Menopause Society. (2017) The 2017 hormone therapy position statement of The North American Menopause Society. *Menopause* **24**(7): 728–753.
4. Sarri G, Davies M, Lumsden MA. (2015) Diagnosis and management of menopause: Summary of NICE guidance. *BMJ* **351**: h5746.
5. The North American Menopause Society. (2015) Nonhormonal management of menopause-associated vasomotor symptoms: 2015 position statement of The North American Menopause Society. *Menopause* **22**(11): 1155–1172; quiz 73–74.
6. Neves ECM, Birkhauser M, Samsioe G, *et al.* (2015) EMAS position statement: The ten point guide to the integral management of menopausal health. *Maturitas* **81**(1): 88–92.
7. Posadzki P, Lee MS, Moon TW, *et al.* (2013) Prevalence of complementary and alternative medicine (CAM) use by menopausal women: A systematic review of surveys. *Maturitas* **75**(1): 34–43.
8. Scheid V. (2007) Traditional Chinese medicine — What are we investigating?: The case of menopause. *Complement Ther Med* **15**(1): 54–68.
9. 罗颂平, 刘雁峰. (2017) 中医妇科学 ('十二五'普通高等教育本科国家级规划教材). 第 3 版. 北京: 人民卫生出版社.
10. 马宝璋. (2012) 中医妇科学 (普通高等教育'十一五'国家级规划教材). 北京: 中国中医药出版社.
11. Buysse DJ, Reynolds CF, 3rd, Monk TH, *et al.* (1989) The Pittsburgh Sleep Quality Index: A new instrument for psychiatric practice and research. *Psychiatry Res* **28**(2): 193–213.
12. Kupperman HS, Wetchler BB, Blatt MH. (1959) Contemporary therapy of the menopausal syndrome. *J Am Med Assoc* **171**: 1627–1637.
13. Heinemann LA, Potthoff P, Schneider HP. (2003) International versions of the Menopause Rating Scale (MRS). *Health Qual Life Outcomes* **1**: 28.
14. Soldatos CR, Dikeos DG, Paparrigopoulos TJ. (2000) Athens Insomnia Scale: Validation of an instrument based on ICD-10 criteria. *J Psychosom Res* **48**(6): 555–560.
15. 李建明. (2012) 睡眠状况自评量表(SRSS) 简介. 中国健康心理学杂志 **20**(12): 1851.
16. Hamilton M. (1960) A rating scale for depression. *J Neurol Neurosurg Psychiatry* **23**: 56–62.
17. Hamilton M. (1959) The assessment of anxiety states by rating. *Br J Med Psychol* **32**(1): 50–55.

18. Ware JJ, Sherbourne C. (1992) The MOS 36-item short-form health survey (SF-36). I. Conceptual framework and item selection. *Med Care* **30**: 473–483.
19. Zung WW. (1971) A rating instrument for anxiety disorders. *Psychosomatics* **12**(6): 371–379.
20. 冯华, 顾晓芳. (2017) 中药内服外洗法用于肾阴虚型围绝经期综合征患者治疗的临床效果. 现代医学 **45**(12): 1779–1780.
21. Greene JG. (1976) A factor analytic study of climacteric symptoms. *J Psychosom Res* **20**(5): 425–430.
22. Hilditch JR, Lewis J, Peter A, *et al.* (2008) A menopause-specific quality of life questionnaire: Development and psychometric properties. *Maturitas* **61**(1–2): 107–121.
23. 李建煌. (2014) 二仙汤加减配合耳穴贴压治疗更年期失眠症的疗效观察.: 广州中医药大学硕士学位论文.
24. Chen HY, Cho WC, Sze SC, *et al.* (2008) Treatment of menopausal symptoms with Er-xian decoction: A systematic review. *Am J Chin Med* **36**(2): 233–244.
25. 王宁, 敖学艳, 杨俊. (2017) 浅析中医和'易筋经'锻炼同时应用于围绝经期女性焦虑症的效用. 心理医生 **23**(30): 300–301.
26. Zhou Q, Tao J, Song H, *et al.* (2016) Chinese herbal medicine Kuntai capsule for treatment of menopausal syndrome: A systematic review of randomized clinical trials. *Complement Ther Med* **29**: 63–71.
27. 张庆云, 王继伟, 余金明. (2013) 坤泰胶囊与雌激素治疗绝经综合征有效性与安全性的荟萃分析. 中华医学杂志 **93**(43): 3445–3449.
28. 李存存, 王晶晶, 陈潮, *et al.* (2013) 坤泰胶囊与激素替代疗法治疗更年期综合征有效性和安全性比较的 Meta 分析. 中国中西医结合杂志 **33**(09): 1183–1190.
29. Gori L, Firenzuoli F. (2007) Ear acupuncture in European traditional medicine. *Evid Based Complement Alternat Med* **4**(Suppl 1): 13–16.
30. Deadman P, Al-Khafaji M, Baker K. (2000) *A Manual of Acupuncture*. Journal of Chinese Medicine Publications, East Sussex, UK.
31. Yang H, Yang J, Wen Z, *et al.* (2012) Effect of combining therapy with traditional chinese medicine-based psychotherapy and herbal medicines in women with menopausal syndrome: A randomized controlled clinical trial. *Evid Based Complement Alternat Med* **2012**: 354145.
32. 成芳平, 王小云, 张春玲, *et al.* (2010) 中医情志疗法治疗绝经综合征的临床研究. 实用医学杂志 **26**(19): 3630–3632.

33. Radloff L. (1977) The CES-D Scale: A self-report depression scale for research in the general population. *Appl Psychol Meas* **1**(3): 385–401.
34. 郝晶, 窦娜, 马素慧, *et al.* (2013) 八段锦气功操对围绝经期妇女生活质量的影响. 中国老年学杂志 (21): 5266–5268.
35. The National Institute of Health and Care Excellence (NICE) Guideline. (2015) Menopause: Diagnosis and management. Available from: https://www.nice.org.uk/guidance/ng23.
36. May BH, Lu C, Xue CC. (2012) Collections of traditional Chinese medical literature as resources for systematic searches. *J Altern Complement Med* **18**(12): 1101–1107.
37. May BH, Lu Y, Lu C, *et al.* (2013) Systematic assessment of the representativeness of published collections of the traditional literature on Chinese medicine. *J Altern Complement Med* **19**(5): 403–409.
38. Scheid V. (2008) Globalising Chinese medical understandings of menopause. *East Asian Sci Technol Soc* **2**(4): 485–506.
39. 周仲瑛. (2007) 中医内科学(普通高等教育'十二五'国家级规划教材). 北京: 中国中医药出版社.
40. 中华中医药学会. (2008) 中医内科常见病诊疗指南•中医疾病部分. 北京: 中国中医药出版社.
41. 中国中医科学院. (2011) 中医循证临床实践指南. 中医内科. 北京: 中国中医药出版社.
42. Avis NE, Stellato R, Crawford S, *et al.* (2001) Is there a menopausal syndrome? Menopausal status and symptoms across racial/ethnic groups. *Soc Sci Med* **52**(3): 345–356.
43. Im EO, Ko Y, Chee W. (2014) Ethnic differences in the clusters of menopausal symptoms. *Health Care Women Int* **35**(5): 549–565.
44. Obermeyer CM, Reher D, Saliba M. (2007) Symptoms, menopause status, and country differences: A comparative analysis from DAMES. *Menopause* **14**(4): 788–797.
45. COMET Initiative. (2019) COMMA (Core Outcomes in Menopause): International collaboration to measure core outcomes in menopause. Available from: http://www.comet-initiative.org/studies/details/917.
46. Davis SR. (2019) The Kupperman Index undressed. *Maturitas* **126**: 90–91.
47. Schulz KF, Altman DG, Moher D. (2010) CONSORT 2010 statement: Updated guidelines for reporting parallel group randomised trials. *PLoS Med* **7**(3): e1000251.

48. Gagnier JJ, Boon H, Rochon P, *et al.* (2006) Reporting randomized, controlled trials of herbal interventions: An elaborated CONSORT statement. *Ann Intern Med* **144**(5): 364–367.
49. MacPherson H, Altman DG, Hammerschlag R, *et al.* (2010) Revised STandards for Reporting Interventions in Clinical Trials of Acupuncture (STRICTA): Extending the CONSORT statement. *J Evid Based Med* **3**(3): 140–155.
50. Cheng CW, Fu SF, Zhou QH, *et al.* (2013) Extending the CONSORT Statement to moxibustion. *J Integr Med* **11**(1): 54–63.
51. Armstrong K. (2012) Methods in comparative effectiveness research. *J Clin Oncol* **30**(34): 4208–4214.

Glossary

Term	Acronym	Definition	Reference
95% confidence interval	95% CI	A measure of the uncertainty around the main finding of a statistical analysis. Estimates of unknown quantities, such as the odds ratio comparing an experimental intervention with a control, are usually presented as a point estimate and a 95% confidence interval. This means that if someone were to keep repeating a study in other samples from the same population, 95% of the confidence intervals from those studies would contain the true value of the unknown quantity. Alternatives to 95%, such as 90% and 99% confidence intervals, are sometimes used. Wider intervals indicate lower precision; narrow intervals, greater precision.	https://training.cochrane.org/handbook
Acupressure		Application of pressure on acupuncture points.	—
Acupuncture	—	The insertion of needles into humans or animals for remedial purposes.	World Health Organization. (2007) WHO International Standard Terminologies of Traditional Medicine in the Western Pacific Region.

(*Continued*)

(*Continued*)

Term	Acronym	Definition	Reference
Allied and Complementary Medicine Database	AMED	Alternative medicine bibliographic database.	https://www.ebsco.com/products/research-databases/allied-and-complementary-medicine-database-amed
Australian New Zealand Clinical Trial Registry	ANZCTR	Clinical trial registry based in Australia.	www.anzctr.org.au/
China National Knowledge Infrastructure	CNKI	Chinese language bibliographic database.	www.cnki.net
Chinese Biomedical Literature Database	CBM	Chinese language bibliographic database.	www.imicams.ac.cn
Chinese Clinical Trial Registry	ChiCTR	Chinese clinical trial registry.	http://www.chictr.org.cn/
Chinese herbal medicine	CHM	—	—
Chinese medicine	CM	—	—
Chongqing VIP Information Company	CQVIP	Chinese language bibliographic database.	www.cqvip.com
ClinicalTrials.gov	—	Clinical trial registry based in the United States.	https://clinicaltrials.gov/
Cochrane Central Register of Controlled Trials	CENTRAL	Bibliographic database that provides a highly concentrated source of reports of controlled trials.	https://community.cochrane.org/editorial-and-publishing-policy-resource/overview-cochrane-library-and-related-content/databases-included-cochrane-library/cochrane-central-register-controlled-trials-central

(*Continued*)

Term	Acronym	Definition	Reference
Combination therapies	—	Two or more Chinese medicines from different therapy groups (e.g., Chinese herbal medicine, acupuncture therapies or other Chinese medicine therapies) administered together.	—
Controlled clinical trials	CCT	A study in which people are allocated to different interventions using methods that are not random.	https://training.cochrane.org/handbook
Convention on International Trade in Endangered Species of Wild Fauna and Flora	CITES	International convention aimed at preventing or regulating trade in threatened and endangered species of plants and animals.	https://www.cites.org/eng/disc/text.php
Cumulative Index of Nursing and Allied Health Literature	CINAHL	Bibliographic database.	https://www.ebscohost.com/nursing/products/cinahl-databases
Effect size	—	A generic term for the estimate of the effect of a treatment in a study.	http://handbook.cochrane.org/
Electroacupuncture	—	Electric stimulation of the acupuncture needle following insertion.	World Health Organization. (2007) WHO International Standard Terminologies of Traditional Medicine in the Western Pacific Region.
European Union Clinical Trials Register	EU-CTR	European clinical trial registry.	https://www.clinicaltrialsregister.eu
Excerpta Medica database	Embase	Bibliographic database.	http://www.elsevier.com/solutions/embase

(*Continued*)

(Continued)

Term	Acronym	Definition	Reference
Grading of Recommendations Assessment, Development and Evaluation	GRADE	Approach used to grade quality of evidence and strength of recommendations.	http://www.gradeworkinggroup.org/
Greene Climacteric Scale	GCS	A scale used to measure bother from menopausal symptoms.	Greene JG. (1976) A factor analytic study of climacteric symptoms. *J Psychosom Res* **20**(5): 425–430.
Hamilton Rating Scale for Anxiety	HAM-A	A scale used to measure anxiety severity.	Hamilton M. (1959) The assessment of anxiety states by rating. *Br J Med Psychol* **32**(1): 50–55.
Hamilton Rating Scale for Depression	HAM-D	A scale used to measure depression severity.	Hamilton M. (1960) A rating scale for depression. *J Neurol Neurosurg Psychiatry* **23:** 56-62.
Health-related quality of life	HRQoL	A conceptual or operational measurement that is commonly used in a health care setting as a means to assess the impact of disease on the person.	—
Heterogeneity	—	Used in a general sense to describe the variation in, or diversity of, participants, interventions and measurement of outcomes across a set of studies, or the variation in internal validity of those studies. Used specifically, as statistical heterogeneity, to describe the degree of variation in the effect estimates from a set of studies. Also used to indicate the presence of	https://training.cochrane.org/handbook

(***Continued***)

Term	Acronym	Definition	Reference
		variability among studies beyond the amount expected due solely to the play of chance.	
Homogeneity	—	Used in a general sense to mean that the participants, interventions and measurement of outcomes are similar across a set of studies. Used specifically to describe the effect estimates from a set of studies where they do not vary more than would be expected by chance.	https://training.cochrane.org/handbook
I^2	—	A measure of study heterogeneity; indicates the percentage of variance in a meta-analysis.	https://training.cochrane.org/handbook
Integrative medicine	—	Chinese herbal medicine combined with pharmacotherapy or other conventional therapy.	—
Mean difference	MD	In meta-analysis, a method used to combine measures on continuous scales, where the mean, standard deviation and sample size in each group are known. The weight given to the difference in means from each study (e.g. how much influence each study has on the overall results of the meta-analysis) is determined by the precision of its estimate of effect; mathematically this is equal to the inverse of the variance. This method assumes that all of the trials have measured the outcome on the same scale.	https://training.cochrane.org/handbook

(*Continued*)

(*Continued*)

Term	Acronym	Definition	Reference
Medical Outcomes Study: 36-Item Short-Form Health Survey	SF-36	A scale used to measure general wellbeing.	Ware JJ, Sherbourne C. (1992) The MOS 36-item short-form health survey (SF-36). I. Conceptual framework and item selection. *Med Care* **30:** 473–483.
Menopause Rating Scale	MRS	A scale used to measure the impact of menopausal symptoms on health-related quality of life.	Heinemann LA, Potthoff P, Schneider HP. (2003) International versions of the Menopause Rating Scale (MRS). *Health Qual Life Outcomes* **1:** 28.
Menopause-specific Quality of Life Questionnaire	MENQOL	A scale used to measure the impact of menopausal symptoms on health-related quality of life.	Hilditch JR, Lewis J, Peter A, *et al.* (2008) A menopause-specific quality of life questionnaire: Development and psychometric properties. *Maturitas* **61**(1–2): 107–121.
Meta-analysis	—	The use of statistical techniques in a systematic review to integrate the results of included studies. Sometimes misused as a synonym for systematic reviews, where the review includes a meta-analysis.	—
Moxibustion	—	A therapeutic procedure involving ignited material (usually moxa) to apply heat to certain points or areas of the body surface for managing disease.	World Health Organization. (2007) WHO International Standard Terminologies of Traditional Medicine in the Western Pacific Region.

(*Continued*)

Term	Acronym	Definition	Reference
Non-controlled studies	—	Observations made on individuals, usually receiving the same intervention, before and after the intervention but with no control group.	https://training.cochrane.org/handbook
Pittsburgh Sleep Quality Index	PSQI	A scale used to assess sleep quality and patterns of sleep.	Buysse DJ, Reynolds CF, 3rd, Monk TH, *et al.* (1989) The Pittsburgh Sleep Quality Index: A new instrument for psychiatric practice and research. *Psychiatry Res* **28**(2): 193–213.
PubMed	PubMed	Bibliographic database.	http://www.ncbi.nlm.nih.gov/pubmed
Randomised controlled trial	RCT	Clinical trial that uses a random method to allocate participants to treatment and control groups.	—
Risk of bias	—	Assessment of clinical trials to indicate if the results may overestimate or underestimate the true effect because of bias in study design or reporting.	https://training.cochrane.org/handbook
Risk ratio (relative risk)	RR	The ratio of risks in two groups. In intervention studies, it is the ratio of the risk in the intervention group to the risk in the control group. A risk ratio of 1 indicates no difference between comparison groups. For undesirable outcomes, a risk ratio that is less than 1 indicates that the intervention was effective in reducing the risk of that outcome.	https://training.cochrane.org/handbook

(*Continued*)

(*Continued*)

Term	Acronym	Definition	Reference
Standardised mean difference	SMD	In meta-analysis, a method used to combine results for continuous scales which measure the same outcome but measure it in different ways (e.g. with different scales). The results of studies are standardised to a uniform scale to allow data to be combined.	https://training.cochrane.org/handbook
Summary of findings	SoF	Presentation of results and rating the quality of evidence based on the GRADE approach.	http://www.gradeworkinggroup.org/
Wanfang database	Wanfang	Chinese language bibliographic database.	www.wanfangdata.com
World Health Organization	WHO	WHO is the directing and coordinating authority for health within the United Nations system. It is responsible for providing leadership on global health matters, shaping the health research agenda, setting norms and standards, articulating evidence-based policy options, providing technical support to countries and monitoring and assessing health trends.	http://www.who.int/about/en/
Zhong Hua Yi Dian 中华医典	ZHYD	*The Zhong Hua Yi Dian [Encyclopaedia of Traditional Chinese Medicine]* is a comprehensive series of electronic books on compact disk. The collection was put together by the Hunan Electronic and Audio-visual Publishing House. It is the	Hu R, ed. (2014) *Zhong Hua Yi Dian* [*Encyclopaedia of Traditional Chinese Medicine*], 5th ed. Hunan Electronic and Audio-Visual Publishing House, Chengsha.

(*Continued*)

Term	Acronym	Definition	Reference
		largest collection of Chinese electronic books and includes the major Chinese ancient works, many of which are from rare manuscripts and are the only existing copies. These books cover the period from ancient times up to the period of the Republic of China (1911–1948).	
Zhong Yi Fang Ji Da Ci Dian 中医方剂大辞典	ZYFJDCD	Compendium of Chinese herbal formulas with over 96,592 entries derived from classical Chinese books. The Nanjing Chinese Medicine Institute compiled the *Zhong Yi Fang Ji Da Ci* Dian and first published it in 1993.	Peng HR, ed. (1994) *Zhong Yi Fang Ji Da Ci Dian* [*Great Compendium of Chinese Medical Formulae*]. People's Medical Publishing House, Beijing.

Index

Vol. 12 *Post-Stroke Shoulder Complications*
Lead Authors: Claire Shuiqing Zhang and Shaonan Liu

Vol. 13 *Post-Stroke Spasticity*
Lead Authors: Claire Shuiqing Zhang and Shaonan Liu

Vol. 14 *Unipolar Depression*
Lead Authors: Yuan Ming Di and Lingling Yang

Vol. 15 *Chronic Heart Failure*
Lead Authors: Claire Shuiqing Zhang and Liuling Ma

Vol. 16 *Atopic Dermatitis*
Lead Authors: Meaghan Coyle and Junfeng Liu

Vol. 17 *Colorectal Cancer*
Lead Authors: Brian H May and Yihong Liu

Vol. 20 *Chronic Cough*
Lead Authors: Johannah Shergis and Yuanbin Chen

Vol. 22 *Urinary Tract Infection*
Lead Authors: Meaghan Coyle and Xindong Qin

Vol. 24 *Menopause*
Lead Authors: Meaghan Coyle and Jian Liu

Forthcoming

Vol. 23 *Episodic Migraine*
Lead Authors: Claire Shuiqing Zhang and Shaohua Lyu

Vol. 29 *Cervical Radiculopathy*
Lead Authors: Claire Shuiqing Zhang and Dihui Zhang

Lightning Source UK Ltd.
Milton Keynes UK
UKHW021059271020
372307UK00001B/46

9 789811 224362